AWAKEN
to Healing Fragrance

The Power of Essential Oil Therapy

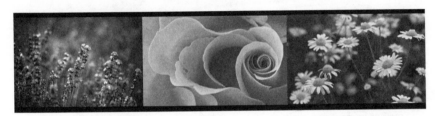

ELIZABETH ANNE JONES

Foreword by Candace Pert, PhD

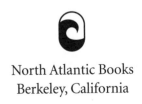

North Atlantic Books
Berkeley, California

Published by
North Atlantic Books
P.O. Box 12327
Berkeley, California 94712

Cover Photos: Left: © istockphoto.com/[ooyoo]
Center: © istockphoto.com/[OlgaLIS]
Right: © istockphoto.com/[fotosav]
Cover and book design by Suzanne Albertson

Printed in the United States of America

Awaken to Healing Fragrance: The Power of Essential Oil Therapy is sponsored by the Society for the Study of Native Arts and Sciences, a nonprofit educational corporation whose goals are to develop an educational and cross-cultural perspective linking various scientific, social, and artistic fields; to nurture a holistic view of arts, sciences, humanities, and healing; and to publish and distribute literature on the relationship of mind, body, and nature.

North Atlantic Books' publications are available through most bookstores. For further information, visit our Web site at www.northatlanticbooks.com or call (800) 733-3000.

Medical Disclaimer: The following information is intended for general information purposes only. Individuals should always see their health care provider before administering any suggestions made in this book. Any application of the material set forth in the following pages is at the reader's discretion and is his or her sole responsibility.

Library of Congress Cataloging-in-Publication Data

Jones, Elizabeth Anne, 1941-
    Awaken to healing fragrance : the power of essential oil therapy /
Elizabeth Anne Jones ; Lawrence E. Jones, contributor ; foreword by Candace Pert.
        p. cm.
    Summary: "Noted aromatherapist Elizabeth Anne Jones explores the value of scent in our lives today and provides a comprehensive look at the past, present, and future of essential oil therapy, focusing on its use in holistic healing and integrative medicine"—Provided by publisher.
    Includes bibliographical references and index.
    ISBN 978-1-55643-875-2
    1. Aromatherapy. 2. Holistic medicine. I. Jones, Lawrence E. II. Title.
    RM666.A68J66 2010
    615'.3219—dc22   2009022209

    1 2 3 4 5 6 7 8 9 SHERIDAN 16 15 14 13 12 11 10

AWAKEN
to Healing Fragrance

T HIS BOOK IS DEDICATED to my dear husband, who has been a devoted partner to me from the very beginning. He has supported me in all the days of writing and contributed some editing and especially his wisdom with chemistry and the GC-MS information in Chapter 14.

This book is in remembrance of my father and mother, who loved history and the arts and had a genuine appreciation of nature. It is also dedicated to my two sons, Alex for his creative yet disciplined mind and Chris for his genuine goodness and humor, and to their two children, Audrey and Sean, my grandchildren, who bring me great fun and delight.

A special dedication is to those unseen spiritual forces who have guided my life and fragrant path with angelic wisdom and gentle empathy.

Contents

PART THREE
Future Prospects for Aromatherapists 253

Foreword

I HAVE ALWAYS BEEN FASCINATED by fragrance. The subject spans the broadest extremes from the most ethereal to the most scientifically concrete. After all, scientists can draw the precise chemical structures of most of the volatile molecules that float through the air and enter our noses, the first step in the sense of smell. The 2004 Nobel Prize was awarded for the discovery that every single olfactory receptor cell inside the nose expresses one and only one of the odorant receptor genes, the mechanism by which we recognize and remember thousands of smells. But understanding the molecular biology of smell doesn't really tell us anything about the power of fragrance, let alone the practice of aromatherapy. How much does learning about phthalocyanine, the chemical in blue paint, tell us about the mystery of how a painting by Rembrandt moves us?

Aromatherapy is mostly uncharted territory in the United States. To understand the powerful link between fragrance and the health of our bodies, one must appreciate how fragrance is the external piece of our molecules of emotion, how we smell not just with our brains but with our entire bodies. Elizabeth Jones, who has taught the mind-body class at the College of Botanical Healing Arts in Santa Cruz for many years, has this deep appreciation as well as an experienced eye (and nose) in relation to essential oil and herbal medicine. Her book captures the mystery as well as the science with a simple, almost poetic style that informs as it pleasures us ("the mind keeps no secrets from the body").

Awaken to Healing Fragrance encompasses the legacy of healing from women in centuries past and present-day science to modern aromatherapy as a powerful, significant (if underappreciated) tool today. The rich stories of how heroines used aromatics to improve the quality and health of their lives blend into case studies of modern women and men.

What interests me as a neuropsychopharmacologist is the way essential oils pass easily through the skin and travel efficiently through the body in a similar fashion to hormones and neuropeptides. The oils find receptor sites on cells to act as catalysts for change within the cell metabolism. The oils are an outside influence on the vital communication network taking place between the nervous, endocrine, and immune systems in the mind-body, what I've called the *bodymind*. The ability of essential oils to harmonize emotions, raise our spirits, and eliminate microbial infections has made them extremely precious and highly sought after throughout human history. Only recently have the molecular and cellular mechanisms of these powerful herbal preparations been studied by scientists.

This book eloquently explores the full scope of how these plant substances can almost instantaneously bridge the physical, emotional, mental, and spiritual realms of human experience. Scientists now know that receptors on all immune cells as well as neurons form ion channels and regulate electrical set points, resulting in changes in cell shape and function with profound concomitant changes in levels of consciousness—from heightened awareness and excitement to reduced awareness and sleep. Essential oils, whose discovery evolved by human selection over thousands of years, can selectively modulate ion channels by dissolving in the fatty membranes much more gently than most pharmaceutical drugs. Their dosage is much more subtle since they can leave the body without liver metabolism being required. Thus, adding an essential oil, say rose *(Rosa damascena)*, to a bodymind experiencing a state of emotional conflict can affect the electrochemical process with a sense of balance and peace by finding the cellular receptor sites that need harmonizing to bring calm to the storm of emotions.

I really appreciate the broad scope of this pioneering author's comprehensive undertaking. Combining historical research, interesting gas chromatographic–mass spectrophotometric analytical documentation of various oils, and discussions of clinical trials on the efficacy of essential oils gives a thorough and inspiring look at this fascinating subject. Elizabeth Jones's love of the subject of aromatherapy, the human body, mind, and spirit shines through all the research. Today, when there is so much disease, pollution, and dysfunction in the Western medical world as hyperactivated cells policing the body for foreign toxins find their way into the brain, it is crucial to find a way home. This book brings us back to nature while holding a compassionate vision of healing that is still grounded in science. Integrative medicine holds the great promise of helping us to understand the unity of the mind and body in order to achieve the greatest state of health possible.

CANDACE B. PERT, PHD
July 17, 2009
Potomac, Maryland

Preface

We call upon all those who have lived upon this earth ... to teach us, and show us the way.

—CHINOOK BLESSING

MANY WOMEN THROUGHOUT HISTORY have used essential oils to empower and heal themselves. Due to available research, only women in the Western world are put forth here, even though there are many examples of feminine heroines in other cultures. The eleven women were chosen because of their documented use of plant energy to sustain, uplift, and bring awareness to their lives. Few possessed outward beauty, but they did have intelligence, moral strength, and a sense of compelling power in what it means to be a woman. All attained a faith in God and looked to him for guidance through the many challenges they each faced. These women of aromatherapy's history had a strong personal presence enhanced by the aromatic oils they used for bathing or massage or perfume. They had an aura of mystery and fascination that drew people to them and enabled them to deeply affect their times and even attain great social status. This aura seemed generated by inner feelings of poise and serenity, of self-assurance and soul beauty. No doubt their spiritual faith, augmented by the use of essential oils, created this inner peace and an ability to maintain and make decisions at crucial moments of their life and at important crossroads in history. Their stories offer some shining examples for modern women and inspiration to use nature's gift of essential oils with conscious deliberation and intuitive spontaneity.

Some modern women who are achieving a great deal in their field are included in this book. One is Patricia Davis, whose life has been devoted to the process of healing with essential oils, crystals, and spiritual painting. She began the first school in England, the London School of Aromatherapy; created a beautiful magazine, *Aromatherapy Quarterly;* and helped to institute the first professional aromatherapy association in the United Kingdom, AOC (Aromatherapy Organisations Council).

Dr. Jane Buckle, an English aromatherapy nurse, has inspired countless American nurses with her clinical aromatherapy trainings to augment their practices with essential oils. She provides clear literature backed up by scientific references.

Another amazing woman is Dr. Candace Pert, whose tireless research of brain chemistry started a revolution for science and the medical world. She is now applying her many skills to HIV research. Her research in the field of psychoneuroimmunology offers a biological, neural basis for our understanding of how the mind and body are interconnected. She offers aromatherapists the clarity and inspiration to use essential oils for healing these systems, both physical and energetic.

Many of my students, present and past, are creative, intelligent men and women who are incorporating essential oils into their lives and careers with a remarkable zeal and diversity. Some of their stories are sprinkled throughout the book.

Introduction

A ROMATHERAPY, OR *essential oil therapy* as I now call this healing modality, is entering a renaissance period as we begin the twenty-first century. Today, countries like Germany, France, England, Australia, Japan, and the United States are undergoing a resurgence of interest in plant medicine. This is partly due to a backlash against the ubiquitous pharmaceutical drugs that can be anti-life (antibiotic) in their severe and sometimes lethal side effects. The female principal of nurturing life is leading the way back to plant therapy, also known as phytotherapy. In the United States, intelligent, holistic men and women who are seeking a natural therapeutic modality for themselves, their families, and their friends embrace the essential oil movement. These oils, derived directly from plants, promote an intense revitalization of body, mind, and spirit. They are pro-life (eubiotic). The use of essential oils offers many unexpected joys since they stimulate the body's cells back to a healthy balance and awaken the mind to a new creativity. The chemical structure of an essential oil is complex, which gives the oil diverse holistic therapeutic properties.

For example, the beautiful Mediterranean plant marjoram *(Origanum majorana)* has a complicated chemistry. Let us give some illustrations of why it is important to know and understand the chemistry of an oil: monoterpenes, some of which make marjoram pain relieving like myrcene and para cymene; alcohols such as terpin-4-ol, which lend an antimicrobial and toning effect; and esters like sabinene hydrate that bring an emotionally relaxing effect. This oil works as a warming capillary dilator, an antibacterial, as well as a soothing, sedating emotional treatment.

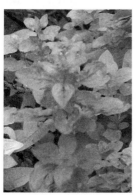

Marjoram

To better understand the roots of the recent discovery of essential oils in industrialized countries, in Part 1 I probe the past to find eleven women in history who used the plants and their oils for mental and physical enhancement. Their use of plant oils offers inspiring examples to guide present-day healers along the essential-oil journey in our petroleum-contaminated water, air, and earth. In our world of high technology stress and polluted resources, the application of essential oils is even more critical to reinforce healthy minds and bodies.

Picture yourself bathing in a pond in a wooded glen where natural spring water is bubbling out of the earth. As you add a blend of Bergamot *(Citrus x bergamia)*, Spruce *(Picea marianna)*, and Lavender *(Lavandula angustifolia)* to the delectable frothy water, your body's immune system and endocrine system receive an immediate boost, and your mind and emotions are delightfully lifted to a new level. The biographical stories relate how much richer and more satisfying the lives of these women were with the beautiful scented chemicals of essential oils. The cadence of each woman's life rings with diversity and a unique ability to overcome adversity. The pace of their eleven lives may differ, but the similarity of interaction with aromatics adds color and energy. Most of the women had prominent stature in their country for their biography to be available. Certainly there were many other women of lowly status who used fragrance for edification and healing of themselves and their families, but their stories were not recorded.

In Part 2 I come into the present day. First the increased scientific knowledge about the olfactory system and how we smell is examined. Then I look at how modern women have a generous range of applications of essential oils from diffusers to spa treatments. Catherine de Médicis of the sixteenth century would adore such variety.

Contemporary essential oil therapists have a sophisticated awareness of essential oil chemistry due to the advances in the field in the last century. The discovery of essential oil chemistry is deepening the comprehension of how the oils work on the body and on the mind. Included is some of Larry Jones's work with GC-MS (gas chromatograph–mass spectrometry)—chemical profiles of the oils—adding a scientific depth and validity to the field.

Examples of case studies done by today's amazing essential oil therapists (often students of the author) are presented according to their focus on physical, emotional, or spiritual aspects of their clients. Then I look at the research and physiological reasons essential oils help us achieve vibrant health today. A vast amount of research, mostly from Europe, speaks to the antibacterial, antiviral, and antifungal actions of essential oils on a cellular level. This leads to the strengthening of the immune system and its many levels of functioning in the body and mind. Its family of white blood cells—phagocytes, natural killer cells, and lymphocytes such as the B and T cells—are potentized by certain essential oils.

The immune system leads into a study of pyschoneuroimmunology, a subject that vibrates with healing truth for today's world. We need to recognize the holistic causes of our diseases and addictions. Since essential oils are so effective at balancing the emotions, centering the mind, and eliminating physical pain, inflammation, and toxicity, their multilevel approach is perfect for mind-body health. The intriguing subject of psychoneuroimmunology continues to be viewed through the holistic haze of essential oils. I begin with a look at scent and how important it is to our lives. I explore the way our olfactory system links up with the limbic brain to understand why scent, emotion, and memory are linked. I tour the endocrine system, finding our hormones are vital to our feelings of wellbeing. Essential oils can mitigate the chemical-hormonal dysfunctions sometimes experienced today. Suggestions on how to use the oils with formulas for immune stimulation and mind balancing are offered.

In Part 3 I turn to the emerging field of energetic medicine, which will play a key role in future healing professions. Studying the integrative approach with herbs and essential oils as indispensable players in the global medicine market is key to creating health worldwide. Next is a tour of an aromatic garden, rich with the potential hydrosols and oils that can be created in the garden stillhouse. Anyone with the land and desire to work a garden will find a blueprint for designing a beautiful fragrant plot. An analysis is presented of some employment opportunities that will be available in the future for essential oil work in professional healing, family health, and community holistic clinics. The possibilities are unlimited and with time will open to many more practical and important uses. Lastly I soar with the molecules of liquid light into a future of living a life of joy and creativity, grounded in spiritual rhythms. The groundwork laid by our historical women will yield much fruit for essential oil therapists today and in the future. In their work with plants for healing and in the rewards of living healthy, ecological lives close to nature, they will experience more happiness and balance.

First let's look at the origins of essential oils. An essential oil represents accumulated solar energy. The sun is vital to an oil's formation, the complex assembly of molecules that creates therapeutic actions in people. The enigma of photosynthesis, which still puzzles scientists, is a complicated parent to essential oil creation and infancy. The tiny sacs of oil that form in the leaf or seed or flower of a plant hold the healing power of that plant. The smell of a beautiful flower grabs your total attention, bringing you into the eternal present, more immediately than any other human sense.

To smell an orange blossom or, better yet, the oil of Neroli *(Citrus x aurantium l. amara)*, which is a concentrated form of the flower's fragrance (a pound of oil is made from about twelve thousand pounds of blossoms), is a heavenly experience! An essential oil results from the distillation of plants: their roots, leaves, heartwood, sap, fruit, flowers, seeds, or bark. The oil offers healing through the fragrant smell and through application to the skin. Both are aimed at internal cellular interaction of the oils as catalysts for the organs and systems of the bodies.

The wild aromatic plant is a product of its surroundings, its terrain. The seed grows according to the soil type, the amount of sunshine and rain, the altitude, the lack of chemical fertilizers, and the love of the farmer. All of these conditions create subspecies of plants or chemotypes throughout the world. It would be a fascinating project to travel the globe and find every genus, species, and variation of Sage (not just *Salvia officinalis)*. To bring back each one, carefully preserved, and examine its plant structure, smell its aromatic leaves, and distill each one for the scientific pleasure of observing it and analyzing its chemistry could be satisfying. The oil extraction by distillation would be governed by the vegetative cycle and harvest time of each plant. Understandably it is vital to the quality of the essential oil that the plant be healthy and organic. Imagine the difference between a plant grown on a hillside overlooking the Mediterranean with fresh sea air and constant sun and one grown on an inner-city plot of shaded land that receives polluted air and water and is fed with chemical pesticides, herbicides, and fertilizers!

Essential oils are distilled from fragrant plants grown in many countries throughout the world. For example, Ravintsara *(Cinnamomum camphora)* comes from Madagascar; Peppermint *(Mentha piperita)* mainly hails from Oregon in the U.S.; Rose *(Rosa damascena)* comes from Bulgaria; and Lemongrass *(Cymbopogon citratus)* grows in India. The oils are plant energy in a focused, liquid form that can be easily used by humans due to their fast absorption through the skin and through the olfactory system. These oils, part of the immune system of the plant, protect it from bacteria, attract pollinating insects, and offer a chemical balance. Marcel Lavabre, in *Aromatherapy Workbook,* discusses how essential oils are contained in the glands, veins, sacs, and glandular hairs of aromatic plants.

The production of essential oils is mostly through a steam-distillation process. Avicenna, an Arabian poet and scientist from about 1000 AD, most significantly discovered this process. Here is a simplified description of this method: Boiling water or steam is driven through several hundred pounds of plant material, releasing the oil from the sacs in the plant. The essential-oil–laden water travels to a pipe at the top of the first tank, often made of stainless steel, where the steam is sent to a second tank filled with cold water. There a coiled pipe circles down, cooling the oil-laden steam and condensing it back to a liquid until the oil floats atop the hydrosol (steam water) and is drawn off to create a pure essential oil. This is like liquid gold to an essential oil therapist! Perhaps the mysterious method of alchemy was associated with these essences in the sixteenth century because the alchemist also dealt with a transmutation process of base metals (instead of plants) into gold. The quality of the oil is affected by the amount of heat, pressure, and time needed to extract the oil. This method of extraction is nonpolluting to the environment and so it offers a sustainable, ecological way of producing "phytopharmaceuticals" for the modern world.

An essential oil has value only if it is pure, complete, and from one plant species. If everyone involved at each stage of the process—from the farmer to the distiller to the importer to the manufacturer to the GC-MS analyzer to the user—has integrity and a desire to create and use a beautiful product, the oil is of the highest quality.

The oils are very complex chemically. A typical essential oil is an amazing mixture of one hundred to four hundred different chemical compounds, created by the parent plant. Any variations in essential oil constituents usually result from the plant's environment: geographical location, elevation, and weather, for example. Each oil has an ideal chemical profile if it has not been adulterated with synthetic solvents and nature-identical man-made substances, both being materials fabricated in a laboratory. The purity issue is explored further in Chapter 14, "The Importance of Chemical Makeup."

Due to the rich variety of nature's chemicals, essential oils have wide-ranging effects on the human body. Most essential oils are time released from the skin to the bloodstream in an average of twenty minutes, as stated by Robert Tisserand and Tony Balacs in *Essential Oil Safety.* During a short sojourn through the body that takes about twenty-four hours, the oils perform many health-producing functions by acting as catalysts at receptor sites of cells. All essential oils are anti-bacterial. Many are immune strengthening, hormone balancing, antiviral, analgesic, anti-inflammatory, and emotionally relaxing or stimulating. Some oils such as Eucalyptus *(Eucalyptus globulus)* and Pine *(Pinus sylvestris)* greatly benefit the respiratory system. Others like Peppermint and Ginger *(Zingiber officinale)* work to balance the digestive system. Grapefruit *(Citrus x paradisi)* and Rosemary *(Rosmarinus officinalis)* stimulate the lymphatic system to clear the body of toxins. The women in history knew nothing about the chemistry of Frankincense *(Boswellia carteri)*, but did experience its wondrous effects on their skin and from the spiritual uplift of their psyches.

Essential oils are lipophilic, meaning they mix best with fatty substances whether it is cold-pressed olive oil or human skin. The Egyptians filled alabaster vases with vegetable oils and added their favorite scents like Myrrh *(Commiphora myrrha)* and Cedarwood *(Cedrus libani)*. They inadvertedly discovered the antibacterial quality of essential oils when they used them to preserve a corpse in the mummification process. During the last century, hundreds of clinical studies have proven the effectiveness of these oils' ability to protect humans against bacterial, viral, or fungal infections. Some specific oils and case studies are examined in Chapter 16, "Essential Oils for the Treatment of Infection."

Essential oils are the soul or essence of their parent plant. You would expect, for example, Rose oil to soothe emotional trauma and elicit feelings of love. What a pleasure to enjoy the cheering, sunny feeling of Orange oil *(Citrus sinensis)* in a bath. The oils work on the whole person, that is, holistically, to heal physically and emotionally. The scent triggers a stimulus of the limbic brain via the olfactory system. The limbic brain is snuggled under the right and left lobes of the cerebral cortex and is the headquarters for memory, moods, and creativity. Today, we are learning more about the mind-body connection and discovering our state of health involves our thoughts and feelings as well as our blood pressure and immune system. In fact, a vital connection exists between the mental and physical states via the neurotransmitters and the hormonal system. Essential oils help to keep these systems balanced and the emotions uplifted. This is something the ancients knew intuitively and we are just rediscovering.

Essential oil therapy seems linked to the destiny of women in the past, present, and future. Women have always been lovers of plants throughout our ancient journey on this planet. First, they gathered herbs from the woods and meadows to create nutritious meals and healing medicines for their families. They sharpened their intuitive powers as they discovered that the divine gifts from the plant world could ease illness and restore vitality. The wisdom was passed down from mother to daughter and healer to apprentice. These women were sources of deep knowledge for their communities. They stayed connected to the cycles of nature and their inner spiritual spark. Women found it more difficult to tap into their innate wisdom as civilization developed in complexity and male preeminence brought a tendency toward the military and science. Being true to themselves often took great courage and focus, which we will see clearly in the lives of the eleven formidable women portrayed in Part 1. They found plant oils to be great allies and derived much strength from using them. There have been, of course, many other unsung essential oil therapists, both female and male, throughout history and in other parts of the world that we would silently like to acknowledge with this book.

Taking these pioneering women as inspiration, this book explores how essential oils can be used to further the healing professions and our families' health, and open us to greater spiritual growth. They also offer a means to balance the male and female energy within each of us. Some essential oils stimulate the logical, the active, the achieving, or the male parts of us. Thyme *(Thymus vulgaris)*, for example, is for strengthening physically, emotionally, and energetically. Other oils elicit the intuitive, the caring, and the emotionally wise or female aspects, such as Clary sage *(Salvia sclarea)*, which soothes menstruation and offers third eye opening and clarity. In the years to come, men and women can enjoy the benefits of this art and science and become more balanced as individuals. Understanding the chemistry of the oils as well as their energetic, spiritual application offers an approach to aromatherapy from both genders' viewpoint. The use of essential oils creates a delicate yet potent relaxed alertness in the human body and mind. We all need such a state to maximize our spiritual receptivity and to create a future world in which we live in global harmony with nature's beauty. The plant oils are a divine gift right under our noses!

This book's purpose is to explore some new realms in antiquity, the present, and the possible future. Essential oil therapy can be used in the treatment of serious ailments, which had previously appeared to lie within

CHAPTER ONE

Hatshepsut, the First Female Pharaoh of Egypt

To look upon her was more beautiful than anything; her splendour and her form were divine; she was a maiden, beautiful and blooming.

—INSCRIPTION ON HATSHEPSUT'S OBELISK

IMAGINE STROLLING ALONG A beautiful stone terrace with a slight breeze brushing your cheek, a breeze that brings the intriguing fragrance of an earthy, rich base note with a slight tinge of bitter orange emanating from a series of trees planted on the terrace. As you gaze at the Nile River and its sinuous shore, the pale blue morning sky, and the silhouettes of elegant birds in flight, you feel grounded and uplifted. This is how Hatshepsut, queen of Egypt, felt as she walked in daily meditation down the avenue of myrrh trees.

Unique in her character, status, and inner life, Hatshepsut is an amazing model of how to live gracefully with aromatics permeating every nuance of life. She relished her olfactory sense as it brought her captivating smells each day of her life. Living at the height of Egyptian culture 3,500 years ago, she used her position as queen and pharaoh to manifest a calm integrity, intelligent innovation, and beauty of form.

Hatshepsut was born about 1500 BC as the eldest daughter of Tuthmosis I and Ahmose (crown princess and sister to Amenophis I), a cheerful and compatible royal pair who reigned in the Eighteenth Dynasty of Egypt. Hatshepsut came from a lineage of great kings. King Ahmose, her great-grandfather, succeeded in reuniting northern and southern Egypt about 1550 BC. He became one of the greatest Egyptian kings and the founder of the New Kingdom, the Eighteenth Dynasty. Hatshepsut's grandfather, cern for aesthetic appearance and cleanliness led Egyptians to make the bath one of the most attractive rooms in any fine house. There women bathed in rare perfumes and then used unguents in the adjoining massage room. Michal Dayagi-Mendel notes in *Perfumes and Cosmetics in the Ancient World,* "The use of oils and ointments was prevalent, then as now, to protect the face and body from sun, dust, and the dryness of the Eastern climate. These perfumed oils were not regarded as luxuries and were used by men and women of all strata of the population."[4] They sensuously anointed the body with oils after bathing too. Among the many paintings in Hatshepsut's magnificent temple at Deir el-Bahri is one of "a lady of the court going through the daily routine of her toilet. She is attended by four maidens, two of whom pour fragrant oil over her body whilst a third massages her shoulder with one hand and, with the other, holds up a Lotus flower for her to smell."[5]

The use of cosmetics in Hatshepsut's time was highly popular, and essential oils were an ingredient in many potions. Women had charming wooden boxes carved with intricate designs. Inside the boxes were jars of henna to rub on their cheeks for a rosy glow, bottles of black kohl to accentuate the beauty of the eyes, and alabaster jars of blended scents to rub all over the body. Archaeologists have unearthed intimate objects bearing Hatshepsut's name, including a pair of golden bracelets and an alabaster eye makeup container with a bronze applicator. She was a human female but a semi-divine pharaoh of Egypt as well.

Near Thebes archaeologists found a turquoise-colored perfume bottle with Hatshepsut's name engraved on the neck, the oldest find of its kind, indicating that perfume bottling likely began in her day. At that time, the Egyptians used opaque glass colored with metallic oxides. In addition, beautiful containers made of granite, diorite, and especially alabaster were carved in lovely animal or lotus shapes to hold the scented oils and keep them cool.

At the great feasts of the nightly royal court, women had an unusual ritual. They wore cone-shaped cakes of fat mixed with oil, perfumes, and herbs. These cakes were created by two different methods. Egyptians lacked our modern still design with the alembic condenser, which Avicenna invented in 1000 AD, so their essential oils were plant extracts. One method was the enfleurage system of extraction, mostly for delicate flowers such as jasmine, lotus, and rose. The petals were spread on a layer of animal fat between two boards; within one day the fat had usually absorbed the fragrance of the flowers. New petals replaced the old every day for six to twelve weeks. At the end of this long process, the result was perfumed pomade. This method is still used today (for example, in India) to extract Tuberose (*Polyanthes tuberosa*). However, now the pomade is washed with alcohol and strained, similar to the modern solvent extraction process.

A second method of extracting plant oil is described by Pedanius Dioscorides, a Greek physician who traveled the ancient world with the Roman army in 1 AD. In his famous *de Materia Medica,* a treatise on seven hundred plant medicines that remained a standard for centuries, Dioscorides instructs: "To make scented ox fat, remove any blood and skin from the fat. Pour over it some old scented wine. Boil together over a slow fire until the fat has lost its own smell and rather smells of the wine.... Then place 2 pints of clean fat in an earthenware pot. Mix with Cyperus [a rhizome] and Balsam wood (to thicken) and finely bruised palm shoots, and sweet flag, and 1 cup of old wine. Bring to a boil three times, remove, and cool for 24 hours. Melt again and sieve through clean linen into a clean pot.... Seal and store."[6]

The ox tallow was then shaped into a cone and affixed to a wig or placed on the crown of the head. The cones melted in the hot banquet rooms and "the fragrant oil bedewed heads and shoulders to smell sweetly and provoke erotic [Jasmine] desires."[7] This custom may seem strange to modern Western women, but it was a wonderful way to receive an aromatherapy treatment for emotional inspiration and moisturized skin. Even today certain Bedouin tribe members carry on the fragrant-cone custom.

The Egyptians are inspirations for us in their goal of living life for spiritual growth. Integral to Egyptian religious observances, fragrance was associated with a search for god. In their pantheon, each god had a certain scent connected with his or her persona. Amun's fragrance was Myrrh. Hatshepsut was devoted to Amun-Re, the fusion of two deities: Amun, the creator of the world, and Re (meaning "sun"), the king of the world. Like other thinkers of her time, Hatshepsut believed in the sacredness of all that lived. This underlying faith gave her reign an atmosphere of serenity and a fearless certainty about the future life. Hatshepsut's mother encouraged a strong sense of religion in her daughter, who recited many prayers, performed rituals, and loved to dance before the altar. The inscription on one of her obelisks at Karnak expresses her devotion and appreciation: "I have made this with a loving heart for my father (Amun).... I have not been forgetful of any projects he has divinely decreed.... He is the one who guides me ... and gives directions."[8]

The priests were usually the perfumers, producing elevating scents for temple worship, rituals, and ceremonies. All over Egypt recipes for perfumed oils and incense were found on the walls in the special scent rooms adjacent to the temples. Aromatic fragrances were given as state tribute and donated to specific temples. The Egyptians believed that their prayers would reach the gods more quickly if wafted by the fragrant blue smoke, which slowly ascended to heaven. In *Perfume*, William Kaufman writes, "The [English] word *perfume* means 'through smoke.'"[9] Incense smoldered at funerals, religious rituals, and the crowning of pharaohs.

Further proof of the importance of scent in the ancient Egyptian religion is that its pantheon included the god of perfume, Nefertum, who inspired the priests to create sacred perfumes. John Steele, my friend, archaeologist, and modern aromatherapist, describes how the priests knew the importance of the biochemical response the human body and mind achieved by inhaling a scent such as Frankincense *(Boswellia carteri)*. They sought to uplift Egyptian citizens, emotionally and spiritually, through the transformational fragrance at large gatherings.

The Egyptians burned Myrrh *(Commiphora myrrha)* every day at noon as part of their sun worship ritual. This fragrance had the emotional effect of energizing, overcoming apathy, and grounding, while at the same time enhancing spiritual awareness. The resinoid is also antiviral and hormone-like, as it balances the thyroid gland. Queen Hatshepsut rubbed Myrrh on the bottom of her feet so she would continually exude a pleasant fragrance for herself and others wherever she went. The oil offered her feet an antiseptic ointment that kept her heels from cracking in the hot sun. As the Myrrh molecules entered her bloodstream, they stimulated the immune system by creating white blood cells or lymphocytes. Energetically, the oil strengthened her spirituality and supported her need to trust those around her. Hatshepsut loved Myrrh because it reminded her of her god, Amun, and it gave her mind and body vitality.

The Egyptians also used essential oils to prepare their dead. They had a preoccupation with the continuation of life after death, believing in the transmigration of the soul (the "Ka"). Preservation of the human likeness through mummification was important so the Ka and the body could reunite and return to the pleasures of life. Careful attention was given to what would be needed in the afterlife in the tomb. The rituals surrounding death made it the leading source of employment in Thebes. Artisans labored in shops all their lives to provide coffins, furniture, goblets, and alabaster vases filled with unguents. The exquisite beauty and care of their work, as shown in the artifacts of King Tutankhamen's tomb, reflect their belief in the continuing evolution of human consciousness, even after death.

Mummification was mainly for the elite due to the expense of the huge amounts of necessary aromatic ointments. First the embalmers removed the brain through the nose and injected Cedarwood oil *(Cedrus atlantica* or *Cedrus libani)* into the head. Next the intestines were detached with an incision by a sharp blade in the side and the stomach cavity was filled with Myrrh and Cassia *(Cassia marilandica),* then sewn closed. The body was placed in natron, a seisquicarbonate of soda found in the desert, for seventy days. "The body was anointed with oils and fats, scented with Myrrh and Cedarwood as melted resin was poured over the entire body to close the pores,"[10] writes Janet Buttles in *The Queens of Egypt.* The body was then wrapped in yards of linen strips and smeared with scented ointments, the strong antiseptic powers of which helped preserve the ancient tissues until even present day. Cedarwood was especially effective for this purpose due to its astringent, drying effect on human tissue. *Juniperus virginiana* is the American cedarwood, an oil that has similar properties to that of *Cedrus atlantica* and *Cedrus libani,* the European and Middle Eastern cedars, respectively.

Cedarwood would also kill all infection, even fungus, and have a soothing, calming action as the deceased one embarked on his or her last journey to the afterlife. In addition, the living used it as a tonic for any chronic complaints or pain. It was especially helpful for coughs and bronchitis. The use of cedarwood in a bath could bring relief from arthritis and a feeling of comfortable composure. It also strengthens the individual's connection with God and brings a sense of balance and control. The Egyptians used cedarwood for durable wooden items such as ships, temple doors, and coffins. The mummified body was laid in a cedarwood coffin, fitted to the size and shape of the body.

Coptic jars made of alabaster, containing the heart, lungs, liver, and gallbladder, were filled with fragrant oils, sealed for future use, and placed in the tomb with the mummified body of a revered Egyptian. When archae-ologists opened the famed King Tutankhamen tomb, the smell of Myrrh and Spikenard permeated the air, adding to the astonishment and awe of the discovering agents.

On the death of her father, twelve-year-old Hatshepsut emerged from the obscurity of the women's palace to marry her half-brother, Tuthmosis II, and became queen consort of Egypt, a role she had been groomed for by her father. Hatshepsut preferred the title "God's wife" (as noted, pharaohs were considered semi-divine). Evelyn Wells reports that by marrying Tuthmosis II, Hatshepsut pledged to be "feminine to a divine degree, to exude fragrance as she walked, and speak in tones that filled the palace with music."[11]

Like her father, Hatshepsut was an innovator. Historians have specu-lated that Tuthmosis I took his young daughter on the royal barge to explore the Nile and introduce her to authorities in major cities in preparation for the time when she would be queen. As the barge traveled north, she learned about a waterway leading from the eastern branch of the Nile to the inland sea and the land of Punt (known today as Somalia), about which she heard stories that intrigued her and made her dream. This red land held the "touch of gold and ivory, the voices of strange animals, the odor of her favorite incense from the citrus-scented myrrh trees that grew in Punt."[12] Perhaps during this journey she resolved to someday send an expedition to Punt.

A few years into his reign, Tuthmosis II died from smallpox. After his death Hatshepsut became the first woman to rule Egypt alone. She car-ried on her father's love of order in the ways of government, architecture, and human relations. Despite having to compete with male relatives to retain her position, she advanced from being ruler regent of Egypt to pharaoh, a position she held for twenty-two years. She decided that she wanted to build and explore during her reign, instead of destroying and conquering. This has been a typical response to power revealed by female sovereigns throughout history, especially those who used essential oils.

The mythological story of Hatshepsut's political ascension is recorded on the walls of her temple at Deir el-Bahri: "Her human father, Tuthmosis I, introduces her to the royal court, nominates her, and has her acclaimed as heir. As soon as her titulature has been announced she undergoes a fur-ther rite of purification [with Myrrh]."[13]

Today our consciousness is opening to the divine feminine. Ancient Egyptian society presented a tribute to the feminine in embracing their female pharaoh, as well as in their emphasis on artistic beauty, morality in daily life, and intuitive healing through the olfactory sense. The close-knit Theban royal family, in which the queen was often the full or half-sister of the king, used the intelligence and political astuteness of their women to rule more effectively. Women were often portrayed in art since they were respected and given more freedom than in most ancient cultures. The Egyptians had a morality and sense of humanity that allowed a woman like Hatshepsut to flourish in such a male-dominated world.

Another feminine value manifested in that culture was the love of gardens. The Egyptians, who greatly appreciated exotic plants and trees, had imported pomegranate and olive trees. On her beautiful temple terraces at Deir el-Bahri, Hatshepsut ordered the planting of twenty-three myrrh trees. Decorating her temple is a relief painted in the most brilliant colors depicting in detail the trade that brought her these precious trees.

Hatshepsut sent a royal expedition of five oared ships to the land of Punt (today, Somalia). Her temple relief shows the supple trees, mysterious animals, and chubby Queen Ety of this foreign country. Punt was rich in precious resins such as the multifaceted Myrrh and the noble Frankincense, which Egypt needed to create incense and their favorite perfume, Kyphi. As noted, incense was burned in great quantity during the daily temple rituals, and Myrrh was used in mummification and in the formulation of perfumes and medicine. For example, "those suffering from sour breath ... were advised to chew little balls of Myrrh to relieve their symptoms."[14]

Neshi, one of Hatshepsut's administrators in charge of the trip, was asked to bring back living myrrh trees, which could not be found in Egypt. The trees, with balled-up roots, were to be replanted in the garden of Amun at Deir el-Bahri. The god Amun smelled like the fragrance of Punt. In addition to myrrh resin and the trees, the ships returned with ebony, cattle, apes, silver, gold, lapis lazuli, and malachite. An inscription in Hatshepsut's temple states: "Never were brought such things to any king since the world was."[15]

Traditionally a king was male. The Egyptian pharaoh was a god on Earth, the messenger between the Egyptian people and their gods. After her coronation, Hatshepsut discarded the feminine dress of her time and chose to wear the typical clothing of a male king: a short kilt, broad collar, head cloth or crown, and false beard. An early statue shows her seated, wearing the kilt and head cloth, but it also clearly shows the slight, soft curves of a young woman. In many later depictions and statues, she wears men's clothing and appears to have a man's body. As the first-known female pharaoh, she must have felt she would be more acceptable to her priests and subjects in the traditional male dress. In addition to the bearded king, she was portrayed as a sphinx and a goddess, but never as a mere woman, except for the one statue of her as the young queen.

Hatshepsut appointed Senemut, a well-known architect of humble parents, to help with building projects. He was equal to her in extraordinary intellect and powerful personality. She had him design and erect two obelisks at the temple of Amun-Re at Karnak. Their twin tips were sheathed in gold foil so they shimmered in the rays of the fierce Egyptian sun. They were engineering marvels on which Hatshepsut had many writings about her life engraved.

Her greatest building was her mortuary temple, Djeser-Djeseru, an architectural masterpiece that fit perfectly into its natural setting. In *The XVIII Dynasty Temple of Deir El-Bahri*, Eduard Naville describes this temple: "The great originality of her complex lay in its organization into a succession of terraces ... which harmonize with the natural amphitheater of the cliffs."[16] The beautiful white stone temple set against the rose-tinted cliffs was the first rock-cut temple in history. Even today its startling, magnificent edifice appears contemporary in design.

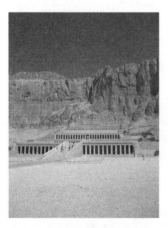

Hatshepsut's final days are shrouded in mystery as she drops abruptly from recorded history. Her name was removed from many of her portraits and monuments. As a result, she was forgotten for almost 2,000 years. The Egyptian expedition of the New York Metropolitan Museum of Art from 1923 to 1928 discovered numerous Hatshepsut and Senemut statues in two large depressions in front of her temple. Archaeologists believe that her jealous stepson and successor, Tuthmosis III, dumped the statues there and ordered her name removed from other

Hatshepsut's temple at
Deir el-Bahri

monuments and statues in an attempt to write his brilliant aunt and step-mother out of Egyptian history. Historians believe she died in 1458 BC and was buried in the Valley of the Kings, although her body has not yet been found. Tuthmosis III did not entirely erase her legacy. Her temple at Deir el-Bahri and her noble inscriptions on its walls can still be seen today. A visitor there can easily conjure up an image of this gracious and wise pharaoh going about her daily activities, and smell the ever-present Myrrh that gave her a balanced, yet inspired feeling, aided her in her creative endeavors, and helped her earn the admiration of those around her.

CHAPTER TWO

Esther, the Persian Queen Who Saved the Jews

Our every act has a universal dimension.
—THE 14TH DALAI LAMA

PICTURE YOURSELF AT A gathering of people about 500 BC, celebrating, eating, and conversing vibrantly in the noontime sun. Before attending this banquet you bathed with your favorite aromatic, Frankincense *(Boswellia carteri)*. The smell of the lingering fragrance on your body empowers you to speak your truth. Even though you must publicly confront the king with a difficult request and reveal to him your secret heritage, the fragrance that you wear in a linen bag around your neck—Patchouli *(Pogostemon cablin)* and Myrrh *(Commiphora myrrha)*—gives you the courage to speak. This was how Esther felt the day she told the king the lives of her people were threatened by his prime minister.

The story of Esther is quite moving in aromatherapy history since essential oils played a vital function in her life. We have only the biblical record of her life in the Old Testament, the book of Esther. Most scholars believe that she lived around 500 BC in Persia. She performed a heroic role in the narrative story of her people, the Jews.

King Ahasuerus, who reigned over a land stretching from India to Ethiopia, containing 127 provinces, sat upon his royal throne in the Shushan palace. Some historians say he was also called Xerxes I, a sovereign who spent his younger days subduing Egypt and Greece. During the years with Esther, his kingdom was in an epoch of peace and abundance. He loved to pass the time at feasts, some even lasting for 180 days. One feast in his garden court had "curtains of white and blue tapestries ... fastened with purple cords of fine linen to silver rings on marble pillars. Gold and silver

couches were placed on a pavement of alabaster, white marble, mother of pearl, and black marble."[1] The king asked for the presence of Queen Vashti to show her beauty before the people. She refused, disobeying his orders. The king became very angry.

Women's lives were absolutely controlled by men in these early times. In the fourth century BC, the Greek philosopher Aristotle spoke for Jewish thinkers of the same period, "The male is by nature superior, and the female inferior, and the one rules and the other is ruled."[2] The wise men of court advised the king to find another queen. They believed Queen Vashti was setting a deplorable example for women throughout the kingdom. A search for attractive virgins and the beautifying oils for women's edification began under the supervision of Hegai, the chief eunuch in charge of the king's harem.

A Jew named Mordecai, among a group of Jews exiled from Jerusalem, lived in the Shushan kingdom of Persia. He was uncle and foster parent to Esther (her Hebrew name was Hadassah), who was orphaned at an early age. She was a beautiful girl of face and figure. When Mordecai learned of the king's search for a new queen, he sent Esther to the royal dwelling of Hegai where women from throughout the land were gathering, eager for the honor of being chosen by their king. Hegai was soon impressed with Esther, whose loveliness, intelligence, and fine character won his favor. He furnished her with seven choice maids and the finest apartment in the harem. She did not mention her nationality or background, as her Uncle Mordecai had instructed.

Esther, like all the girls, underwent the prescribed treatment for women:

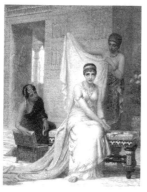

Esther

six months with the oil of Myrrh and the attar of Rose *(Rosa damascena),* and then six months with the balm and perfume of Spikenard *(Nardostachys grandiflora),* Aloe *(Aloe vera),* Sandalwood *(Santalum album),* and especially Frankincense. These treatments were designed to purify the women and make them acceptable as ordained by law. In the first century AD, the Jewish philosopher Philo wrote, "The soul has ... a dwelling, partly women's quarters, partly men's quarters. Now for the men there is a place where properly

dwell the masculine thoughts [these are] wise, sound, just, prudent, pious, and filled with freedom and boldness, and kin to wisdom.... And the female sex is irrational and akin to bestial passions, fear, sorrow, pleasure and desire from which ensue incurable weakness and indescribable diseases."[3]

The essential oils used in the yearlong treatment were administered for internal purging and emotional cleansing, as well as beautifying the skin. Women were also considered unclean due to their monthly menstruation. They were given baths and massages, and "it was the custom of the women to carry, beneath their clothes, a small linen bag containing Myrrh and other fragrant substances. This was usually suspended from a cord around the neck and lay in the hollow between the breasts. Here, the solidified Myrrh would release its fragrance from the warmth of the body and this would be enjoyed both by the wearer and by those in close contact."[4]

Frankincense of the Burseraceae family worked to purify all mucous membranes, whether in the mouth, lungs, or uterus. The oil of Frankincense comes from the gum of the tree in brittle, round drops or tears. Like myrrh, frankincense grew on the rocky hillsides and in the desert ravines of southern Arabia. Its value was on a par with gold, as illustrated in the famous story of the three kings from the east who offered baby Jesus gifts of Myrrh, Frankincense, and gold. Frankincense was bitter to the taste but had a rich, balsamic odor when heated. It was used as a tonic for the uterus and helped to regulate all secretions. Like the Egyptians, Persian women used it to rejuvenate skin, smooth wrinkles, and reduce inflammation. Emotionally, it slowed breathing and calmed the mind, so was a real aid for the "flighty" women of Persia. As in the Egyptian temples of the past and the Catholic Church today, Frankincense elevated the mind to the higher self and emotionally broke obsessional ties with the past.

Precedents in Hebrew history for using aromatic oils came from both Moses and Solomon. Moses was given directions for making holy anointing oil in the wilderness. He had learned about the oils in Egypt. "The Lord said to Moses: take the following fine spices: . . . liquid myrrh, half as much . . . fragrant cinnamon . . . fragrant cane . . . cassia and . . . olive oil. Make these into 'a sacred anointing oil, a fragrant blend, the work of a perfumer.' It shall be the sacred anointing oil."[5] King Solomon actively traded in spices as depicted in the story of the Queen of Sheba. The Song of Solomon lyrically describes all of the fragrant flowers, spices, and trees that grew in Israel in 1000 BC.

A garden you are, my sister, my bride.
    a garden walled in, a fountain well sealed;
A pomegranate orchard with precious fruits,
    a garden of henna with spikenard,
    spikenard and saffron, calamus and cinnamon,
    with all the trees of frankincense,
    myrrh and aloes, with all the chief spices.
You are a garden fountain, a well of living water,
    flowing streams from Lebanon.[6]

In Palestine, perfumes were usually produced with a base of olive oil. Three different methods were used to produce the finished fragrant essence: pressing, enfleurage, or hot steeping. For pressing, the herbs or plant material were chopped, mixed with olive oil, and then placed in a folded cloth with loops at both ends. In each loop a rod was inserted. With two people, each one holding one of the rods, the cloth was twisted in opposite directions, thus pressing the contents. The process was moderately successful since much of the plant material was not exuded.

Enfleurage—using animal fat to extract the fragrance—is described in Chapter 1, "Hatshepsut, The First Female Pharaoh of Egypt." Attar of Rose originated in Persia and was produced on a large scale in the sixth century BC. "Skilled perfumers working in the cosmetics department of the royal women's quarters followed Hegai's method in mixing Attar of Roses with Myrrh. They also used his recipe in combining pungent concoctions of herbs with honey, thereafter kneading the liquid [oils] into a sticky, but snowy-white, mass of the best hog fat. Applications of this perfumed grease made the skin as soft and supple as silk."[7]

Hot steeping (maceration) was the method most commonly used. The oil was pretreated with a solution of astringent materials like lime, then mixed with wine or water in which the plant parts and resin had steeped. A tomb painting from Thebes that depicts a perfumer's process shows first the grinding of the aromatic materials with a mortar and pestle. The components are mixed with the oil in a large basin, then the liquid is heated to 149°F in vats of boiling water (the double-boiler method). They did not use an open flame because the fragrant molecules would have evaporated. After the heated mixture was left to stand for several days, the florals were strained off and fresh ones added. When it was aromatically strong, it was strained one last time and decanted into containers. Artists created beau-

tiful vessels of glass, ivory, and metals like copper; alabaster was preferred because it kept the oil cold. The perfume was then stored in a cool, shady place.

Back in the Shushan palace, after twelve months of consecrating their souls and beautifying their faces and bodies with essential oil treatments, the girls visited the king for his approval. As described in the Modern Language version of *The Layman's Parallel Bible,* "When the turn came for Esther ... to go to the king, she requested nothing but what Hegai, the king's eunuch in charge of the women, suggested, and Esther won the hearts of all who saw her.... the king felt more love for Esther than for all the women. She gained more attachment and kindness from him than did all the girls, so that he placed the royal crown on her head and made her queen in the place of Vashti."[8]

Mordecai sat outside the royal gate to stay abreast of how Esther was faring. One day he overheard two guards plotting to kill the king. Mordecai told Esther about the conspiracy and she passed the word on to King Ahauseurus, whose investigation resulting in the hanging of the two guards.

The king had promoted Haman, the son of Hammedatha, higher than all the princes. Haman wore a three-cornered prime minister's hat wherever he went. One day he passed Mordecai, who refused to bow to him, saying "I am a Jew, I bow only to God."[9] Angry at the lack of respect, Haman began scheming to destroy the Jews. He announced to the king, "There is a race scattered and dispersed among the peoples in the provinces of your realm who ... do not observe the king's laws, so that it is not expedient for your majesty to tolerate them."[10] The king agreed to pursue Haman's evil plan. His first act was to send royal letters to all the governors in the provinces ordering them to kill all of the Jews—young, old, children, and women. He chose the number *14* out of his hat and set the fourteenth day of Adar (late February or early March) as the day of punishment. There was deep mourning and weeping among the Jews.

Queen Esther was told the shocking news by her maids. She sent a messenger to Mordecai saying she had not seen the king in thirty days, but to gather all the Shushan Jews and have them fast for three days and three nights. She pondered her course of action. She knew that only the king could save her people, yet it took great courage for her to approach him. No one, not even the queen, could lawfully summon the king without him first requesting it. Esther bathed and had a massage with essential oils (no

CHAPTER THREE

Cleopatra, the Queen of Kings

Age cannot wither her, nor custom stale her infinite variety.
—WILLIAM SHAKESPEARE, *ANTONY AND CLEOPATRA*

SEE YOURSELF GAZING at the beauty of an Egyptian palace while sitting in the women's section on a gilded chair and anticipating an aromatic bath. As your women servants help you disrobe, a cascade of fragrance descends upon you like a shimmering waterfall of Cinnamon *(Cinnamomum verum)*, Cardamom *(Elettaria cardamomum)*, Jasmine *(Jasminum grandiflorum)*, Sandalwood *(Santalum album)*, and Lime *(Citrus x aurantifolia)*. To your delight the panoply of scent plays hide and seek with your olfactory receptors. Sometimes the Jasmine emerges as a strong single note and sometimes it blends into a symphony of cinnamon-lime musical notes. The total effect makes you feel alert, excited, and sensually awake. This was the experience of Queen Cleopatra VII as she bathed in a fragrant milk bath, preparing to meet the man of her destiny, Antony.

Cleopatra VII was born in 69 BC, the third child of King Ptolemy Auletes XI of Egypt. The Ptolemy kings were descendants of Alexander the Great from Macedonia, so Cleopatra was largely of Greek descent and her mother was Jewish from Palestine. Cleopatra lived in Alexandria, the lovely city Alexander the Great founded in 336 BC. These were the twilight days for the Egyptian kings. The Ptolemaic Empire had once extended north into Asia Minor and Syria to the East, but had now dwindled to Egypt itself, and the kingdoms conquered by Alexander had already fallen to the Romans. The Ptolemy's strength was failing and the Roman Empire was rising.

Lucy Hughes-Hallett wrote, "Egypt was certainly the most feminine country of the Ancient world, especially compared to the starkness and rigidity of Roman life."[1] The Egyptian family had freedom, kindness, and intimacy. Egyptian women were not shut up at home like Roman wives were; they were free to move about the country, own property, and express themselves in different trades. An Egyptian wife accompanied her husband as an equal and created a moral influence. Egypt was economically rich, but politically unstable, so Cleopatra's father, Auletes, felt insecure about his national status. He taught his daughter to seek a strong political alliance with Rome. He also offered his favorite daughter, Cleopatra, training with the most learned and cultured men of Alexandria. She grew in charm, grace, and intellect.

When she was seventeen, Cleopatra's father, King Ptolemy XI, died (52 BC). Cleopatra and her twelve-year-old brother, Dionysus, were married; Dionysus became King Ptolemy XIII and Cleopatra was his queen. According to Egyptian law, throughout her reign Cleopatra was obligated to have a consort who was either a brother or a son. Ever since the god Osiris had married his sister, Isis, the brother and sister who ascended the throne were obligated to marry. Cleopatra was the forceful part of the pair, alluring and ambitious; Dionysus was completely overshadowed by his brilliant sister. When she became co-regent, there was anarchy abroad and famine at home.

In 48 BC a Roman general, Julius Caesar, arrived in Alexandria. He brought with him 3,200 legionnaires and 800 cavalry, and soon there was rioting in the streets of Alexandria. Ptolemy XIII had gone to Pelusium and Caesar placed himself in the royal palace and started giving out orders. Cleopatra wanted in on the deal making. She had herself smuggled in through enemy lines rolled in a carpet. She was delivered to Caesar and dramatically rolled out from the carpet in his presence. He was not struck so much by her physical beauty as by her charming intellectual mind, her graceful voice, and her body well-anointed with perfume oil. They became lovers. On his return Ptolemy XIII realized this and stormed out screaming that he had been betrayed. He tried to arouse the Alexandrian mob but was captured by Caesar's guards and returned to the palace. Due to Caesar's enchantment with Cleopatra and upon her urging, he forced Ptolemy XIII to again share the throne with his sister. Ptolemy XIII drowned in the Nile while he was trying to flee the Alexandrian War between Pothinus, an influential regent and eunuch in Ptolemy XIII's court, and Caesar. Cleopatra's rise to the throne was a dangerous and bloody episode in her life.

Cleopatra's greatest assets were her large, bluish mauve eyes, her beautiful musical voice, and her poise. The latter was partly the result of her daily extensive bathing and her use of all the fragrant oils available at that time. She used Rosemary, Lavender, Spikenard, Myrrh, and Jasmine in milk to create a tranquil aromatic moment designed to strengthen her mind, refresh her body, and empower her personality for courageous acts.

Rosemary oil *(Rosmarinus officinalis)* of the Lamiaceae family, with all its vitality and mind-stimulating qualities, was certainly one of the favorites of this vigorous queen. She could inhale it for enhancement of memory or rub it on her skin for aching joints and painful muscles. She valued its regenerative quality, its boost for the heart and liver, its ability to act as a protector, and its work for clear thinking. She no doubt used it in her bath and had a servant pour it on her hair since it stimulated her scalp and gave her hair a special luster. It helped her become a leader of cunning and vision.

Cleopatra truly loved and revered perfume, and used it with great discre-

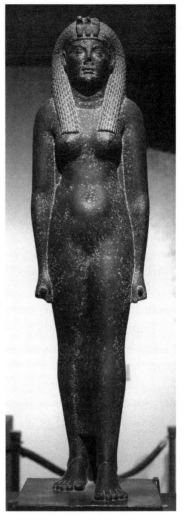

Cleopatra

tion and taste. At that time the city of Alexandria was a veritable rose garden of perfume markets and booths. The Egyptians gave the olfactory sense a primary human significance. For hundreds of years priests kept the secret formulas of scents, which were prepared in fragrance workshops attached to the back of every temple where only the priests entered. Inscriptions of formulas can still be found on the walls. One such room is clearly visible today at the great temple of Edfu, begun by King Ptolemy III in 237 BC about sixty miles south of Luxor. If we walk into this ancient perfume laboratory in total darkness, a flickering light would reveal the many hieroglyphics, recording of the creative formulas of perfumes and unguents. The priests kept their treasured scents in beautifully carved boxes of wood or ivory and in jars made of onyx or alabaster. By 80 BC, the average Egyptian citizen was a connoisseur of fragrance and could find at least a hundred different oils in the marketplace. They especially loved Jasmine, Saffron, Rose, Lavender, Cedar, Cinnamon, Ginger, Coriander, Flag broom, Lily, and Lotus.

Scent was often used to bring about an altered state of consciousness, especially at Alexandrian cafes where people sat discussing philosophy and religion in rooms filled with essential oil fragrance. The Egyptian god Nefertum, the lord of oils and unguents, was known for his transformational, life-giving powers. His influence was especially important on the voyage into the afterworld, according to contemporary aromatherapist John Steele, where one's personal fragrance denoted one's soul status. The *unguentari* (perfumers) of Cleopatra's time were learned chemists as well as artists. As described by Richard Le Gallienne, "These traders in perfumes were not tarnished by their street transactions, but became affiliated with the mysterious, the elusive, and the aristocratic sides of life. They partook in all the divine and noble associations of perfume."[2]

Shakespeare describes Cleopatra as a woman whose "age cannot wither her, nor custom stale her infinite variety."[3] Even though her face was not gorgeous, she fit the Egyptian norm of feminine beauty. She spent much time at her toilet and was always beautifully perfumed. She even wrote a "famous book on beautification in 1 AD which has not survived, but is extensively quoted by various authors from the Roman period and even later."[4]

Cleanliness and personal appearance were highly regarded by the Egyptians. Deodorants were important in this hot climate. To repel body odor, they put little balls of myrrh or balsam incense where the limbs met the body. They often used an ointment of Frankincense and honey as a moisturizer or for a burn. Since they had a healthy diet and did not eat sugar, they had little tooth decay. They chewed fennel seeds for their breath and Frankincense to keep their teeth clean. They used Juniper berry oil to color graying hair and stimulate the scalp.

In *An Ancient Egyptian Herbal,* Lise Manniche describes a recipe for wrinkles found on a papyrus: gum of frankincense, wax, fresh Moringa oil, and cyprus grass is ground finely and mixed with fermented plant juice.

Apply daily.[5] "The almond shape of the black Egyptian eyes was underlined with an application of black kohl or green malachite,"[6] writes Manniche. According to Michal Dayagi-Mendels, the kohl, "prepared from sunflower soot, charred almond shells, and frankincense,"[7] was also considered preventive medicine for eye diseases. Little distinction was made between a medicinal remedy and a cosmetic.

After Ptolemy XIII's death, Cleopatra became the sole ruler of Egypt. Caesar had restored her position, but now she had to marry her brother, Ptolemy XIV, who was eleven years old, an act necessary to please the citizens of Alexandria and the Egyptian priests. Caesar was so smitten with Cleopatra's intelligence and her inheritance of Egypt's vast resources that he was committed to a relationship with her. He also found her perfumes to be incredible aphrodisiacs.

One of her favorite perfumes was Jasmine *(Jasminum grandiflorum)* of the Oleaceae family, known for its powerful effect on the reproductive organs and its aphrodisiac qualities, especially as a stimulant for transforming the physical act of reproduction into a more spiritual experience. It must have been an aid to Cleopatra in her two main love relationships (Julius Caesar and Mark Antony) and in childbirth. Once labor started, it strengthened the uterine contractions and brought a bonding of mother and child. It was wonderful when diluted as a massage oil in the pelvic area to balance a woman's hormones and create a regular menstrual cycle. Jasmine also boosted Cleopatra's confidence and warmed her emotions when she felt depressed. Just the perfect fragrance for a meeting with Julius Caesar!

After Cleopatra and Julius Caesar became lovers, they spent many days on a luxuriously furnished houseboat on the Nile. They stopped in Dander where Cleopatra was worshipped as a pharaoh. Caesar left the boat to attend to important business in Syria just a few weeks before the birth of their son, Caesarion (Ptolemy Caesar), who was born on June 23, 47 BC, and always adored by Cleopatra. In July of 46 BC, Caesar returned to Rome with Cleopatra and her entourage. He was given many honors and a ten-year dictatorship; celebrations lasted from September to October. The conservative Republicans were shocked when he established Cleopatra in his home. They were upset by her title, "the new Isis," and her lifestyle of luxury. Caesar openly claimed Caesarion as his son, even though Roman laws forbade bigamy (Caesar was already married) and marriages to foreigners.

The end came for Caesar on the Ides of March in 44 BC by a conspiracy of senators who thought he and Cleopatra were a threat to the republic's well-being. After Caesar's murder, Cleopatra fled from Rome and returned home to Alexandria. She felt her life, as well as that of her son, was in great danger. Her dream of ruling both the Roman Empire and Egypt died slowly. After her return to Alexandria, she had her consort, Ptolemy XIV, assassinated and established Caesarion, only four years old, as her co-regent. Egypt was suffering from plagues and famine, and the Nile canals had been neglected during her absence, which caused the harvest to be inadequate. She began the work of revitalizing her beloved Egypt. After a few more years under her guiding hand, this is how Lucy Hughes-Hallett describes the country: "Egypt was the only self-contained country of the ancient world: her agriculture was flourishing, her industry prosperous, her commerce widespread, her schools famous, and her artistic life vigorous under Cleopatra's reign."[8]

Unlike the legend built about her, Cleopatra spent most of her life celibate, and chose her two loves with a shrewd eye to the political advantages they offered her. "She appears to have been a tactful and efficient ruler, a tough negotiator, and a thrifty manager."[9] During her reign, the country was internally at peace and the economy was strong. She closely watched the changes in Rome, in particular who would become the next emperor. After Brutus and Cassius were killed, she noted that Antony, Octavian, and Lepidus were triumphant. Since Octavian and Antony had divided up the civilized world into West and East, Cleopatra decided that she and her son's future were linked with Mark Antony.

When Antony visited the trading port of Tarsus, he sent for Cleopatra. She knew about his limited strategic abilities, his blue blood, the drinking, the womanizing, and his ambitious nature. In 41 BC she arrived in her royal galley with its silver oars and purple sails. She was magnificently and aromatically adorned, reclining beneath an awning of gold. "The banks of the river, Cydnus were even scented with incense and Kyphi, the wonderful perfume compounded according to the sacred books of sixteen ingredients, which were being burned in bronze bowls on her galley and the boats of her suite."[10] Cleopatra used all her abilities to charm and lure Antony, including aromatherapy. In Shakespeare's *Antony and Cleopatra*, Enobarus describes her arrival in Tarsus:

The barge she sat in, like a burnished throne
Burn'd on the water; the poop was beaten gold
Purple the sails, and so perfumed that
The winds were lovesick …
From the barge
A strange invisible perfume hits the sense
Of the adjacent wharfs.[11]

The perfume Shakespeare referred to was Kyphi. This expensive offering was described by Plutarch in *Treatise on Isis and Osiris* as honey, wine, raisins, galangal, resin, myrrh, aspalathus, sessile, lemongrass, asphalt, fig and sorrel leaves, juniper, cardamom, and sweet rush. The French chemist Loret claims that henna, peppermint, calamus, and cyperus were part of the exquisite mixture, the world's first perfume. According to Plutarch, Kyphi "lulled one to sleep, allayed anxieties and brightened dreams."[12]

This all mesmerized Antony; he looked upon Cleopatra with ecstasy as she dined on the galley at the most luxurious banquet he had ever experienced. The Greek historian, Athenaeus, wrote in 220 AD that red rose petals were used to cover the floors of the royal apartment up to eighteen inches deep! Antony loved the idea of a blue-blooded Ptolemy woman mating with his own aristocratic inheritance. His current wife, Fulvia, was merely middle class. The day after Cleopatra's arrival, Antony agreed to help her strengthen her power on the throne of the Ptolemies and spend the winter in Alexandria. Later she offered Antony the position of king of Egypt, and the Egyptian fleet, the finest in the world, was to be at his disposal—if he became her husband. She needed the bond with Rome for its strength and its army.

Antony and Cleopatra were married in 36 BC. She bore him three children (two were twins). Antony loved her. She was an able colleague and a cultured companion; she possessed the glamour of ancient royalty and wealth. She also knew the key to love: "She must always appear beautiful and amiable, exhale a perfume of lotus flowers and ambrosia, and have the aroma of love."[13] Cleopatra planted the aphrodisiac lotus in their garden. In Egypt gardens had shade, scent, and water. Painted pergolas were covered with vines. Glorious water landscapes were created with the sweet blue lotus *(Nymphaea coerulea)* as a focal point, floating on the water's surface. The lotus was a sacred flower, "symbolizing the purity of the spiritual life of man, for as the flowers have their roots in earth and water, but float above in the sunlight, so the soul of man rises above the earth life."[14]

In the spring of 40 BC, Mark Antony returned to Rome. He sought reconciliation with Octavian that autumn by marrying Octavian's sister, Octavia. She was a beautiful and intelligent woman who had recently been widowed. Antony told Octavia she would be of more use to him at home in Rome, keeping peace with her brother, Octavian. The first thing Antony did when reaching Antioch was send for Cleopatra. He needed her support in a campaign against the Parthians. He gave her much land (Cyprus, Phoenicia, Coele-Syria, Judea, and Arabia), which enabled Egypt to build ships with the lumber from the Cilician coast (modern Turkey). Egypt did build a large fleet

In 30 BC Antony led a successful campaign into Armenia, which filled his purse as well, giving him additional land. He celebrated with a parade through Alexandria with Cleopatra as "the new Isis." This was a fulfillment of his dream of a Greco-Roman rule. At a public, political ceremony a few days later, Antony proclaimed his children with Cleopatra to be kings and queens. Cleopatra was called "the queen of kings," and Caesarion (Ptolemy XV), her official co-ruler, became "the king of kings" in the Donations of Alexandria, a magnificent ceremony. Cleopatra was close to becoming empress of the world.

Antony put Cleopatra's face on the silver *denarius,* a Roman coin that circulated throughout the Mediterranean. This broadcast his relationship with the Egyptian queen to the Western part of the world. In 30 BC Antony finally divorced Octavia, which prompted Octavian to formally declared war against Cleopatra, although Antony was not mentioned. Most Romans hated and feared "the new Isis" and were afraid Antony and Cleopatra would begin world conquest and co-rule from Alexandria. Octavian, who later became Caesar Augustus, decided he must destroy the two lovers. Antony and Cleopatra were defeated at Actium in 30 BC, where Antony urged her to leave on a ship with the Egyptian treasury on board. They both returned to Alexandria and there took a defensive stand. When that failed, Antony committed suicide by falling on his sword. Cleopatra could have seduced Octavian, but she chose instead to show her deep love for Antony by her final act: Faced by the cold and unmoved Octavian, she took her life with an asp, which was considered a divine messenger from the gods. The Egyptian religion declared that death by snakebite would secure immortality. She died on August 12, 30 BC, at the age of thirty-nine. After Cleopatra's death, Caesarion was strangled and her other children were raised by Antony's former wife, Octavia. Octavian's victory in Egypt was significant for the development of civilization; Rome, not Egypt, now dominated over the Greco-Egyptian alliance of the East.

Even though her life ended in tragedy, the love and strength of Cleopatra has been remembered throughout time. As the last pharaoh of Egypt, her great schemes failed, but her ambition, capability, and remarkable charm left a great impression on history. Cleopatra saw herself as the goddess Isis, awesome but kind. She was also a mathematician and excellent businessperson. Cleopatra, like Isis, revealed courage and resourcefulness at every dramatic twist of her life's path. Although she used the power of oils like Jasmine, her real aphrodisiac was power. She looked men straight in the eye with a sense of equality. "The death of Cleopatra brought to an end the grandeur of Egypt with its then unparalleled appreciation of beauty and good living."[15] Her work as an aromatherapist was invaluable as a statement of the empowering effects of perfumed oils on the body and mind.

CHAPTER FOUR

Women in the Life of Jesus

Love is the strongest force the world possesses.

—MAHATMA GANDHI

IMAGINE YOURSELF WALKING on a dusty road beside a charming man whose faith in you inspires unimagined confidence and joy. As you walk through the countryside of arid desert and open fields, he encourages you to be glad for the simple things in life like honesty, health, and love. He suggests you share these gifts with those less fortunate. Just as you decide to take his advice, you pass some lovely bushes and a haunting fragrance permeates your olfactory consciousness. The exquisite smell of rose will forever be imbued with the feeling of gratitude you feel for having known such a man. This was the experience of those in the Women's Evangelistic Corps, a group that traveled with Jesus and the apostles in 20 AD.

Jesus was a majestic spiritual teacher who came to our planet to enhance the revelation of God to every soul who lived then and in future times. Even though his being was of divine origin, he wanted to live on earth as an average man so he could relate best to the common people. He often reached out to the outcasts or powerless in his society. He grew up in a humble Jewish family as the oldest son, losing his father, Joseph, at an early age. Before beginning his public ministry, he helped his mother, Mary, raise his brothers and sisters.

Jesus was born into a world that was experiencing a revival of spiritual thinking and religious living. Roman political and social systems, the Greek language and culture, and the influence of Jewish religious and moral teachings acted as unifying forces. For the first time, the entire Mediterranean world was a coordinated empire with good roads, abundant trade and transportation, and internal peace. Merchants traveled with camels and horses over routes such as the Spice Road, while the armies of Egypt, India, Assyria, Parthia, Babylonia, Rome, China, and Malaysia swept compatibly over Palestine. Essential oils, spices, and herbs safely flowed throughout this region along these caravan routes.

Jesus especially related to the plight of women during his life. Women enjoyed a limited freedom throughout the Roman Empire, yet they had an even more restricted status in Palestine. However, family loyalty and affection of the Jews transcended that of the gentile world. The city of Jerusalem brought unity to the Jewish people as their center of worship and some self-government under Herod's overlordship.

Jesus honored the women in his life and time. This was a radical step considering the status of Jewish women in this time. Palestinian Hebrew women were among the poorest in the world. They had no inheritance rights and could not own land. Jewish women received no education and were married as soon as they could bear children, around the age of twelve or thirteen. The Jews felt that burning the records of their sacred book, the Torah, was better than delivering it into the hands of a woman. Jewish rabbis began every temple meeting with the words, "Blessed art thou, O Lord, for thou hast not made me a woman."[1] Women of respect stayed hidden at home. In public a woman could speak to no man, not even her husband. A woman was subordinated first to her father and then to her husband. Public affairs were the domain of men only. Women were not allowed to travel. For Jesus to elevate women to religious leaders in a public arena was an amazing, compassionate act in those times. Many of the stories about the courageous women who were loyal to the master were lost to history shortly after his death.

The story of Nalda shows how Jesus disregarded all of these patriarchal rules and acknowledged women as people, daughters of God with souls. In one of his most famous and touching public encounters with a woman, Jesus met Nalda at Jacob's well in the Samaritan town of Sycar. He and the twelve apostles had been preaching for some weeks and arrived there very tired. The apostles, who considered a Samaritan town as enemy territory, went to look for accommodations. Jesus sat alone by the well and asked a woman, Nalda, to draw water for his thirst. Nalda was shocked that a Jewish man would speak to her in public. In exchange for her cup, he offered her a symbolic drink of the living water that becomes a "well of refreshment, springing up even to eternal life."[2]

Women were subordinated first to their fathers and then to their husbands. One week of the month (during her menses), she was unclean, and anything she touched during that time, including food or other people, was considered contaminated.

In another encounter, as Jesus walked through the narrow streets of Capernaum, he suddenly said, "Someone touched me.... for I perceived that living energy has gone forth from me."[3] He looked around and saw a woman who came and knelt at his feet. She said, "For years I have been afflicted with a scourging hemorrhage."[4] She spoke of having seen many doctors, spending all her money, and feeling ostracized in her community. She told Jesus, "I touched the border of your garment, and I was made whole."[5] Jesus took her by the hand, lifting her up, saying, "Daughter, your faith has made you whole; go in peace."[6] He touched her in love, showing how he was unafraid of any uncleanness. He knew how painful it must be to be cast aside by the social mores that disregarded her individuality due to a physical illness.

Another woman who meant a great deal to Jesus was his childhood friend, Mary, the sister of Lazarus. She had the courage to publicly bestow an essential oil treatment on the man she loved and whom she considered a family friend. The event took place after a feast at the home of

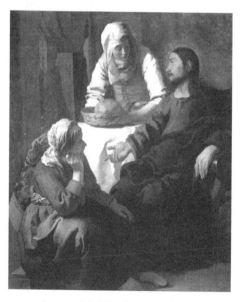

Jesus with Martha and Mary

Simon, one of the most prominent citizens of Bethany. Jesus had chosen the small village of Bethany as the place where he would raise Lazarus from the dead because almost every man, woman, and child who lived there believed, as Jesus taught, that they were the children of a loving God. Near the end of the feast, Mary, accompanied by her sister, Martha, walked forward from a group of women onlookers. She was carrying a large alabaster vase of a very rare and expensive essential oil, Spikenard *(Nardostachys grandiflora)*. The scene is described in the Bible (John 12:3): "Then Mary, taking a pound of costly perfume made of purest [Spike]nard, anointed the feet of Jesus and dried His feet with her hair. So the house was filled with the fragrance of the perfume."[7] All those present were amazed at what Mary had done.

The essential oil Mary used came from Spikenard (sometimes called "mountain nard") of the Valerianaceae family and found in the high mountains (11,000–17,000 feet) of the Himalayas, such as Botan and Nepal in India. According to Roy Genders, "Jatamansi is a Hindu word signifying a 'lock of hair' for the most fragrant part of the plant is that portion of the stem just above the root which is covered with fibres from the petioles of the withered leaves. These hair-like filaments are formed so closely together that they have the appearance of a lock of hair."[8]

The most sought after oil by the Romans, Spikenard was considered valuable as a perfume for the hair. Today it is steam-distilled from the hairy stems and has a strong odor reminiscent of Patchouli and Valerian with a faint background of musk. A desirable aspect of Spikenard is that the longer it is kept, the more potent becomes its odor. In *de Materia Medica,* the Greek physician Dioscorides described Spikenard as a warming and drying oil, good for treating nausea, indigestion, and inflammation. It was also known to be very calming emotionally, yet it also intensified feelings of devotion toward God or a spiritual teacher. Patricia Davis finds that Spikenard exemplifies the "spirit of generosity."[9]

Mary's Spikenard would have been mixed with olive oil since Jewish law required that sacred oils—often used by priests for anointing a tabernacle or burning on the alter as incense—be blended with a carrier oil. When Mary finished anointing the feet of Jesus, Judas Iscariot murmured to Andrew that Mary should be reprimanded for such waste, for Spikenard was very precious. Jesus was touched by her act of aromatic devotion and put his hand on Mary's head, saying to everyone present that they should not rebuke her, seeing that her action came from her heart. He remarked that the ointment could have been sold to give alms to the poor, but the poor would always be there to minister to: According to the version of this incident in *The Urantia Book*, Jesus foresaw Mary's place in history: "... I shall not always be with you; I go soon to my Father ... In the ages to come, wherever this gospel shall be preached throughout the whole world, what she has done will be spoken of in memory of her."[10]

Even though her act was extravagant, Mary loved Jesus and wanted to bestow this offering upon him while he lived instead of at his burial. In spite of the risk of public disapproval, she felt empowered to act. The energy of the plant was like a balm to the pain in her heart caused by the thought of the immanent departure of Jesus. She had the hearty approval of her brother, Lazarus, and her sister, Martha, since she had saved the money for a long time to buy the cruse of Spikenard. Once again a woman received courage through the act of bestowing an essential oil—in this case not on herself but on a beloved friend.

Earlier in his life Jesus—along with Peter, James, and John—was invited for a social dinner at the home of another Simon, a Pharisee of Jerusalem. During a banquet, the Pharisees customarily left the doors open so street beggars could come in and stand behind the guests' couches to receive extra food. One person who entered was a woman who had formerly been the keeper of a high-class brothel. She had closed her infamous place of business and convinced the majority of her female partners to accept the gospel and make ethical improvements in their lifestyle. Even though she had become a believer in the gospel of Jesus, she had been compelled by the disdainful Pharisees to wear her hair down as a badge of her harlotry. The Bible states in Mark 14:3, "While he was at Bethany in the home of Simon the leper as he was sitting at the table, a woman came with an alabaster jar of pure [spike]nard perfume, very valuable and, breaking the jar, she poured the ointment on his head."[11]

According to the version of this incident in *The Urantia Book*, the woman also began to anoint the feet of Jesus with the flask of perfumed lotion mixed with her tears of gratitude, wiping his feet with her long hair. She continued crying and kissing his feet. Simon was shocked to see Jesus allowing a notorious sinner touch him like this. Jesus said to Simon, "My head with oil you neglected to anoint, but she has anointed my feet with the precious lotions. . . . because her many sins have been forgiven and this has led her to love much."[12] Jesus then told her not to be depressed by the insensitive and unkind attitude of her surrounding peers, but to live in the light and joy of God's kingdom. Jesus made clear to the Pharisees that when mighty transformations are made in the mind and spirit, even the most humble soul and the most dastardly sinner are welcome in the spiritual kingdom. Jesus said it was better by far to be a soul in progress with a small but growing faith than to possess a great intellect with its dead accumulation of knowledge and spiritual unbelief.

Jesus loved women because he could see into their hearts and souls, and how they suffered in the male-dominated world around them. Using fragrant plant oils offered women an opportunity to give, to serve, and to be strengthened. The New Testament has a paucity of information about the women who followed Jesus, yet we know from Luke 8:1–5 that women spent time with him, traveling throughout the countryside into the towns of Galilee and Samaria. Even the apostles used these plant oils, as reported by Mark in the Bible: "So they [the apostles] went out and preached that men should repent. They expelled many demons; and many sick they anointed with oil and healed."[13]

Of all the audacious things Jesus did during his life, the most astonishing was gathering a group of twelve women to further the work of his ministry. At the time women were not allowed to read the Torah at synagogue due to their periodic "uncleanness," and they had to sit in a separate upstairs gallery in the synagogue. Women were educated only in household tasks and food preparation. Only the wife of a rabbi was educated in reading. Women could not teach the law or be witnesses in Jewish courts. In a country ruled by the religious elite, this rendered them invisible and powerless. Yet on January 16, 29 AD, Jesus said, "On the morrow, we will set apart ten women.... Susanna, the daughter of the former chazan of the Nazareth synagogue; Joanna, the wife of Chuza, the steward of Herod Antipas; Elizabeth, the daughter of a wealthy Jew of Tiberias; Martha, the elder sister of Andrew and Peter; Rachel, the sister-in-law of Jude, the Master's brother in the flesh; Nasanta, the daughter of Elman, the Syrian physician; Milcha, a cousin of the Apostle Thomas; Ruth, the eldest daughter of Mathew Levi; Celta, the daughter of a Roman centurion; and Agaman, a widow of Damascus. Subsequently, Jesus added two other women to this group— Mary Magdalene and Rebecca, the daughter of Joseph of Arimathea."[14] This group of twelve women became known as the Women's Evangelistic

Corps. Jesus authorized them to create their own organization and directed Judas to provide money for their equipment and pack animals.

The story of the women of Jesus is continued in *The Urantia Book:* "... they [the twelve apostles] were literally stunned when he proposed formally to commission these ten women as religious teachers and even to permit their traveling about with them. The whole country was stirred up by this proceeding, the enemies of Jesus made great capital out of this move, but everywhere the women believers in the good news stood staunchly behind their chosen sisters and voiced no uncertain approval of this tardy acknowledgment of woman's place in religious work."[15]

Jesus announced the emancipation proclamation, which set women free for all time, even though Paul later limited women in the Christian church. The Urantia Book explains: "... no more was man to look upon woman as his spiritual inferior."[16] The women elected Susanna as their leader and Joanna as their treasurer. Soon they were self-sufficient and created their own earnings. Women who had not even been allowed on the main floor of a synagogue were now authorized teachers of the new gospel. These women were able to minister most effectively to their downcast sisters in Magdala, for example, where the apostles were not allowed to go. The women could visit the sick and offer fragrant oils, herbs, and food to the inmates in this evil resort. There they found Mary Magdalene, who became their strongest teacher. The twelve apostles, recovering from their initial horror at the formation of the Women's Evangelistic Corps, began to see the wisdom of Jesus in making this decision and often enjoyed traveling with their female counterparts. Although the story of the Women's Corps does not specifically mention the use of healing with essential oils, the women certainly carried them while ministering to the sick, and their aroma added to the upliftment of their grace-filled message wherever they went.

The twelve women surely carried with them the red petals of rose *(Rosa gallica)* of the Rosaceae family, native to Persia and one of the oldest plants known to humans. Jeanne Rose writes, "In Persia, such large quantities of rose water were produced that canals were filled with it, and on hot, sunny days, an oily scum would rise to the surface and be captured in small vials."[17] Rose water was in great demand throughout the East due to its valuable astringent qualities. Women might have used it to stem hemorrhage. Due to the rose's ability to retain its perfume, even when dried, it later earned the name "the apothecary's rose" in the Middle Ages and was used to heal lung disease. It was also valuable for the heart, as a tonic for sluggish blood circulation. Emotionally, Rose was soothing for dark feelings like jealousy, depression, and grief. Spiritually, it was believed to open the heart chakra to radiate more love. The heart is the middle ground where the spiritual and physical are united. Appropriately, the heart is associated with Jesus, who was a living example of spiritual energy uniting with physical reality. The Rose, either *Rosa gallica* or *Rosa damascena,* is symbolically his scent. (*Rosa damascena* is an absolute, using modern solvent extraction methods.) The fragrance of Rose is known to enhance the truth, beauty, and goodness of anyone fortunate enough to use the oil or smell the flower.

The women of Jesus spent much time healing people of physical and spiritual infirmities, using the herbs and oils of prominence at that time. They certainly addressed some physical problems common to people of all ages: headache, toothache, indigestion, arthritic pain, infection, colds, flu, PMS (premenstrual syndrome) and depression. Dioscorides, who traveled throughout the Mediterranean with Roman troops, was one of the first in the Western world to document the therapeutic application of over seven hundred plants. A contemporary of Jesus, his *de Materia Medica* was widely used until the 1800s. These are some of the plants described by Dioscorides and promoted by the Women's Evangelistic Corps:

> **Hyssop** *(Hyssopus officinalis):* for respiratory infections, as a laxative, and for purification.
> **Marjoram** *(Origanum majorana):* for rheumatic pains, grief, and toothaches.
> **Frankincense** *(Boswellia carteri):* for the nervous and endocrine system.
> **Peppermint** *(Mentha piperita):* for digestive upsets, cooling, and infection.
> **Myrrh** *(Commiphora myrrha):* for gum and skin infections, and as an immune stimulant.

These plants were used in both herbal and oil ointment forms. The oil form was infused oils, meaning they were created in vegetable oils like olive oil. The distilled oils we use today are more powerful in their aroma and concentration than those used around 1 AD.

The women who surrounded Jesus during his lifetime felt a loving devotion for this extraordinary friend. In the last moments of his life, as Jesus hung on the cross, all the apostles had fled but one, yet (according to *The Urantia Book*) the Women's Evangelistic Corps were "all present, and not one either denied or betrayed him."[18] During one of his last appearances before a gathering of women, including Mary Magdalene, Jesus said, "Peace be upon you. In the fellowship of the kingdom there shall be neither Jew nor gentile, rich nor poor, free nor bond, man nor woman. You also are called to publish the good news of the liberty of mankind through the gospel of sonship with God in the kingdom of heaven. Go to all the world proclaiming this gospel and confirming believers in the faith thereof. And while you do this, forget not to minister to the sick and strengthen those who are fainthearted and fear-ridden. And I will be with you always, even to the ends of the earth."[19]

In the person of Jesus, we can see the development of both male and female characteristics into one harmonious personality. His strength, his honesty, his practicality blended with his divine insight. His compassion and his gentleness made him a balanced human being. He had the graciousness and the "aroma of friendliness that emanates from a love-saturated soul."[20] Men and women today can use the model of this integrated person to reveal how more equilibrium can be created between the two genders and into each individual psyche. He revealed the true purpose of our lives: to grow in our spiritual understanding and love of God. Through the scent of rose, the heart fragrance, we can unite our physical and spiritual selves.

CHAPTER FIVE

Zenobia, the Syrian Queen of the Palmyrene Empire

The desert always waits, ready to let us know who we are—the place of self-discovery.

—RUTH BURGESS

I N YOUR MIND'S EYE, see yourself perched on a rock in a desert landscape outside of Palmyra, in the middle of today's Syria, watching the sun plummet like a ball of fire into a dry, arid void. It is the year 298 AD. Against a darkening sky, you see the beautiful white Greek columns of Palmyra's buildings. Suddenly you hear the thundering sound of galloping horses and you see an amazing female dressed in a helmet and armored vest, leading a troop of warriors. As this military queen rides near you, you smell an intriguing fragrance of Clovebud *(Syzgium aromaticum)*, Thyme *(Thymus vulgaris)*, and Lemon *(Citrus x limon)*. It gives a sense of power and stamina. You know that a stunning person is commanding such an army.

This beautiful, courageous woman combined female virtues with male strengths during a time when few women dared to express their beliefs, much less act on them. Zenobia was the daughter of a general, Julius Aurelius Zenobius; she was born in 241 AD in the city of Palmyra. This magnificent city built in the middle of the vast Syrian desert was part of the Roman Empire for 200 years. Its origins go back to the second millennium BC. The desert city, located between Roman Syria and Persian Babylonia, was built near an oasis watered by the Efqa spring. Its citizens were a mixture of Aramaic and Arabic stock; most were former Bedouins. Palmyra was a center of ancient world trade for exotic oils from southern Arabia, the Far East, and the Mediterranean world. Tradition says it was built by Solomon on the spot where David killed Goliath. The city was on a route that linked the Euphrates River to the cities of the Mediterranean like Antioch to the north and Gaza to the south. "Palmyra, as the channel of East Indian oils, grew in wealth, but not in strength," writes William Wright.[1] About 50 BC Mark Antony tried to plunder her merchant princes. Under Septimius Severus, at the end of the second century AD, Palmyra was raised to the status of a Roman colony. From 100 AD on, the relations between Rome and Palmyra were cordial. Palmyra ministered to the Roman desire for the luxury of fragrant oils and Rome pledged to uphold the safety and stability of the merchant city. The trade in spices, aromatics, and silk created the wealth of Palmyra.

Zenobia was raised in Palmyra, amidst the beauty of the Greek and Roman architecture, and was married at the early age of fourteen to the senator and self-proclaimed king of Palmyra, the widower Septimius Odaenathus. The Roman Emperor valued him for suppressing the revolt of two pretenders, and he became a hero to the East when he stopped the Persian invasion of Syria. Inscriptions on stones at Palmyra, written in Aramaic and Greek, give Odaenathus status as "chief of Palmyra" and describe his line of descendants; the stones date back to 251 AD. Other inscriptions call him Roman senator, consul, and governor of the Roman province of Syria. Odaenathus was returning from victory when his cousin, Maeonius, murdered him in 267 AD. The teenage son of Odaenathus and Zenobia, Vaballathus, became king of Palmyra while Zenobia stood behind him as regent. Vaballathus received the title "illustrious king of kings," which he inherited from his father, Odaenathus. Zenobia became the true director of Palmyra's policies and deeds. This situation was similar to that of Hatshepsut and Tuthmosis III as described in Chapter 1.

Zenobia's ambition proved to be far greater than her husband's. "Zenobia is perhaps the only female whose superior genius broke through the servile indolence imposed on her sex by the climate and traditions of Asia," wrote Roman historian Edward Gibbon in *The History of the Decline and Fall of the Roman Empire*.[2] Claiming her ancestral history was from the Macedonian kings of Egypt, she felt a kinship with Cleopatra, whom she equaled in intelligence and surpassed in beauty, courage, and chastity. Zenobia had a dark complexion, pearly white teeth, and large black eyes that sparkled with a fiery sweetness. Her voice was strong and melodious. She spoke Latin, Greek, Syrian, and Egyptian. She had studied the history of her people in the Orient as well as Homer and Plato. She shared Odaenathus's love of hunting the wild beasts of the desert like lions and panthers. According to Gibbon, she disdained the use of a carriage and rode on horseback. As leader of her troops, she always wore a military habit and as their captain often marched several miles ahead on foot. The most reliable source on Zenobia is the Greek historian Zosimus, who wrote *Historia Augusta* in 500 AD.

Like Cleopatra, Zenobia had a love affair with fragrant oils. One of her favorites was the stimulating, spicy, and penetrating Clove *(Syzygium aromaticum)* from the Myrtaceae family, which came over the spice route that ran through Palmyra from China. Today clove comes from Zanzibar and Sri Lanka. The tree reaches a height of fifty feet and remains in bearing up to one hundred years. The buds are picked in August through December. The closed buds are pinkish yellow when picked, and later turn dark red as they are spread out on mats to dry. The essential oil is best from the clove buds, which is not as hot and toxic as oil from the bark. Clove oil is high in eugenol (a phenol); its use requires care since it can irritate skin and mucous membranes. Its antibacterial qualities were known to prevent disease. Its benefits to the digestive system were renowned for relieving gas, vomiting, diarrhea, and intestinal spasms. It also is a classic as an analgesic for tooth pain.

Zenobia would sprinkled a few drops of Clove oil into her bath water and sometimes on her food. It gave her a tingling feeling of strength and health. She frequented the perfumer's bazaar at a market in Palmyra where scents of aromatic gums like Frankincense from Oman, Myrrh from Yemen, and Balsam from southern Arabia mingled with floral aromas like Rose and Lupine to delight the nose and intoxicate the brain. She loved Cinnamon from Indonesia, Costus and Spikenard from Bactra, Sandalwood from North India, and Nutmeg from Ceylon. As noted in Richard Stoneman's *Palmyra and Its Empire,* she also used a renowned Greek perfume called Megaleion, named for its inventor Megallus, who lived in the time of Alexander. His perfume, made with a base of the celebrated oil of Balanos from the date-like fruit of a thorny desert tree, included Myrrh, Cassia, Cinnamon, and burnt resin. Megaleion was a famous unguent for its rejuvenating qualities when applied to the face, which was helpful in the desert air.

According to Richard Stoneman, "These aromatics were the most expensive items the Romans imported from the East to feed their sybaritic tastes."[3] Romans burned the aromatic incense to win the favor of their gods and used the oils at the time of death. Roman emperor Nero burned so much incense after the death of his second wife, Poppaea Sabina, that a whole year's crop of frankincense was consumed. In the first century AD, Pliny the Elder wrote, "Arabian fortune has been caused by the luxury of mankind [Roman], even in the hour of death, when they burn incense over the departed, the products they had originally understood to be created for the Gods."[4]

For 250 years, both before and during Zenobia's life, Palmyra emerged as an architectural splendor. Most buildings were built of local marble with long colonnades linked by richly ornamented capitals atop large columns. The Temple of Bel was the first public building in 1 AD and even today is impressive with its Athenian design. When the Roman emperor Hadrian visited the city in 129 AD during the height of its brilliance and wealth, he granted Palmyra the rights of a free city within the Roman Empire. Its streets were paved and clean; water fountains were interspersed between the palaces and temples. A vibrant, ethnically Semitic mixture from every Middle and Far Eastern country, the people dressed in many colorful, ethnic costumes, and rode on elephants, camels, and Arabian horses.[5] On Palmyrene tombstones, pictures of both camels and ships are inscribed because the camel was the true ship of the desert; the economic trade of the city depended on the camel. Palmyra's raison d'être was the spring, Efqa, which created this oasis in the desert. The wealth of the trading sheiks

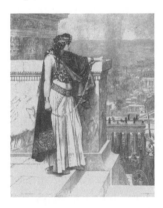

offered the resources to build the beautiful edifices of Palmyra. The people of Palmyra felt the control of Rome, which taxed the perfumes in bulk and the perfumer paid a further tax. The city appeared to be a Roman city with its forum, senate, amphitheater, temple, and market, lacking only a public bath, yet internally the city held onto the culture of its various Arabian tribes, at least thirty in number.

After the death of Odaenathus, Zenobia and her son became rulers of this unique city. It was astounding that a female ruler could

Queen Zenobia's last look upon Palmyra

rise to power in the extremely patriarchal ancient Arabian world. She ruled partly through the support of her husband's friends, the sheiks of Palmyra. One of her models was the Syrian Queen Sammuramat, who, famous for her beauty and wisdom, conquered many lands and introduced religious reforms in 812 BC. A myth developed that after a long and prosperous reign, Queen Sammuramat vanished from the earth in the shape of a dove. Zenobia also had the support of neighboring Arabian, Jewish, and Armenian tribes. She attended the parties of the military; she could drink with the best of her generals and then ride off with them to exercise or to battle. The queen dazzled her people with her beauty and her noble bearing on a horse. During the eighteenth century, Catherine the Great of Russia, who created a military and intellectual court, liked to compare herself to Zenobia.

For her court Zenobia had a city palace and, near the spring, a country palace—both of exquisite architecture. Her country palace stood on a vast plain. To the north stretched a wild country inhabited by the wild animals she enjoyed hunting. To the south the view included cultivated fields, flowing canals of water, light bridges, arbors, statues, and rich foliage. The palace had arches, pinnacles, domes, towers, and fountains. William Ware wrote, "The fountains took many fantastic forms ... like an enormous elephant of stone disgorges from his uplifted trunk a vast, but graceful shower, sometimes charged with the most exquisite perfumes and which are diffused into the air through every part of the palace."[6] She surrounded herself with images of her distant relative, Cleopatra, according to Ware: "The walls and ceilings and carpets in her palace represented the scenes of the life and reign of the great queen of Egypt."[7] To fully invoke the presence of Cleopatra, Zenobia filled her rooms with the fragrance of Frankincense, Juniper, and Rose.

The oil of Juniper *(Juniperus communis)* of the Cupressaceae family seemed to resonate with Zenobia. Derived from the berries of a juniper shrub, the oil gives off a powerful, no-nonsense scent like this queen. It is a diuretic and detoxifying agent for a body laden with too much alcohol or food. It regulates the appetite and is a tonic for the kidneys and liver. Wanda Sellar claims, "Its [Juniper's] ability to throw off poisons by purifying the blood ... and eliminating uric acid ... in cases of arthritis, rheumatism, and gout" made it a valuable oil.[8] Mentally, Juniper clears and stimulates thoughts, especially in challenging situations, so Zenobia would have enjoyed the effect of the oil in her military and intellectual pursuits.

She appreciated its strong purifying effect on the body and on the atmosphere of her palace.

At her court Zenobia had young girls who acted as foot masseuses and officiated at the hot perfumed bath, as Alexander Baron accounted in his historical novel *Queen of the East*. The Arabians revived the aromatic arts as Rome slipped into decline and Europe began to stumble through the Dark Ages. Later, around 1000 AD, the Arabian physician Avicenna made the important discovery that a coiled pipe in a vat of cold water facilitated the process of distillation. He first used the condenser devise to distill rose oil, which was a favorite in Arabia.

The city of Damascus was named after the damask rose, which was grown in every garden in Syria. According to Roy Genders, "The country takes its name from the word *suri*, meaning 'land of roses.'"[9] Today in Persia, marketers of roses cry, "Buy my roses. The rose was a thorn; from the sweat of the Prophet, it blossomed."[10] This is a reference to Mohammed, whose sweat, when he was uplifted to heaven, fell back to the earth and from it sprang a rose. Even today in northern Persia, people deodorize their apartments by burning fragrant woods and gums, and every Friday after bathing, the body is anointed with fine-smelling perfumes.

"The Persians, of all eastern peoples, have brought the preservation of flowers to a fine art," wrote Roy Genders.[11] They gathered the buds of fragrant flowers like roses, stored them in sealed earthenware jars, and buried them in a garden. Then, in an off-season, the rose buds were dug up for special occasions and placed in water to fragrance a room.

The tradition of aromatics was intense in Syria from such legends as that of Antiochus Epiphanes, king of Syria from 175 to 163 BC, as described by Athenaeus: "Antiochus ordered that two hundred women, stripped to the waist, carry golden sprinklers filled with expensive perfumes to disperse over the crowd. Then, boys marched in, dressed in purple tunics, each bearing a golden dish containing very expensive Saffron, Frankincense, and Myrrh. All participants in the games were showered with perfumes of Spikenard and Cinnamon brought a thousand miles from the Himalayas. Every guest at the games was given a crown of interwoven twigs of frankincense and myrrh."[12]

Zenobia surrounded herself with the intellectuals of the day: orators, philosophers, religious leaders, and historians. She reclined on a couch next to a large table covered with her writing materials and the work of

her favorite authors. She ordered that her sons be instructed in the Latin language and arrayed them in the imperial purple. "She spoke Egyptian perfectly and was so versed in the history of Alexandria and the East that she made an abridgment of Oriental history," wrote Trebellius Pollio in the fourth century.[13] The most famous member of her court was Cassius Longinus, a Greek philosopher who had been a Syrian student in the Athenian Plato Academy. He was summoned to Zenobia's court to teach her Greek and to conduct her diplomacy with Rome in that language. Eunapius, also writing in the fourth century, describes Cassius Longinus as "a living library and a walking museum."[14] People of her court loved nothing better than to recline on seats around a fountain scented with sweet-smelling water and listen to Longinus share some of the great passages of Greek and Roman literature. Longinus stated, "... the benevolence of the Supreme God cannot be sustained without the admission of the reality of a future life."[15] Even in Greek mythology the concept of fragrance was included in the afterlife. The Greek's idea of heaven was the elysian fields, a golden city with gates of cinnamon. About the walls flowed a river of perfume deep enough to swim in and with an odorous mist hovering over it. Inside this golden city, over three hundred fountains cascaded the sweetest essences. Longinus must have enjoyed relating these tales while sitting next to Zenobia's fragrant fountains.

There is much speculation about Zenobia's religious beliefs. At the time a belief in the divine nature of Jesus was replacing the idolatry of the Greek gods. In 33 AD Paul was blinded by a light and converted to Christianity on his way to Damascus, some one hundred miles southwest of Palmyra. Paul made Antioch, which was northwest of Palmyra, near the Mediterranean, his center of Christianity. These religious events led to the development of a solar religion at Palmyra that was later transferred to Rome. The text of Zosimus brought by Aurelian from Palmyra to Rome states that the "astral religion of the great desert city recognized a supreme God, residing in the highest heavens, and a solar god, his visible image and agent."[16]

By 272 AD Zenobia had become a respected heroine to her people. She lived in a splendid palace in one of the most magnificent cities of the East, surrounded by a court of writers and dignitaries. She was waited on by aged eunuchs and served loyally by an army of Bedouin soldiers. She was clad in the finest silk brocades and wore the most powerful essential oils

of the time. The reverse side of a coin struck of Zenobia portrays Selene, the moon goddess, which reflects the queen's admiration for Cleopatra. Rome was now afflicted by barbarian invasions from the north and had no strong leaders in the East. Zenobia, encouraged by her advisors, decided to move ambitiously and invade some surrounding countries. She initially felt she was allied with Rome and would keep peace in the countries of the East. Her troops fought south through Bostra. After this success, she gained control of Antioch and eventually the Eastern third of the Roman Empire.

A coin issued from two Roman mints, Antioch (270 AD) and Alexandria (271 AD), shows Aurelian, the new Emperor, on one side, and a young Vaballathus on the other side. This indicates that the Palmyrenes first gained control of Antioch, then of Alexandria in Egypt. Zenobia may have originally hoped for partnership with Rome, but she was guilty of not consulting them first. She had not anticipated the raw aggression of Aurelian. He was not nearly as compliant as his predecessor, Gallienus, who had supported Odaenathus. Aurelian was a foot soldier called to be Emperor by the army due to the onslaughts on the Roman Empire, especially to the north. Within the first year of his reign, Aurelian had subdued the Goths, the Germans, and the Vandals in Europe. Now he could turn his attention to the threat of the beautiful, valiant Zenobia in the East. Zosimus gave a full written account of the Aurelian campaign against the Palmyrenes.

The time was at hand for another decisive battle between the East and West, as the one between Cleopatra and Octavian. Aurelian had courage, brute strength, and military superiority on his side. Zenobia had refinement, culture, popularity with her people, the tradition of the warrior queen, and her desert Bedouin troops on her side. Her call to arms brought thousands of rugged desert tribes to the sandy plains of Tadmor. They were ready to protect their beautiful queen and to keep intact the routes of commerce that made them wealthy. She visited the camps daily on her Arabian steed, with a helmet on her head and her arms bare. In *An Account of Palmyra and Zenobia,* William Wright describes Zenobia: "Her martial bearing and knowledge of war kindled their [her troops'] military ardour and enthusiastic confidence."[17] The battle took place near Antioch in early 272 AD. Due to special maneuvers, Aurelian tired her troops and then brought in fresh infantry to crush her army. He instructed his cavalry to wait until the Palmyrenes attacked, then he pretended to flee but turned around and chased the heavily armored Palmyrene army in the heat. The

Theodora, Empress of the Byzantine Empire

Beauty is life when life unveils her holy face.

—Kahlil Gibran

Imagine yourself sitting with a throng of people in the hippodrome of Constantinople about 536 AD. The people are cheering the newly wedded emperor, Justinian, and his lovely wife. She seems so confident and happy, speaking to the crowd about her plan to be an empress for the people's rights. As the crowd applauds and roars, she sends forth a waft of perfumed incense directly toward you. A sense of joy and hope comes with the smell of Lemongrass *(Cymbopogon citratus)* and Sandalwood *(Santalum album)*. You feel her warmth and commitment with every delicious inhalation.

Theodora, the wife of Emperor Justinian, arose from a humble beginning, according to our main ancient source, *Anekdota (Secret History)* by Procopius. She was born in Cyprus about 508 AD and her parents came to Constantinople soon after her birth, seeking a better life in the large, wealthy city. Her mother, Comito, was an actor and prostitute; her father, Acacius, was a trainer of circus animals, especially the bears that appeared in the hippodrome, where events like Rome's Circus Maximus were held. Acacius was hired by the Green Party to perform with animals during the intermission between the chariot races. An exciting spectacle, this was also a political arena and a precursor to democracy since the people could express their likes or dislikes of public issues at the games. Both Theodora's mother and her father belonged to the lowest social strata. The Greens, who drew support from traders and artisans, supported Monophysitism, a belief in the divinity of Jesus. The Blue Party was more conservative and represented suburban landowners and the Orthodox Church. Both parties served as safety valves for popular discontent and as a means to pressure authorities at the hippodrome. Theodora's family lived beneath the stairs of the hippodrome and could hear the rumblings of chariots and the roar of the crowds in their home.

Constantinople was the capital of a dying Roman Empire during Theodora's life. Constantine had proudly established the city as the capital of the Roman Empire in 330 BC, choosing the location between the Black Sea and the Mediterranean Sea with its magnificent harbor. The major population and economic sites had shifted from Rome in the West to the eastern half of the Empire. Constantine also embraced Christianity as the empire's main religion. The Christian church became rich, influential, and public, so he built the beautiful Hagia Sophia as the city's most famous building. This church represents the supreme masterpiece of Byzantium architecture. The city was a copy of old Rome with its senate, city prefect, palace, and hippodrome. Greek was the everyday language in the government and in the army. There was chronic unemployment, homelessness, and poverty next to great wealth: Constantinople was a center of luxury trades including perfumery. During Justinian's time, the city imported Frankincense, Myrrh, and other aromatic oils through the straits of Bab-el-Mandeb at the mouth of the Red Sea.

The use of essential oils was especially popular at the public baths where water was provided by aqueducts as in Rome. Public baths were established by the state to promote the health and comfort of the citizens. Roy Genders describes the Roman baths: "The baths or thermae of ancient Rome were the most important feature of the city's social life and, like the perfume shops of Athens, were the meeting place for the fashionable coteries of the day."[1] In Rome during the time of the emperors Agrippa, Nero, Titus, and Diocletian, the baths could accommodate two thousand to eighteen thousand people at one time.

Justinian (Theodora's husband to be) loved to frequent the baths. The beautiful bath buildings in Constantinople were constructed with gilded and vaulted ceilings, marble walls, and mosaic pavement. They had three large rooms: In the central room, the tepidarium (warm room), bathers warmed themselves in preparation for the caldarium (hot room), and the frigidarium (cold room). Smaller rooms included the sweating room, the oil-anointing room, and the room for wiping and drying off. On entering patrons took off their clothes and proceeded to the unguent shop (unctuarium), where oils were chosen for every part of the body. Some popular unguents, placed in a small jar known as an *ampoule*, were made from roses, bitter almonds, and narcissus. After being freely anointed with strong oils, he was covered with sand or powder. Then he went to the sphoeristerium, an immense hall where he engaged in gymnastic exercise. Then he would go to the various temperature bathing rooms where he took his place on a marble bench, placed below the surface of the water. There were also immense basins for swimming. While here, an attendant scraped the skin with an ivory knife, called a *strigilis*, by which all impurities were detached. In *The Toilet in Ancient and Modern Times*, James Cooley describes the scene: "After leaving the bath, he was thoroughly cleansed from head to foot by pails of water poured over him. Then he went to the cold bath (frigidarium) to brace the pores. He was then dried with cotton and linen cloths.... The attendants came out of the unctuarium, carrying little alabaster vases full of perfumed oils which they rubbed over every part of his body, even to the soles of his feet."[2] The baths were extremely popular because they provided an arena for meeting friends, discussing the issues of the day, and being uplifted by the fragrant oils.

The unguents were made with a base of vegetable oil (olive, almond, sesame) or animal fat. The fragrant plant material was allowed to steep in the oil for days and then strained out. Fixatives of milk, honey, and salts were added. Poor people used a castor-oil base. Resins such as Frankincense, Benzoin, and Myrrh were dissolved directly in the vegetable oil base.[3]

The baths were mainly for men, especially after Hadrian's edict in 200 AD, which decreed separate bathing hours for each sex. Therefore, Theodora learned the value of fragrant bathing at home. Her mother, Comito, bathed her three daughters, Comito, Anastasia, and Theodora, and rubbed their skin with scented unguents. She also taught them how to read and write Greek and Latin.[4]

One day after their father died and they lost their home beneath the seats at the hippodrome, the three children were sent out into the arena to beg mercy for themselves. Their mother had bathed them with essential oils and dressed them in their best clothes. The little girls addressed the crowds of the Blue Party with their story, and were so well received that they were given a new home on the Blue side of the hippodrome. This was Theodora's first experience in how essential oils could elevate her presence at an important moment. Throughout her life, even after marrying

Justinian, Theodora was a fervent supporter of the Blues.

As soon as they were old enough, Theodora's mother put her children on stage. Theodora played a slave attendant for her older sister. Theater was considered very immoral in the sixth century, and by the end of the seventh century the church had banned it. As a young girl of fourteen, Theodora was sold to a brothel of Maxuma and stayed there for two years. In *Empress of the Dusk,* John Vandercook describes Theodora's typical routine: "She spent much time bathing and in the long luxuriously pleasant task of anointing, shaving, and tinting her body."[5] She also applied the oils to her legs and feet because she had heard the story of the Greek cynic, Diogenes, who was reputed to have said, "When you anoint your head with perfume ... it flies off into the air and only the birds obtain any benefit. But when applied to the legs and feet, the scent envelopes the whole body and gradually ascends to the nose."[6] Theodora wished to smell the aromatics as long as possible, perhaps to lift her spirits. Procopius, the Byzantine historian, describes her (marred by his personal prejudices) as a shameless prostitute with a difficult life. She had one illegitimate daughter for whom she later arranged a good marriage. This was to be her only child.[7]

As an actor Theodora became famous playing the lead role in *Leda and the Swan,* in which she stripped off her clothes (complete nudity was banned) and lay on her back while some attendants scattered barley on her abdomen. Geese, playing the god Zeus in disguise, picked up the barley with their bills. For the first time Theodora could afford to buy expensive essential oil perfumes from Damascus, like Rose and Sandalwood. Sandalwood *(Santalum album)* of the Santalaceae family, one of the principal commodities shipped from India to the Roman world, is distilled from a parasitic evergreen that attaches its roots to other trees and eventually reaches a height of forty feet. In India Sandalwood was used to build temples and entrance gates that still stand today. The highly scented wood is used as incense in Hindu religious ceremonies. Theodora loved the essential oil for its balancing action on dry, sensitive skin. Its relaxing, soothing effect on nerves and hormones helped her remain calm. Sandalwood also acts as an antiseptic for acne and infected wounds, and as an emollient for baby's skin. It is useful for healing urinary tract and respiratory infections. The young Aphrodite, goddess of love, appreciated its aphrodisiac effect.

By the age of twenty Theodora was Byzantium's most famous courtesan. She was extremely clever, had a biting wit, and was very popular as an actor. In *Justinian and Theodora*, Robert Browning wrote, "She faced life with a wholly independent daring."[8] After an adventurous journey to Cyrene, North Africa, as the mistress of Hecebolus, Theodora fled to Alexandria, where she met a famous religious man, Severus of Antioch, on the Monophysite path. She believed Christ had been pure spirit and all God; in contrast, the belief of the Orthodox Church was that Christ was both man and God. Theodora later influenced Justinian to reconcile the Monophysite path with the Orthodox Church. In this new phase of her life, Theodora probably discovered another aspect of Sandalwood: its spiritually elevating effect on the mind. It opens the crown chakra and helps meditation by quieting the chatter of the mind. It must have been useful to Theodora as spiritual inspiration.

Due to this religious experience, Theodora renounced her former way of living. Back in Byzantium, she gave up her acting career and her role as a prostitute to lead a quiet, contemplative, and chaste life. She settled in a small house near the palace, making her living by spinning wool. She was introduced to Justinian by a Blue Party ballet dancer, Macedonia. When he came to meet her in her little home, looking radiant as she humbly spun her wool, they immediately fell in love and she became his mistress. Robert Browning wrote, "She was still, by all accounts, strikingly beautiful, though her countenance bore the marks of her eventful life. Nature and experience had given her a quick and ready wit, an unfailing memory and a talent for public appearances. Her self-confidence was boundless, and she feared no man."[9] Part of this was due to the empowering effect of her use of essential oils. Justinian, a solitary man, showered Theodora with all the wealth of the ruler of the Roman world. She adjusted to the luxury of palace life with feline ease. "She found full sensual pleasure in the long formalities of her bath, in the texture of her gowns, and in the possession of rare unguents and jewels," wrote John Vandercook.[10]

Justinian issued an edict in Latin stating that actors who have abandoned their former life may contract a legal marriage. He then married Theodora in 525 at the beautiful church of Hagia Sophia with its soaring domes. Her older sister, Comito, married the master of soldiers, an old friend of Justinian. When Justinian's ruling uncle, Justin, died, Justinian and Theodora were crowned emperor and empress. They made their way to the hippodrome and received the acclamations of their joyful subjects. Anointed in oils and jewels, standing with Justinian before the huge crowd,

Theodora gave her finest performance at the same place where she had begun her life living under the seats. This was an amazing social coup for the formerly downtrodden, unacceptable actor and prostitute.

Justinian was a compulsive worker on state affairs; he was steady and patient with his plans, which were carefully thought out for years ahead. Yet at crucial moments his courage floundered. According to Robert Browning, "Theodora was his ideal complement. She had every social grace, she lived for the present, and she never lost her head in a crisis. He was devoted to her, and their confidence in each other was absolute."[11]

In the fifth year of their reign, the mob became discontented by the emperor's neutrality during the chariot races. As the emperor arrived at the hippodrome, a riot broke out between the Greens and the Blues. The Greens left the hippodrome and began a rebellion that escalated into a full-scale revolt. The mob forced opened the prison and let out thousands of criminals. They yelled, *"Nika"* ("victory"), as they almost toppled the regime. Justinian went before them, admitted his shame and guilt, and promised to pardon both factions. Theodora knew the crowd had lost respect for him. A fire was started and burned the Hagia Sophia church, the senate chamber, the public baths, and the hospital. On the sixth day of the riot, the Greens nominated a new emperor, Hypatius, and Justinian prepared to flee, but Theodora refused to leave the city. They summoned a dozen counselors.

Theodora spent the day in her bath with soft clouds of fragrance filling her chambers, creating psychological rest and contemplation, providing serenity and vitality for mind and body. Then she applied the oils directly to her body in the fashion followed by the Greeks: Rosemary to her ear lobes, Sandalwood to her forehead, Rose to her chest, Jasmine to her stomach, Lemongrass to her thighs, and Lavender—of which she was so fond—to her hands and feet. Then her attendant rubbed her body, blending the beautiful body fragrances. Kathryn Degraff describes Theodora during this ritual: "...she anticipated and rehearsed the moment ahead and her awareness of herself as a woman reached its height. This feeling of womanhood, carefully nurtured and enhanced by the use of perfume, was the source of her power."[12]

She chose Lemongrass *(Cymbopogon citratus)* of the Poaceae family for its invigorating effect on her body and mind. A grass that grows prolifically in Indian and an Indian favorite for hundreds of years, lemongrass balances

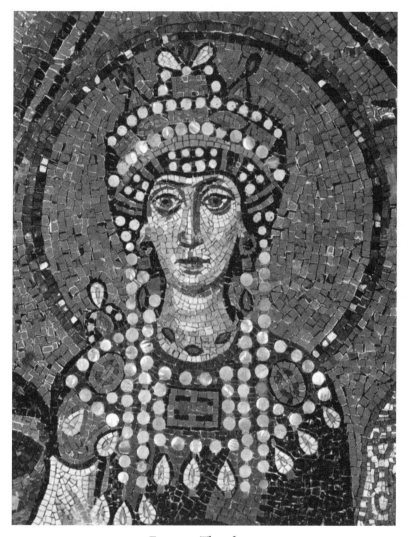

Empress Theodora

excessive sweating, so it is a natural deodorant. Due to the lemon scent of its aldehyde, citral, it gives a revitalizing yet calming boost to the parasympathetic nerves. It acts as a good tonic for the body, speeding recovery from an illness and encouraging appetite. It is excellent for relieving aching muscles and pain, and for stimulating circulation, so this was a good choice for Theodora's thighs. Mentally, Lemongrass energizes and gives an exhausted mind new vitality, something she needed at this moment of crisis.

After her toilet Theodora dressed in the full magnificence of her position as empress, in silks and jewels, to appear before the counselors. Then she proudly said to her husband, "You can seek exile, but I find it a pitiful thing. For my own part, I who have known the glory of the purple, if death seeks me, he will find me here."[13] She had a plan to reestablish order at any cost and ordered the palace troops to shoot anyone rioting at the hippodrome. Thanks to Theodora's resolute council and the aid of Belisarius, Justinian's general, and Narses, the revolt was put down. The city was saved and the reign of the Justinian and Theodora continued. People heard about the council meeting and were amazed at the valor of their empress. Such generous and public praise of a woman had no counterpart in Roman history. Justinian, who loved his wife, in all sincere humility published the story of her refusal to leave. According to one historian, "... Theodora had Justinian's ear while he was still the heir-in-waiting, but it was the 'Nika' revolt which demonstrated her steel."[14]

Theodora enjoyed the imperial power that her marriage gave her, but sometimes the small group of bureaucrats who ran the empire had trouble accepting this strong and unorthodox queen. She presented herself as a friend of the unfortunate, remembering her difficult beginnings. She shut down brothels in the capital and moved the prostitutes into a convent. She intervened on behalf of women who were wronged with legislation that Justinian had passed. An inscription in the church of Saints Sergius and Bacchus in Constantinople proclaims "God crowned Theodora with a mind that is adorned with piety and whose constant toil lies in unsparing efforts to nourish the destitute."[15]

Justinian, probably at Theodora's urging, forbade exposure of unwanted infants, who were usually girls. He eased the punishment for adultery, forbidding a husband to kill his wife. He made it illegal for a woman to be put in jail where guards might violate her; instead, she could go to a nunnery. A woman gained the right to hold property, a right previously held only by men. It is certain that Theodora's counsel influenced Justinian to create many legal edicts that enhanced the promulgation of women's rights.

After the revolt Justinian and Theodora began rebuilding Constantinople, starting with a new design for the Hagia Sophia church. From 532 to 537 the imperial architects, Anthemius and Isidous, designed and built a fireproof building that survives today. This was just the beginning of Justinian's daring program of expansion. He also insisted upon caesaropapism, the supremacy of the emperor over the church in matters of organization and even dogma. His greatest accomplishment was the codification of Roman law, called Corpus Juris Civilis, which gave unity to the centralized state and influenced all subsequent legal history.

Theodora's ambition was fulfilled when a great naval fleet was created, and Generals Belisarius and Narses took back the lost provinces of Africa and reclaimed Italy. Mosaics at the Church of San Vitalein in the Italian town of Ravenna show Justinian and Theodora in all their splendor as they restored faith in the Byzantine Empire. Remembering her earliest years, Theodore passed laws to protect the poor. She remained true to her religious beliefs and established the Monophysite branch of Christianity in Constantinople. She was an advocate for women's rights long before it became acceptable. Cheerfulness, hope, and success replaced the old mood of despair and decay in this part of the Mediterranean world. Justinian and Theodora became very popular rulers.

Theodora died of breast cancer in 548 AD when she was in her early forties. Justinian greatly mourned the loss of his courageous partner. At the end of his life, Justinian converted to Monophysitism, perhaps due to his many lengthy discussions with his devout wife. This woman, born to poverty and with little formal education, managed by her intelligence, grace, and faith to positively affect the lives of thousands of her fellow citizens. Through bathing in essential oils and creating a quiet time to make decisions, she found the courage to confront the difficult social problems that existed in the last days of the Roman Empire. She was an outstanding woman who left her mark on her era.

CHAPTER SEVEN

Trota, the Wise Woman of Medicine

The physician is only nature's assistant.

—GALEN

DREAM YOU ARE LIVING in southern Italy about 1115 AD, walking in a beautiful garden with an interesting woman who is talking and snipping plants as you go. The Mediterranean sun pours down on your head, filling you with vibrancy and well-being. This climate seems ideal for growing the multitude of healing botanicals before you. You embrace the pleasurable smells and sights. This woman beside you, Trota, describes some of her female patients who need help with menstruation and childbirth. She cuts sprigs of pennyroyal *(Mentha pulegium)*, sage *(Salvia officinalis)*, and peppermint *(Mentha piperita)*. Then you walk to a shady part of the garden where she harvests some violet *(Viola odorata)* and wormwood *(Artemisia absinthium)*. You reemerge into the sun to pick some rose *(Rosa damascena)* for the incredibly fragrant bouquet of plants Trota will use in her work as a female healer and teacher.

In the eleventh and twelfth centuries, medical ideas, research, and observations were centered in the flourishing city of Salerno, Italy. Physicians from all over Europe and the Mediterranean world went there to learn. The city, located south of Rome, was luxurious as a trade and agricultural center. The Salernitans had an abundant supply of medicinal plants from their local crops; additional herbs were available from foreign trade, as well as resins, spices, and minerals; all became integral parts of their medical system.

There was a culture of water in Salerno due to the construction of three aqueducts during Roman times. Spring water also came down the hills and replenished the wells. The opulence of the city provided public fountains and baths. Bathing, both publicly and privately, was quite popular. Of course, the Mediterranean was nearby.

The medical school of Salerno during the twelfth century was an informal community of masters and pupils who developed formal methods of instruction and investigation. Founded around the year 1000, it was the first nonreligious medical school. Greek, Arabic, and Jewish texts were freely studied. These texts reflected the population of Salerno, which consisted of the dominant Lombards, a Germanic people who had migrated to the area in the sixth century, Greeks, Romans, Jews, and Muslims from northern Africa. The learned doctors of Salerno, at the most famous Western medical school of the Middle Ages, maintained high standards of surgery, teaching anatomy and surgical techniques by dissection of animals. They brought a unity between surgery and medicine. The school was shut down by Napoleon's decree in 1811.

From the eleventh to the thirteenth century, women in Salerno were allowed to learn and practice medicine alongside men. Licenses to practice medicine were granted by the state. Because the church had no say in the matter, the profession became more available to women. Most of the women healers who practiced medicine and midwifery during the Middle Ages left no written records of their activities. Throughout Europe women were excluded from formal medical education and thus from the lucrative practice of medicine. One of the few exceptions was an Italian woman who was to become renowned as a healer, teacher, and writer, not only in her lifetime but also for centuries after her death. Stories of a Norman traveler who had been in Salerno describe a woman who had attained great medical knowledge.

This woman was Trota, known as *magistracy mulier sapiens* ("the wise woman teacher"). We do not know personal facts about her, such as her birth, her family, and her death. Her practice is included in the classical texts of Salvatore de Renzi, *Collectio Salernitana,* published from 1852 until 1859. Some of her manuscripts are found in museums throughout Europe. We know Trota wrote *Practical Medicine According to Trota (Practica Secundum Trotam),* which includes seventy-one remedies for everything from gynecological and obstetric conditions to problems of the eye, foot, and spleen. She gives advice on how to treat a fever, a toothache, or hemorrhoids, and, of course, there are recipes for cosmetics.

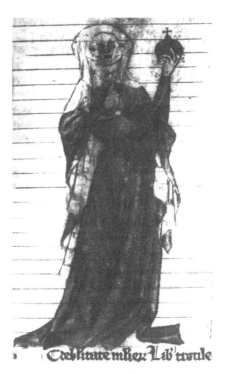

Trota of Salerno

It is amazing how Trota gained literacy and wrote in Latin when most women of Salerno married, had children, and received very little education. Yet the door was open to a woman seeking more knowledge. She must have been a very intelligent, dedicated, dynamic person to accomplish so much. She must have loved plants and attained great botanical learning as revealed in her remedies. She was a skilled diagnostician who used all her senses. She discussed pulse and urine analysis, as well as observation of a patient's face and words. She had the courage to learn and to write down her findings.

On the Treatment of Illnesses, a massive book written in the second half of the twelfth century by seven leading Salernitan medical writers, including Trota, also verifies her importance. Her writings reveal considerable expertise on gastrointestinal disorders and ophthalmology. This quotation, attributed to her, explains the true motivation for her work: "Women, on account of modesty, dare not reveal the difficulties of their sicknesses to a male doctor. Therefore I, pitying their misfortunes, began to study carefully the sicknesses which most frequently trouble the female sex."[1] This is why she chose to focus on gynecology, obstetrics, cosmetics, and skin disease.

Evidence of her medical practice is also apparent in *Treatments for Women (De Curis Mulierum)*, in which remedies from *Practical Medicine According to Trota* appear, showing her authorship for both. Her advice is practical—based on oral tradition and a medicine based on international trade. With references to remedies of Salernitan masters and the larger realm of medical practice being developed there, in *Treatments for Women* Trota was creatively expanding the field of medicine. She begins with the concept of determining if a woman is too hot or too cold. Galen believed men tended to be hot and women cold. Trota believed women could be either, and this imbalance could be the cause of many symptoms and diseases.

If a woman suffered from heat, Trota recommended cooling herbs of marshmallow, violet, and rose to be rubbed on the body as massage oil or fumigated into her uterus. The properties of Violet made it one of her favorite treatments. Excessive heat led to swelling and inflammation of the skin, which an oil infused with the violet flower or leaf could cool down. It was useful to disperse general congestion in the body, especially the respiratory system. Heat was often experienced in the liver and Violet oil acted as a decongestant. If the woman were too cold, Trota suggested that warming oils and plants such as Clovebud *(Syzgium aromaticum)*, Spikenard *(Nardostachys grandiflora)*, Storax *(Liquidambar orientalis)*, and Nutmeg *(Myristica fragrans)* be placed in an eggshell and set upon a few hot coals for fumigation.

In these remedies Trota used local herbs and flowers for the cooling action and imported spices from India for the warming effect. We certainly must classify her as an aromatherapist because almost all of her remedies dealt with aromatic substances, even if they were in herbal incense form. She recommended Spikenard fumigation after a bath for a woman who experienced difficulty giving birth. To help women remain celibate (for religious reasons), she recommended anointing a piece of cotton with pennyroyal and then inserting it into the vagina. This dissipated the desire due to the purgative effect of the large amount of the chemical family of ketones in pennyroyal.

For relief from itching, Trota recommended: "Hence, we should anoint these parts with an unguent which is good against burns caused by fire or hot water, and for excoriations of this kind. Take one apple, [Armenian] bole, mastic, frankincense, oil, warm wine, wax, and tallow, and prepare them thus. We should place the apple, cleaned of both the exterior and interior rind and ground, on the fire in a pot with the oil, wax, and tallow; and when they have boiled, we put in the mastic and frankincense, both of which have been powdered. Afterward, it should be strained through a cloth. Note that if anyone because of any burn has been anointed with this ointment, on the anointed place, there ought to be put a leaf of ivy cooked in wine or vinegar, or a leaf of gladden. This remedy is decent."[2]

For gout of the mouth, Trota recommended: "... wash the mouth with warm wine, rubbing the teeth well, and this in the morning and the same thing in the evening. Later we spread rose oil during the night and she will be freed in a short time."[3] Probably the Rose oil she referred to was made from roses infused in a vegetable oil (perhaps almond), not a steam-distilled oil or a solvent extraction that we use today.

For pain of the vagina after birth, Trota recommended: "... take rue, mugwort, and camphor, grind them well and, having prepared them with pennyroyal oil and warmed them in a pot, wrap them in a cloth and insert as a suppository."[4] She recommends Pennyroyal oil as an emmenagogue to treat delayed menses. It is a dangerous oral toxin and abortive in pregnancy. Pennyroyal is also recommended to relieve pelvic congestion and as a tonic for the liver and the spleen. It cools the body and is an analgesic for headaches and for pain in the muscles or joints. The large number of ketones in it places it on a rarely used list by modern essential oil therapists.

To treat cancer, Trota recommended: "We anoint it with this ointment: Take Frankincense, Mastic, wax, oil, Greek pitch, Galbanum, aloe, Wormwood, mugwort, pellitory-of-the-wall, Rue, and Sage. ... Let the herbs be ground and let the oil be poured in and mixed upon the fire, and when it is exceedingly hot, strain the oil and place it again upon the fire, and when it begins to boil let the wax be added. Afterward let the other things, which have been powdered and cooked, be strained and added. The sign of thorough cooking is when a drop placed upon marble stays there and hardens."[5] Her directions are very clear and specific, making them useful for future generations.

Trota often included sage *(Salvia officinalis)* in her prescriptions, which was grown in most medieval gardens, either in a monastery or at home. The Romans valued it so highly they called it *herba sacra* ("sacred herb") for its use in respiratory infections, digestive complaints, and menstrual difficulties. It is still included in the *British Herbal Pharmacopoeia* as a specific remedy for inflammations, especially of the mouth, tongue, and throat. Sage serves as a source of natural antioxidants, which may be why Trota used it in her cancer treatment. Her directions are very clear and specific, making them very useful for future generations.

Besides her incredible botanical wisdom, Trota's treatments show a high level of care and attention to detail. Trota trained her students to be observant, to conduct a thorough examination, and to listen to what patients had to say about their ailments: "When you reach the patient, ask where her pain is, then feel her pulse, touch her skin to see if she has a fever, ask if she has a chill, and when the pain began and if it is worse at night. Watch her facial expression, test the softness of her abdomen, ask if she passes urine freely, look carefully at the urine; examine her body for sensitive spots, and if you find nothing, ask what other doctors she has consulted and what their diagnosis was. Ask if she ever had a similar attack and when. Then, having found the cause of her trouble, it will be easy to determine the Treatment."[6] This is like the intake exam that modern day essential oil therapists do for their clients.

Trota also believed in making her patients physically and emotionally comfortable, recommending warm herbal baths, special diets, scented oils massaged into the skin, and plenty of convalescent rest to aid the healing process. In *Treatments for Women* there is a story of how she cured a young woman of gas in her uterus. The woman was just about to be operated on when Trota was called in "as a master." She took the woman home with her and treated the "wind" in her uterus with baths and external applications and recommended that she rest. This showed her compassion for patients and her willingness to go the second mile for them. She wrote about a healthy diet and the effects of emotional stress. She discussed birth control, problems of infertility, breech birth, sex, and celibacy, always with the underlying tone of hygiene. Until the sixteenth century, people trusted her honesty and her sensible, humane ideas.

Most medical ideas in the eleventh century could be traced back to Hippocrates and Galen. Hippocrates, who is fondly considered "the father of medicine," lived from 460 to 361 BC. He was a highly skilled, successful, and ethical physician. He conceived of the four humors as the cause of disease: blood, phlegm, black bile, and yellow bile. The four humors are also associated with the four qualities (hot, cold, moist, and dry), the four elements (earth, air, fire, and water) and the four temperaments (sanguine, phlegmatic, choleric, and melancholy). Health is the result of the harmonious balance of the four humors. There was a Hippocratic preference for mild and simple remedies based on a healthy diet ("food is the best medicine"). See the table below, The Four Humors as the Cause of Disease. The concept of the four humors led physicians into bleeding and purging. Yet medicine owes Hippocrates a great debt. Perhaps this is why present-day physicians say the Hippocratic oath. The Hippocratic tradition included gynecological material that made up one-fifth of its vast collection of writing; this influenced Trota.

The Four Humors as the Cause of Disease

4 Temperaments	4 Elements	4 Humors	4 Seasons	4 Qualities
Melancholy	Earth	Black bile	Autumn	Cold & Dry
Sanguine	Air	Blood	Spring	Hot & Moist
Choleric	Fire	Yellow bile	Summer	Hot & Dry
Phlegmatic	Water	Phlegm	Winter	Cold & Moist

Galen (130–215 AD) was a Greek physician who left Asia Minor to practice medicine in Rome. When he died, he left three hundred writings with only one devoted to women's medicine. His writings were lengthy and unclear. He based his work on the Hippocratic principles of the four humors with a rigid, complex system of plant medicines. Often his remedies had compound remedies with as many as thirty-six different herbs, viper's flesh, and minerals that needed to mature for twelve years. He became the patron saint of the medieval medical school and paralyzed European medical thinking until 1628. According to Galen, women were colder than men and the absence of menstruation led to disease. He was a strong believer in bloodletting and purging to restore equilibrium.

In the seventh century, the Arabs overran northern Africa. They asserted Muslim supremacy over the Mediterranean world and a treasury of Greek and Roman medical texts, which they stored in the House of Wisdom in Baghdad. These texts were translated into Arabic. Avicenna (980–1037), a talented Arab physician from Persia and a devoted student of Galen, wrote the famous *Canon of Medicine,* five volumes summarizing all the known medical knowledge of the civilized world—Greeks, Europeans, Arabs, Indians, and Chinese—with mathematical accuracy. He did much to promote the benefits of aromatic oils and wrote a whole book about Rose oil, his favorite. He developed the apparatus and method of alembic distillation with a condenser for the extraction of essential oils. He used the method of investigating plants described by Dioscorides (the Greek doctor who traveled with Roman troops in 1 AD), adding eight hundred new plants with their potency, dosage, and toxicity to *de Materia Medica.* His *Canon* became a standard text for most medieval medical schools.

In 1070 Archbishop Alfanus of Salerno invited Constantine the African to Italy. He stayed at the Benedictine Abbey of Monte Cassino, north of Salerno, where he became a monk and translated his valuable Arabic medical texts into Latin. He translated twenty works, including Avicenna's on pharmaceuticals, diets, fevers, cancer, sexual intercourse, leprosy, and depression. A very important translated work was *Viaticum,* seven books on etiology and therapeutics. In one of these translations, Constantine describes Trota performing a cesarean section to save a child's life. The availability of the translations of these Arabic volumes eventually change the direction of Salernitan medicine.

Conditions of Women, which was part of the Trotula trilogy, was greatly influenced by Galen, Hippocrates, and Constantine. This book plus the *Practical Medicine According to Trota* and *Treatments for Women* were grouped together to form the Trotula ensemble, which became the most important specialized texts in medieval Western Europe for at least five hundred years. Trota was held in such respect that when she died, her casket was followed by a procession of mourners two miles long. She is also credited with writing *Concerning the Diseases of Women (Passionibus Mulierum Curandorum),* also known as *Trotula Major.*[7]

Conditions of Women begins with a philosophical discussion of how God created man and woman: God created man to be stronger with heat and dryness and woman to be the weaker one in coldness and humility. "Therefore, because women are by nature weaker than men and because they are most frequently afflicted in childbirth, diseases very often abound in them especially around the organs devoted to the work of nature.... Therefore, their misfortune ... ought to be pitied.... And so with God's help, I have labored assiduously to gather ... the more worthy parts of the books of Hippocrates and Galen . . . to discuss the causes of their diseases, their symptoms and their cures."[8] Trota described women's menstruation as a necessary purging of her body every month in accordance with Galen and Hippocrates before him. Like Hildegard of Bingen, who is described in Chapter 8, Trota viewed menses as a positive process, similar to the Beng ethnic group in the Ivory Coast. In Alma Gottlieb's study of the Beng, an elder describes menses: "Menstrual blood is like the flower; it must emerge before the fruit—baby—can be born."[9] The *Viaticum* showed the similarities between the menses and the resin exuded from trees.

Trota said, "The best remedy [for menstruation] is that the hands and feet of the woman be rubbed moderately with Laurel oil and that there be applied to the nose those things which have a foul odor, such as opopanax, castoreum, pitch, burnt wool, burnt linen cloth, and burnt leather. On the other hand, their vaginas ought to be anointed with those oils and hot ointments, which have a sweet odor, such as Orrisroot oil, Roman chamomile oil, Musk oil, and Spikenard oil. Let cupping glasses be applied on the inguinal area and the pubic area. The women ought also to be anointed inside and out with oils and ointments of good smell."[10] There is incredible emphasis on fragrant plants and oils in most of these remedies.

For a woman who has difficulty giving birth, Trota advised that she should "be bathed in water in which mallow, fenugreek, linseed, and barley have been cooked. Let her sides, belly, hips, and vagina be anointed with oil of Violets or Rose oil. Let her be rubbed vigorously."[11] Trota also suggest the woman drink mint and wormwood tea, and that sneezing be provoked by placing frankincense powder in the nostrils. Finally, the woman should be encouraged to get up and slowly walk throughout the house.

Trota's book *On Women's Cosmetics* gave a very detailed look at preparing and applying skincare products in a head-to-toe order. The recipes relied on local ingredients such as herbs and animal products as well as imported oils such as that of Clove, Cinnamon, Nutmeg, and Galangal. It also recommended mineral substances such as arsenic, sulfur, natron, and white lead for whitening skin and teeth. Bathing was an important, elaborate ritual.

Trota suggests, "In order that a woman might become very soft and smooth and without hairs from her head down, first of all let her go to the baths, and if she is not accustomed to do so, let there be made for her a steam bath in this manner. Take burning hot tiles and stones and let hot water be poured in so that steam is produced. And let the woman sit upon it well covered with cloths so that she sweats. Afterward let her also anoint herself all over with this depilatory, which is made from well-sifted quicklime. If the skin is burned from the depilatory, take Rose or Violet oil with juice of leek, and mix them until the heat is sedated."[12]

Trota continues, "When she combs her hair, let her have this powder. Take some dried roses, clove, nutmeg, watercress, and galangal. Let all these powdered; be mixed with Rose water. With this water let her sprinkle her hair and comb it . . . so that her hair will smell better."[13]

Trota's remedies were much simpler than the Galenic compound recipes; they were easier to use and included more effective herbs. There was a major difference between Galen's bedside manner and Trota's. Galen taught his students to be lofty and arrogant practitioners (with their lofty medical compounds), always using one-upmanship with the patients. Trota taught gentleness and sincere sympathy for the sick clients. Her medicine was more direct and touch oriented.

Trota's name is on *Concerning the Diseases of Women, Conditions of Women,* and *On Women's Cosmetics.* Trota was a common Italian name in the eleventh century and Trotula literally mean "little Trota." The famed women's healer named Trota was definitely a master of medicine *(magistra)* who taught as well as practiced. Her name attached to the books made them "authentic women's medicine." The 126 manuscripts of the Latin Trotula were circulated in Europe from the late twelfth century to the late sixteenth century. The three books were fused into a single work that was extremely popular among European doctors, midwives, and women in general. The book had no peer for hygiene, medical treatments, and beautification. In the 1400s, it was translated into Dutch, French, and German. By the 1500s, there were six different versions of the Trotula ensemble. New chapters and recipes were added. In 1544, at Strasbourg, Austria, George Kraut reorganized all materials into one smoothly ordered book with sixty-one chapters and called it the work of a single, feminine author. This book became one of the "pillars on which later medieval culture was built, being present in the libraries of physicians, surgeons, monks, philosophers, theologians, and princes from Italy to Ireland, Spain to Poland."[14]

Through the plague of the 1300s and the witch burning of the twelfth, thirteenth, and fourteenth centuries, Trota's writings were very sensible and humane. She discussed with complete frankness birth control, birthing, and the problems of infertility. She told how to sew up tears suffered in childbirth and she gave clear directions for repositioning a breech birth. She wrote on sex, celibacy, and how to pretend to be a virgin. Her womanly understanding of female needs in illness and childbirth made her a folk heroine. Her love of aromatic herbs and oils gives modern essential oil therapists many imaginative ideas on how to combine both the plant material and the distilled essential oils.

Sadly, the opportunities open to Trota and her northern sister in the health field, Hildegard de Bingen, were not to endure. The door closed for women healing in public by the end of the twelfth century. The church emerged as a new authority in the world of medicine. Women were no longer able to study medicine and become teachers, although Salerno was one of the last cities to oppose female education. Women inspired confusion and fear in the medieval male, but so did the prospect of illness and suffering. The unreliability and cost of professional treatment ensured that women of all types, from housewives to professors, would continue to provide basic medical care to the community.

Trota represented the woman healer of the distant future. She personified the balance that modern women need as health care and essential oil professionals. She showed a trust in her intuition, a knowledge of science, an awareness of suffering, a sense of service, a love of botanical medicine, and the ability to choose compassion. She also seemed to possess a fluid religious belief structure, rare in her time, that made her open to creative medical solutions for an individual. Eventually, in centuries to come, some shining examples of female healers would emerge: nurses, doctors, alternative health practitioners, and midwives. The example and the writings of Trota were inspirations for all.

CHAPTER EIGHT

Hildegard of Bingen, Prophetess of the Rhine

I saw a stranger today.
I put food for him in the eating-place
And drink in the drinking-place
And music in the listening-place.

—Saint Teresa of Avila

IMAGINE BEING TRANSPORTED in 1150 AD to the German convent of a captivating woman of intensity and valor. Hildegard has the aura of a holy woman combined with practicality. Her eyes sparkle as she tells you about her book, *Physica,* describing the importance of the natural world for human health. She asks you to step out into the garden with her to gather food for dinner. She brings in some root crops, including a fennel bulb, which becomes the main course. As you help her prepare the meal, you hear some beautiful medieval chants in the background, sung by other nuns living there. The fragrance of lavender *(Lavandula angustifolia)* permeates the convent and gives you a feeling of peace and spiritual upliftment.

Hildegard was one of the most remarkable women of the Middle Ages and one of the first to present a whole healing system of botanicals in writing. She was born in 1098 into a noble family in Germany at Bermersheim in Rheinesse, the tenth child, and began her visionary life at the age of five. Her accomplishments were immense for any time, but especially for a medieval woman in the German patriarchal society. She not only wrote down her incredible inner life, but she also was very active externally, founding a convent at Rupertsberg, on the Rhine River near Bingen. Going forth as a monastic troubleshooter, she became an important visiting preacher and healer in her country. At a time when few women even wrote letters, Hildegard produced extensive writings on the subjects of theology, natural history, music, poetry, cosmology, and plant medicine. They all radiate a visionary beauty and intellectual power. "The whole of her life was inspired by and dedicated to God and she . . . reminds us of the sanctity of all life," wrote Flona Bowie.[1]

After her first inner vision and due to her precarious health, when Hildegard was eight years old her parents, Hildebert and Mechthilde, dedicated their daughter to the service of God. They took the radical step of enclosing her in the cell of an anchoress, Jutta, at the local Benedictine monastery. Jutta was the daughter of Stephan of Spanheim and lived the life of spiritual purity in a cell near the church of the Benedictine monks at Disibodenberg. Flona Bowie continued the story: "The women were to be hidden from the world in two small spartan cells for the good of their souls and for the greater glory of God."[2] Perhaps this was a blessing since Jutta was understanding of Hildegard's visions and always listened to her ideas, later supporting her in writing them down. Jutta taught Hildegard to read and write by instructing her young student in the recitation of the Psalter. Later Hildegard said she was "taught by an 'indocta mulier' (unlearned woman) and, consequently, that any insight she gained into theological or secular matters was divinely inspired."[3] Hildegard had little formal education. At age fifteen she took the habit of a Benedictine nun. The reputation of the sanctuary of Jutta and her students spread in their community, so other women came to join them in the recluse's cell. When Jutta died in 1136, Hildegard was chosen to be the head of the community of nuns, the provost of the convent. She owed a great spiritual debt to Jutta for her patience and encouragement.

When Hildegard was forty-two, "a blinding light of exceptional brilliance flowed through my entire brain. And so it kindled my whole heart and breast like a flame. . . . And suddenly I understood the meaning of the psalter [Bible]. . . ."[4] She also received a command: "O fragile one, ash of ash, and corruption of corruption, say and write what you see and hear."[5] Because Hildegard doubted herself and was truly afraid, she refused to write for a long time and became ill. When she began writing down her visions, the illness lifted and she wrote *Scivias*.

Hildegard recognized the link between her visions, which brought on migraine headaches, and her state of health. Perhaps this was the first time

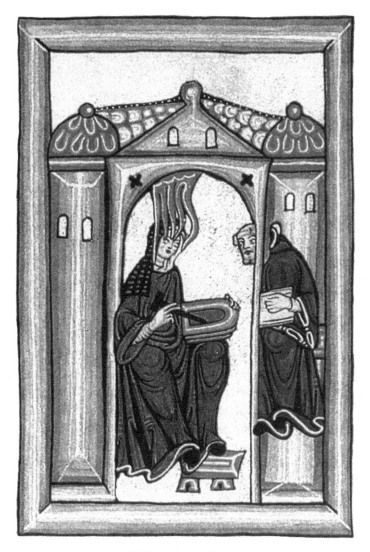

Hildegard von Bingen

she realized the important mind-body connection in relation to illness that she later expounded on in her writings on plant medicine. Her closest friend, teacher, and trusted assistant, the monk Volmar of Disibodenberg, helped her with the transcription of her visions and communicated about them to the abbot. He remained with her until his death in 1173. In 1141 she received the divine word to reveal the content of her visions. As leader of her own community, a new physical and spiritual strength invigorated her, replacing the weakness of her youth.

For ten years, from 1141 to 1151, Hildegard worked on *Scivias* (an abbreviation for *Scito vias Domini,* or Know the Ways of the Lord), in which she had a new understanding of the writing of the prophets and the Gospels, based on direct inspiration from the "living light." She had twenty-six visions in all and told of creation as an event similar to the uniting of man and woman. She received much information on the feminine aspect of God. In *A History of Their Own,* Bonnie Anderson and Judith Zinsser state, "She [Hildegard] envisioned the Creator as feminine, nurturing and sustaining the fruits of the union. She saw Jesus and described how humanity could be saved on a Day of Judgment—an endless day when the movements of the sun and stars ceased, when fire would not burn, when air would be thin and water forever calm."[6] She also brought forth beautiful songs in praise of God and the saints without any musical instruction.

Perhaps, due to her isolation and lack of public education, Hildegard was not indoctrinated in women's supposed inferiority. This allowed her creativity to blossom. As her confidence and reputation spread, she found a divine light illuminated her mental life. Her visions came as a light, a nonspatial light she called "the reflection of the Living Light." She wrote, "I see so great a brightness that my soul trembles."[7] The ability to see things with her soul was constantly present. The light would produce images that sometimes were accompanied by a voice that spoke in Latin. Hildegard faithfully recorded every word. She saw herself as a prophet in proclaiming the truths that God wished illuminated for humanity. Her friend, Richards von Stade, assisted her in translating and refining her Latin prose. Other nuns of the community helped copy the manuscript, the illuminations, and the illustrations that she had designed. She did need the support from church authorities to cautiously begin her public ministry. News of her work reached Pope Eugenius III, who sent an ecclesiastical delegation to Disibodenberg to meet her and inspect her writings. The pope was pleased and in 1147 authorized Hildegard to publish all that she had learned from the holy spirit.

Hildegard was born into a stable social hierarchy in which everyone knew their place: kings, dukes, clergy, monks, nuns, and the mass of ordinary people who worked. The growing interdependence of popes and kings soon created a new wave of reform. This was a movement based on the conflict between secular and religious power. During Hildegard's lifetime, dozens of popes and antipopes were elected to the See of Peter in Rome. The twelfth century became a time of battles between local lords and the German king, the time of the Crusades, and the time of conflicts between the crown and the pope. It was a time of turmoil. Hildegard sympathized with the church reformers and wanted an improvement of the morality of church officials, who seemed mostly interested in their privileges, not the people they were to serve. Hildegard began leaving the convent to teach and preach throughout the Rhineland. Her act of writing took her from emotional depression to spiritual leadership. In a culture where official theology was defined by papal decrees and scholastic debate, Hildegard managed to freely speak her mind. Hildegard reminded corrupt clergymen that God had been forced to choose an inferior mouthpiece, such as herself, because they had fallen to such depths.

After a period of illness and then a vision, Hildegard received a message to leave Disibodenberg with her sisters and found a new community where Saint Rupert lived. The nuns and their families resisted the move; some clergymen called her possessed. She took to her bed and lay there semiconscious until the abbot changed his mind and agreed to her plan. She rose from her bed, healthy once again. They journeyed one day on the River Nahe to Rupertsberg, where she and twenty nuns began construction of their new home. The early years at Rupertsberg were very difficult and the sisters lived in poverty. Hildegard faced substandard accommodations, the loss of revenue, and internal dissension. With faith in God and stalwart perseverance, she overcame many of the problems. By 1158 and after many struggles, she succeeded in obtaining a charter for the distribution of assets from the monks at Disibodenberg to the nuns at Rupertsberg. Their material struggle was over.

To provide for the needs of her monastic community, Hildegard began writing the poetry and music for their religious services. She wrote seventy beautiful and original hymn sequences and responsaries that are extremely enjoyable in musical performance or recording even to our modern ear. Sabina Flanagan describes the ambitious project: "Worked into song cycles, these hymns and sequences were to form the mature 'Symphonia armonie celestium revelationum' (Symphony of the Harmony of Celestial Revelations)."[8]

After another long illness, which seemed to precede all of her major decisions, Hildegard began her first serious preaching tour. Her fear and worry seemed to produce a physical illness before allowing her faith to produce a breakthrough decision. At the age of sixty, after so many cloistered years, she began to preach the word of God in villages along the River Main, traveling on horseback or walking. She gave advice to lay and clergy figures. She preached to monastic communities in Würzburg and Kitzingen.[9]

Her main concern was reforming the clergy on whom the direction of the church and the education of the public depended. She felt the ecclesiastical leadership had failed, and her prophetic role was primarily for them. God had chosen a *paupercula forma* (poor weak woman) to offer inspiration for the misguided, immoral conduct of the clergy. Such a journey was unheard of for a woman, but Hildegard felt impelled by her inner voice. Flona Bowie states, "She felt confident enough to address the most exalted lay and religious leaders of her day."[10] Popes and emperors believed her to be a divine prophet, a woman receiving revelation that she recorded and expressed for her contemporaries. She was greatly acknowledged in her time.

Hildegard was holistic and ecological in her approach to life. She was a prophetic seer whose images were based on physical reality; technically, she was not a mystic at all. Nowhere was this more obvious than in the scientific works that she wrote in her early years at Rupertsberg. She first wrote *Physica (The Book of Simple Medicine)*, which summarized the natural science of her times; the work was broken into four parts on animals, two parts on herbs and trees, and three parts on gems and metals. In this book she lists about three hundred herbs, relating the best time to pick them and their medicinal uses. A companion book, *The Book of Composite Medicine: Causes and Cures*, analyzes two hundred diseases and their cures, including actual proportions for ingredients used in the formulas.

Both books reveal her knowledge of classical authors like Pliny and twelfth-century medical sources in Salerno, Italy. The medical descriptions of many plants focused on their four cardinal properties: hot, dry, wet, or cold. For example, broom is very hot, Hildegard wrote. "Let those suffering from leprosy express the juice and smear it on the sores of affliction."[11] She uses the system of the four elements and the four humors (as described in Chapter 7, "Trota, the Wise Woman of Medicine"), which dates back to the time of the ancient Greeks (Hippocrates). This model greatly influenced Islamic medicine like Avicenna's *Canon of Medicine,* written about the same time, and has much in common with the ayurvedic system of India. Hildegard's herbal methods bring Western systems to an equal level of sophistication with the Eastern systems that are becoming popular today. Like the eastern systems, she believed in preventive medicine. She wrote that the best protection against disease could be found in examining the lifestyle of the patient and helping him or her choose a proper diet and a positive mental attitude towards life.

In medieval times a Benedictine monastery was often like a modern destination spa for the ill and afflicted. Jeanne Achterberg in *Woman as Healer* writes, "Hildegard's practical knowledge of medicines included the function of 485 plants, each of which she believed to be a God-given remedy."[12] Most of her remedies are easy to prepare and consist of herbal teas, wines, syrups, herbal oils (similar to the Egyptian method of soaking plant material in olive oil), salves, and powders. She proposed sound principals for a balanced diet as a keystone of her healing system. There are three foods she highly recommends: chestnuts, spelt grain, and fennel. She called fennel God's greatest gift in the plant world.

Fennel *(Foeniculum vulgare)* of the Apiaceae family remains an important essential oil in aromatherapy today. Hildegard urged using it daily to promote good digestion. She said it assisted the body in throwing off accumulated toxins and waste products, furnishing good blood circulation. She wrote, "It gives us a healthy skin. a happy disposition, clear eyes, a pleasant body odor, and good digestion."[13] As a tonic for the digestive system, Fennel relieves hiccups, nausea, colic, constipation, and vomiting. Rubbing the oil on the stomach or drinking fennel tea can neutralize stomach acid, with the fennel acting as an antacid. The phytoestrogen in Fennel stimulates the hormonal system, which helps prevent PMS in women, slows the aging process, and glides a woman through menopause. Hildegard retained a high level of energy past the age of eighty, probably due in part to her use of Fennel and other herbs.

During the twelfth century nuns were regarded as knowledgeable in medical matters such as midwifery and herbalism. People came to monasteries seeking cures by natural or supernatural means. Hildegard was sought after as a healer, exorcist, and psychotherapist. Women were not excluded from the practice of medicine until the thirteenth century, when the burning of witches began and lasted for four hundred years. Hildegard grew an herb garden at the convent and greatly depended on herbal therapy for herself and others. She gathered her knowledge of disease and healing plants from observation, the study of medical texts, and the traditional folk medicine of her German countryside. In a letter to Bernard of Clairvaux (1146), she wrote, "I am an uneducated mortal and am in no way learned in things concerning the external world, but taught from within by means of my soul."[14]

Hildegard showed us that we too must trust our inner wisdom and that spiritual force is the real healing power. Guided by her intuition, which she had grown to trust implicitly, and her sharp observational powers, she built up great medical knowledge. This information is not claimed as only a direct transmission from "the living light." She recommends a balanced diet, the alleviation of stress, and the making of moral decisions.

According to Hildegard, disease came from the disruptions of the body's equilibrium and suggested insights way ahead of her time. She was one of the first to point out physiological truths like the circulation of blood, the link between sugar and diabetes, the development of the female reproductive system, and the nerve action of the brain. She used herbs and essential oils as one of the main ways to restore the body's equilibrium.

Hildegard especially loved lavender. She is credited with making the first lavender water in her still in the convent garden. She advised using lavender to relieve liver and lung pain and congestion, which she knew too often manifested simultaneously. In *Liber Vitae Meritorum (The Book of Life's Merits)*, Hildegard wrote, "I am a soothing herb. I dwell in the dew and in the air and in all greenness. My heart fills to overflowing and I give help to others. I lift up the broken-hearted and lead them to wholeness. Since I am the balm for every pain with a loving eye, I observe the demands of life and feel myself a part of it all."[15]

The essential oil of Lavender of the Lamiaceae family is amazing in the diversity of its attributes. It has a sedative action on the heart, being very effective at reducing high blood pressure. It soothes nerves, headaches, and tension in the central nervous system. Hildegard believed that Lavender refreshes and frees the spirit as the nervous system relaxes. It relieves colds, sinusitis, and bronchitis when drinking the oil in a mixture of wine, honey, and water, or when inhaling it in a steam. It is great for relief from painful periods and PMS, and for reducing stress. As Hildegard reported, Lavender helps the liver with bile production and the digestion of fats. Emotionally it brings calm and balance. She wrote, "Lavender wine will provide the person with pure knowledge and a clear understanding."[16]

The aim of medical practice at that time was to find a balance among the elements of dryness, cold, moistness, and heat, as well as with the corresponding elements of air, earth, water, and fire. Using oils and herbal remedies could bring a person's predisposition into harmony, which would allow him to better perform the work that God had planned for him. Wighard Strehlow wrote, "The plants give off the fragrance of their flowers. The precious stones reflect their brilliance to others. Every creature yearns for a loving embrace. The whole of nature serves humanity, and in this service offers her bounty."[17]

Sometimes Hildegard used communal prayer and ascetic practices to help relieve mental instability. She used plant images in writing about the mind and soul. In *The Book of Life's Merits*, written from 1158 to 1163, she describes thirty-five vices and outlines the penance for each. About apathy she wrote, "I saw a fifth image in the form of a woman at whose back a tree was standing, wholly dried up and without leaves and by whose branches the woman was embraced.... Her feet were of wood. She had no other clothes but the branches going around her. And wicked spirits coming with a very fetid black cloud swarmed over her, at which she lay lamenting."[18] The paralyzing effects of apathy, or an inability to turn to God, are very similar to modern-day depression. This is another mind-body analogy. In a more positive analogy between a human mind and plant life, Hildegard writes: "The soul also affects the brain, because it understands the things not only of earth, but of heaven when it knows God wisely. And it pours itself through all of our parts, since it has bestowed on the whole body, the vigor of the marrow and of the veins and of all the limbs, just as the tree gives sap and greenness from the root to all its branches. Will is like the flowers on the tree, mind like the first fruit bursting forth. But reason or wisdom is like the fruit in the fullness of maturity."[19]

Hildegard was explicit in describing the relationship between the mind and the body. She saw a direct connection between spiritual protective factors like hope, joy, and affection, and a strong immune system. She recognized the greatest health-destroying factor to be an excess of harmful body juices developed from overeating, nutritional poisons, environmental poisons, and emotional poisons. Worrying, rushing, stress, sadness, and anger can increase black bile, a blood poison. For such emotional problems Hildegard recommended preventive measures like fasting, the heat of a sauna, bathing, exercise, and, of course, a healthy diet. "A healthy way of life is characterized by the general Christian attitude of moderation in all things, eating, sexuality, sleeping, and movement," she wrote.[20] Her medical insights are astounding and profound for her time, with great meaning for present-day medical research and practice.

In 1163 Hildegard began her third, final, and most accomplished visionary work, *The Book of Divine Works*. Two years later she established and restored a second monastery across the Rhine at Eibingen. She visited the community twice a week but experienced problems with some of the nuns there. By one account, she had a strong will "combined with a dazzling array of spiritual and intellectual gifts, a courage hardened by decades of struggle, and a prophetic persona."[21] In the last year of her life Hildegard found herself in opposition to the local church officials of Mainz. Only her reputation and her acknowledged ties to the divine gave her the authority to oppose the male ecclesiastical hierarchy. By the next century women such as Hildegard had completely lost their opportunity for intellectual pursuit, medical achievement, and spiritual power.

Hildegard died on September 17, 1179, peacefully and in the heart of her community. In 1324 Pope John XXII gave permission for her to be canonized as a saint in the Catholic Church. Her feast is celebrated in the German calendar on the anniversary of her death. Today she is so popular in Germany that several groups practice her cures and medical advice with great success. Dr. Wighard Strehlow and Dr. Gottfried Hertzka have spent the last forty years testing over five hundred of Hildegard's remedies. They have found her methods of treatment to be a great success for thousands of patients. Although she was more an herbalist than an aromatherapist, her influence in the healing of the body, mind, and spirit with plant energy created a lasting model that survives in the present. Hildegard's insights into the unity of creation and the goodness of the natural world make her especially important for us today. She was a mouthpiece, a "feather on the Breath of God,"[22] to teach her fellow brothers and sisters and glorify the creator. What an astonishing life!

CHAPTER NINE

Catherine de Médicis, Queen of France

A beautiful flower would grow from bloodstained soil.

—Nostradamus

YOU ARE ENTERING an elegant French castle with ornately carved stone walls. You pass the wooden doors of many mysterious rooms until you find one open with a glimpse of young princesses and princes dressing for a ball. The smell of Jasmine *(Jasminum grandiflorum)* and Patchouli *(Pogostemon cablin)* floats over their excited voices. The fragrance reveals the sensual frivolity and royal camaraderie of the queen's children. Finally you come to a large ballroom where a small, beautifully dressed woman is orchestrating the evening's events. She appears intelligent and commanding, yet somehow quite alone in the large group gathering there. Catherine is creating an Italian play and dance for her courtiers and her children.

Catherine de Médicis had a most extraordinary life of extreme difficulties and exalted opportunities. Throughout the highs and the lows, she trusted her intuition, which led her to use essential oils for supporting the amazing stamina she needed to endure. She spent her early years in humility and her last years emotionally alone, but in between this Italian princess became the crafty regent of France during a moving, turbulent time in French history. Like Isabella of Spain and Elizabeth I of England, Catherine played the part of a queen, a faithful servant, a female Machiavellian incarnation of the national monarchy.

Catherine was born in 1519 into the richest nonroyal family in Europe, but without any emotional security since her mother, a French princess, Madeleine de la Tour d'Auvergne, died soon after her birth. Her father,

Lorenzo de Médicis, a lazy grandson of Lorenzo the Magnificent, who founded the famous merchant family in Italy, died five days after her birth. The seeds for her future life sprouted in her Italian childhood. She was related to two popes, Leo X and Clement VII. Even her roots were in essential oil therapy; the Médicis family had amassed a fortune in the spice trade, bringing oils from the Far East. Since Catherine was the last of the family line, she was brought up in Florence with two illegitimate cousins and a governor. During a massacre by some Médicis foes, eight-year-old Catherine was rushed out the back door, nearly evading death to hide in a convent, The Murate, near Florence. The three years she lived there were the happiest of her entire life; the nuns showed her great kindness and strengthened her faith in God. They also taught her Greek and Latin, making her one of the best-educated woman of her time. Pope Clement III, who was her uncle, arranged a marriage for her with Henry II of France, even though Catherine wished to marry her cousin, Ippolito. The union with Henry II was to bring political prestige to Italy. Her childhood, except the years at the convent, was spent being a political pawn with little love or nurturance.

France at this time was a kingdom of abundance with twenty-five million inhabitants (England had a population of four million), manor houses, factories, mines, thriving cities, vineyards, and great fields of grain. Catherine journeyed to France in 1533 to marry Henry II when they were both fourteen years old. According to George Young in *The Medici*, Catherine was described by the Venetian ambassador in Rome as "small and slender, with fair hair, thin and not pretty in the face, but with fine eyes peculiar to all the Medici."[1] The wedding, the most magnificent the sixteenth century had seen with gifts of rare splendor, is depicted in a painting by Giorgio Vassari that hangs today at the Palazzio Vechio in Florence.

Due to her small stature, Catherine wore the world's first high heels at her wedding to appear taller. This was just the beginning of many fashion and cultural innovations she would offer to Western civilization. Catherine brought with her the Italian perfumer René le Florentin, who was famous for his Florentine flair with fragrance. The alchemist Cosimo Ruggieri and the astrologer Lorenzo Ruggieri, brothers who served as counselors to Catherine at key moments in her life, were also in her entourage. They too used oils in their "magical" alchemy. The fact that she brought these three men with her from Italy reveals that she already valued essential oils at an early age.

She entered the life of the French court of Francis I (Henry II's father), who was a patron of the arts, literature, and beautiful women. To him, "a court without ladies is like a garden without flowers."[2] The French court at this time was the most scintillating gathering on earth and the envy of all visitors. Catherine understood right away that she was a suspicious foreigner to many and that she must be self-effacing and submissive in this new world. She was bright and keen to learn mathematics, natural history, astronomy, and dance, and she was especially interested in astrology. In spite of her ugliness, she won over Francis I with her intelligence and spunkiness. He was her only friend since the nobles looked on her as "the Italian woman." She loved riding horses sidesaddle, which started a whole new style for French women.

Her new husband was a dull man, scarred by spending four years of his childhood in a Spanish prison under Charles V, making him serious and repressed. An older woman (twenty years his senior), Diane de Poitiers, consoled him, mothered him, and became his mistress for twenty years. Diane had the cold, lofty beauty of a goddess and the mind of a power-hungry businesswoman. Although Catherine was genuinely in love with her husband, she was always polite to Diane, keeping her jealous thoughts to herself. Both women used fragrance for their own needs.

Henry became heir to the throne when his brother died. After Catherine remained barren for ten years, her unpopularity with the French people became greater than ever. Her enemies went to King Francis I and suggested that he find a more accomplished and fertile wife for his son. She tried many herbal and essential oil potions. She made an herbal douche of hyssop *(Hyssopus officinalis)*, citronella *(Cymbopogan nardus)*, oregano *(Origanum vulgare)*, valerian *(Valeriana officinalis)*, and wormwood *(Artemisia absinthium)*. She took hot baths perfumed with Juniper *(Juniperus communis)*, Bay laurel *(Laurus nobilis)*, Basil *(Ocimum basilicum)*, Thyme *(Thymus vulgaris)*, and Rosemary *(Rosmarinus officinalis)*. She made pilgrimages to the shrine of Our Lady of Conception outside of Paris. After months of uncertainty and torment, she went to Francis I and on her knees begged him not to send her away. Being a gracious king, Francis raised her up, dried her tears, and said, "Have no fear, my daughter. Since God willed that you should be the wife of the Dauphin, perhaps it will please him in this matter to grant you and me the gift we so long for."[3] She asked Cosimo Ruggieri to make perfumes of aphrodisiacs such as Jasmine

(Jasminum grandiflorum), and with that she put it all in God's hands. Finally in the tenth year of her marriage, she gave birth to her first son.

In the following years Catherine gave birth to a total of ten children; five were sickly and three died in infancy. Of the eldest, Francis, Ralph Roeder has written: "Smuggled into being, he came from the womb a warped little creature about whom the invisible caul of another world seemed to cling, and for years he was only half awake to this one."[4] In childhood a series of ailments stunted his growth. Even so, he became engaged and married Mary Stuart, who later became Queen of Scots. Since Mary spent many of her young years growing up in the nursery with the future Francis II, she learned the value of fragrant oils from Catherine and later took the knowledge back to the British Isles when her young king passed away. Catherine loved to heal and had a stock of medicinal herbs and oils for her children and friends. Later she was accused of using some of these natural remedies as poisons for political enemies, but most historians find no validity in these rumors.

Francis I, having been an exceedingly popular king but excessive in habits such as partying and sexual exploits, died of syphilis in 1547. Henry II became king, although he did not know how to govern. In his role as a father, he was patient, gentle, and devoted. Catherine was queen, but Diane de Poitiers was the first lady of France, even receiving the royal jewels. Diane gave Henry political advice and had him dismiss all of his father's more moderate advisors in favor of the Guise family, a group of radical pro-Catholic Germans who sought power in France. Henry was a slave to Diane, giving her Château de Chenonceaux, the castle she had redone in her favorite colors, black and white. Diane used a famous lotion she called "The Secret of Diane," and she took daily baths in clear, cold water with essential oils, dreaming of the Greek goddess Diana.[5] Through Diane's influence, Henry ordered the murder of many

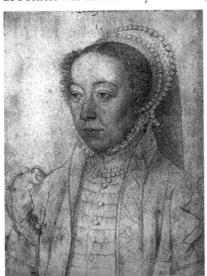

Catherine de Médicis

heretics who believed in the new doctrine of Calvinism. The growing belief in this Protestant doctrine clashed with traditional Catholicism and haunted the life of Catherine and her children.

Catherine brought to the French court a cosmopolitan atmosphere and delighted in promoting Italy in her adopted country. She made the Italian pageants part of the French court, and daily dance classes became a requirement of the courtesans. According to Ralph Roeder, she brought "the pomp and the color of Italian luxury. She imported her gowns from Italy. She patronized Italian artists, humanists and perfumers"[6] such as Nostradamus and René le Florentin. The perfumer René occupied a shop on the Pont au Change in Paris, which became a meeting place for the fashionably elite. René created fragrances, lotions, and balms that enchanted Catherine. When he introduced a new fragrance, the whole court took time to appraise its qualities. His perfumes were made entirely of essential oils unlike today's commercial perfumes that are 95 percent petrochemicals. "... René's shop continued to serve the beaux and belles of Paris for many years, at least until the end of the seventeenth century,"[7] wrote Roy Genders. Catherine even imported Italian artisans to make perfumed gloves and her favorite small cut-glass perfume bottles. In her day the fountains of Paris on festive occasions had perfume added to their splendor. A 1548 receipt was found for six golden crowns, paid by the city of Paris to the perfumer Georges Marteau "for aromatic herbs and plants to perfume the waters of public fountains."[8]

Many French noblemen considered Catherine to be merely a Florentine shopkeeper, but Catherine distracted herself from her jealousy of Diane by becoming adept at music, the arts, and literature. Diane allowed Henry to go to Catherine's bed so he could create children for France, and a bond of parenting did grow between the three adults. This strange dysfunctional family was united by their concern for the royal children. The two oldest daughters, Elizabeth and Claude, suffered a variety of illnesses in childhood but became vivacious and charming adults. Elizabeth, the oldest daughter and Catherine's favorite, married the future King Henry II of Spain in 1559. Claude, the second daughter, married Charles III of Lorraine (a Guise). Catherine sought high and politically advantageous marriages for all of her children. She became regent for a royal heir in the tradition of Zenobia.

Twelve years after becoming king, Henry received a severe blow to his eyes in a jousting match. Chamomile and rhubarb oil were initially rubbed on the wound, but it was not cleansed again and the infection grew until it brought death to the king, just as Nostradamus had predicted to Catherine. She was inarticulate with grief as her oldest son became King Francis II at the age of fifteen and she became regent for a royal heir in the tradition of Hatshepsut and Zenobia. Henry left France with a huge debt, a reduced army, and an increase in the power of the Calvinists (also known as Huguenots). Catherine's political instincts rallied against the Guises, who were trying to take charge of all fiscal, military, and diplomatic affairs. Then Francis II became ill and died in 1560. Catherine appeared before the Privy Council and said, "Since it has pleased God to deprive me of my [husband and my] elder son, I mean to submit to the Divine will and to assist and serve the King, my second son [Charles IX of France, ten years old].... I have decided to keep him beside me, and to rule the State as a devoted mother must do."[9]

Catherine was compensated in her grief to realize that she had the natural ability to rule in matters of state. She felt a surge of delight in wielding her new authority. No one expected political genius to emerge from the humble, self-effacing woman she was during her first forty years. Perhaps it was the Patchouli oil *(Pogostemon cablin)* of the Lamiaceae family that was imported and distilled from the leaves of a bush in India. She constantly used this oil to keep her earthbound, awake, and forceful. She loved it in her daily toilette blended in one of Rene's perfumes or by itself. It has astringent and diuretic properties that help alleviate water retention and promote weight reduction; both were something Catherine had to watch. The oil has a masculine character that she found useful in solidifying her new sense of political power. She found its grounding effect on the mind and body of vital importance after taking the reins of the French government. She liked its persistent and voluptuous fragrance, which was akin to her own personality. The oil tuned her immune system and balanced her central nervous system, which allowed her to cunningly bring warring forces together for the purposes of peace.

While visiting Florence, Italy, a few years ago, I found the Officina Profumo Farmaceutica di Santa Maria Novella, one of the oldest pharmacies in the world, established by the fathers of the Dominican Order in 1221. In their garden, the fathers began to cultivate the herbs that they needed to prepare medications, balms, and creams for the monastery's little infirmary. As I walked through the rooms of the pharmacy, I noticed many ancient bottles, books, mortar and pestle sets, and scales that had been used for close to eight hundred years in their medicinal and cosmetic preparations. I picked up a bottle called "Eau de Cologne" that was for sale. I was amazed to read the history of this formula: The "Water of the Queen" was produced for Catherine de Médicis who, as queen of France, made its precious perfume famous in her adopted country. This complex formula included the oil of Patchouli, along with Amber (a resin), Caycanthus, Honeysuckle, Cuba, Hay, Frangipani, Freesia, Mimosa, Gardenia, Carnation, Broom, Iris, Lavender, Imperial Lavender, Magnolia, Pomegranate, Lily of the valley, Musk, Opoponax, Peau d'Espagne (used by tanners to scent chamois), potpourri, Rose, Russian cologne, Sandalwood, Tuberose, Vanilla, Verbena, Vetiver, Violet, and Orange blossom.

The French Religious Wars between the Royalists and the Huguenots began in 1562 and Catherine knew an armed force would not achieve pacification. She believed theological arguments were a waste of time. She was a student of Machiavelli, who advised "to steer a middle path."[10] She wanted to let people pray to God in the way they pleased, seeking compassion for them rather than repression. She wrote a revealing letter to Elizabeth, her eldest daughter in Spain: "You may rest certain that I shall govern myself in such a manner that God and the world will be pleased with me, since my principal aim is to honor God in everything and to preserve my authority, not for myself, but for the conservation of this kingdom and the welfare of all your brothers. . . . God has taken my beloved from me and your brother, and left me with four little children and a divided kingdom, where there is not one man I can trust, who is not governed by private passion."[11] This letter gives a glimpse of how Catherine assumed the many responsibilities of her position with lifelong loneliness.

Charles I, Catherine's second son, had a quick and capable mind and enjoyed writing poetry. His real nature seemed to be docile with a natural goodness that made him a wise monarch but his nerves subjected him to uncontrollable fits of temper. He married Anne of Austria and loved her deeply. Then the antagonism between the brothers—Charles and Henry III, who was absolutely Catherine's favorite son—and the rumor of a plot to kill her and her children created their dreadful and revengeful decisions. During the horrible bloody night of the Saint Bartholomew's Day Massacre, August 24, 1572, more than fifty thousand Huguenots were killed. King Charles I was put in command, and he dared not show his mother and brother his jealous fear. He personally killed many that night; he never recovered emotionally and died in 1574 from tuberculosis. This night showed the failure of Catherine's policies and she was overcome with anxiety. She became a prisoner of the pope and the Catholics ruled temporarily. After this night, the religious civil wars were resumed.

Marguerite, Catherine's youngest daughter, was a beautiful, charming, high-spirited girl who started her love life early. Catherine always felt the need to discipline her. Catherine had her drink tea made of herbal lavender *(Lavandula angustifolia)* and French sorrel *(Rumex scutatus)* to cool her "hot boiling blood." She loved music and was an excellent writer. Catherine negotiated a marriage for her with Henri, King of Navarre and heir to the spiritual and political leadership of the Huguenot movement from his mother, Jeanne d'Albret. Some writers claim Catherine sent Jeanne a pair of poisoned gloves via her personal perfumer René le Florentin, but an autopsy showed she died from natural causes. The political marriage between Margot (for short) and Henri took place in 1572. Henri, who had red hair and eyes of sweetness, later became one of the most popular kings of France, Henri IV, as he successfully implemented the religious policies of reconciliation for which Catherine prepared the way.

Catherine was the most skillful person of state at that time in Europe, maintaining always an awareness of the French relationship with other major powers. She mourned the death of her daughter, Elizabeth, who died during childbirth as the Spanish queen. On a busy day she wrote twenty letters and seemed indefatigable. She encouraged her youngest son, Francis, the Duke of Alençon, to court Elizabeth I in England. Elizabeth was fond of the short, scrawny man with the enormous nose, calling him "her frog," but lost interest due to religious and political pressures at home. Catherine traveled constantly throughout France, walked briskly when engaged in conversation, and she ate with a healthy appetite. After Henry II's death, she expelled Diane de Poitiers from Château de Chenonceaux, which Catherine loved as a fairytale castle, to a smaller, less desirable one called Château de Chaumont.

Catherine drew up a program of government that was a masterpiece based on her fifteen years of experience. If followed it would have brought salvation to a France that was financially and spiritually bankrupt from all the religious wars. She was still a political genius; she had the Médicis trait that knew the importance of power and the ability to compromise. She reorganized a council to include eight men who supported her policy of national unity. According to William Crain, "In Balzac's brilliant study *[Le Secret des Ruggieri]*, she is the enigmatic 'Mona Lisa' ... with a virile and implacable nature. Florence never produced a more singular piece of mosaic than this woman."[12]

She called Henry III back from Poland to become the new king of France. She imagined him to be a brilliant, heroic figure. Catherine mourned the death of Charles, but was delighted that her beloved Henry was at last to be king. Henry was a flamboyant mixture: a gracious presence and a natural legislator, a breeder of pet apes, a dancer who went to balls every night dressed in mulberry satin, and the founder of cultural academies. He was a good, yet unfaithful husband, in love with the beauty of both males and females, a transvestite, a self-flagellating monk, a serious politician, and a mystical, sensual eccentric. This infamous son had cosmetics and perfumes dating back to the time of Poppaea, the wife of Nero (first century AD). He had a dressing table with several hundred perfume bottles in all shapes and colors. He brought musk back from Poland and formed a group of young men called the *les mignons* ("the dainty ones") who were quite effeminate. They loved the delicate scent of Violet for their nightly parties. Henry used aromatherapy at this time for sensual extravaganzas and religious mortifications. He often wore a morbidly black cape with a wide ebony collar adorned with carved, ivory skulls.

Catherine is accredited with fostering the advancement of ballet in France, which evolved from the Italian court pageants. In 1555 Balthasar de Beaujoyeulx, an Italian violinist, came to Paris. His ability to organize fetes at the royal court was encouraged by Catherine, and his most important work, *Le Ballet Comique de la Reine*, was performed in 1581. It was considered the first *ballet de cour* ("court ballet"). Catherine asked Balthasar to write down the music and hired artists to draw pictures of the event. She sent the pictures to all the courts of Europe, which were so impressed they sought ballet masters from France. The language of ballet became French. At the time Italy was more interested in opera, England in drama.

The earliest book on perfume, *Les Secrets de Maistre Alexis de Piedmont*, was written in French and appeared in 1580. Its strange recipes were possibly taken from the alchemy lab of Cosimo Ruggiero, who was an active member of Catherine's court until the end. To perfume an apartment, Master Alexis suggests using musk (from the Asian deer), ambergris (from the sperm whale), civet (from the large cat), benzoin (from a tree resin), storax, calamus, and aloe. He advises making a powder of these ingredients, covering the powder with damask rose water, and placing the mixture near a fire. It will then release its delicious perfume throughout the apartment. According to Roy Genders, the sixteenth-century book also has many recipes for sachets, often made with damask rose petals and orrisroot.[13]

To reveal how perfumery and alchemy were closely intertwined, renowned French author Alexandre Dumas describes René's perfume shop located on the Pont Saint-Michel near the time of Catherine's death. He sold perfumes, unguents, and cosmetics in his shop. Roy Genders describes the shop as having a staircase that leads to a small chamber containing "a stove, alembics, retorts and crucibles, the necessary tools of an alchemist's laboratory. In the front part of the room were ibises from Egypt; mummies; death's heads with eyeless sockets. From the ceiling hung a stuffed crocodile.... The room was lit by two silver lamps supplied with fragrant oil which cast their yellow flame over the eerie place and its contents."[14] In spite of its aura of sorcery, René's shop continued to provide the elite of Paris with beautiful fragrances until the end of the seventeenth century.

The court could not take Henry III seriously. His extravagances made him the comic king of France. The country grew weary of its government's impotence in restoring peace, prosperity, honor, and greatness. The Calvinists took advantage of the distracted king and demanded freedom for John Calvin's Protestant Reformed Church, while Catholic zealots took up arms in every province. Henry, under the influence of the Jesuits, sought allegiance with the Catholics. Catherine wanted tolerance of both religions and disapproved of his taking sides. In 1577 the war finally ended and a policy of compassion was restored with the rights of both religions asserted. This was a victory for Catherine, but her darling Henry increasingly alienated her. The atmosphere of Henry's court was Roman decadence; he often appeared at feasts dressed as a woman in snowy white and pink and accompanied by laughing goddesses. This neurotic son created much anxiety for his mother, who took statesmanship seriously. Henry respected his mother but dismissed her council and thwarted her as he played at being king.

In her fifty-ninth year, 1578, hobbled by obesity and rheumatism, Catherine undertook another journey through France to take Marguerite back to Navarre. Shakespeare's *Love's Labor Lost* was based on this trip. The two queens spent hours having aromatherapy massages and baths in Bordeaux. Catherine knew France was in peril and she wanted the intelligent and well-balanced Henri of Navarre and Marguerite to take up the monarchy. Catherine single-handedly negotiated a fragile peace with Henri, signing the Articles of Nerac. When Catherine took the long trip home to Paris, she rode on her mule from town to town "like a doctor, in order to bring the message of peace to her people as a cure for their many ills."[15] She was complimented and praised wherever she went. On her return to Paris, she found the monarchy in shambles.

Everyone was amazed at Catherine's patience and endurance. By the age of sixty-seven she was no longer able to ride a horse, but she took long walks. Her mental energy was still acute, perhaps from the Basil essential oil she used for bathing. The oil of Basil *(Ocimum basilicum)* of the Lamiaceae family was held in high esteem in Greece. *Basil* means "king" in the Greek language. India also considered the oil sacred and used it in ayurvedic medicine. Catherine no doubt loved its stimulating and go-getting effect. She must have appreciated how it sharpens the senses and the concentration, clarifying the intellect while strengthening the nervous system. In her bath it helped to relieve tired, tight, overworked muscles. It is first rate for headaches, especially the migraines she must have endured at some of the difficult impasses in her life. It also has a refreshing, tonic action on congested, sluggish skin, which Catherine had from sometimes overeating. Basil also minimizes uric acid to relieve gout, a condition that plagued Catherine. Catherine kept her mind keen and confidant by bathing in the sharp, spicy fragrant oil, even near the end of her life.

When her youngest son Francis, the Duke of Alençon, died, Catherine seemed to draw strength from her faith in God and from her perfumers and alchemists, who used the essential oils that offered physical and mental fortitude. Henri of Navarre said to her near the end, "Madame, you grow strong on these troubles. If you had peace, you would not know how to live."[16] The brave old woman worried so for her adopted country, nearing seventy years, ill with gout and rheumatism. She reveled in memories of her happier days when she cultivated the arts, adding to the Louvre and improving the Palace of the Tuileries with her sculptors, painters, goldsmiths, and perfumers. She was a keen gardener at Château de Chenonceaux.

Besides Catherine's influence on French architecture, the arts, ballet, and religious policy, she was central to the development of the French perfume industry, which owes her a great deal since she sent Renato Toubarelli from Florence to found the first laboratory of perfume in Grasse. Thanks to her the making of perfume has been a thriving industry in Grasse for four centuries, giving work to everyone from the peasants who gather the flowers in the fields to the learned artists of perfume who create their ethereal potions. The geography and the climate made Grasse the ideal garden. Roses are gathered in winter, lavender blooms like heather across the hills, and English geraniums are in perpetual blossom. Today Grasse has fifty distilleries and 60,000 acres planted with flowers. Richard Le Gallienne describes Grasse in *The Romance of Perfume:* "It [the beginning of the perfume industry] was an involuntary good deed of Catherine which in its creation of generations of happy people counterbalances her part in the St. Bartholomew's [Day] Massacre."[17] She brought the perfume industry firmly into the French consciousness to later develop into the world's most sophisticated fragrant center.

Catherine had a tremendous influence on women of her time, encouraging them to use essential oils for their pleasure and well-being. By consulting with those who combine magic, alchemy, and plant oils, she gave aromatherapy a certain prestige at a time when women were burned to death for being healers. As the regent mother, she had personal immunity from the suffering many women experienced from the late 1300s to the late 1600s in Europe, for their interest and practice of plant medicine and midwifery. As doctors became licensed and women were excluded from medieval schools and the profession, the persecution became worse. Jeanne Achterberg writes, "It was widely believed that wise women who used herbs for cures did so only through a pact with the devil. In Germany in the 1500s women could be accused of witchcraft for owning oil and ointment, even though these were common medicaments of the time—on any pharmacist's shelf or in any women's pharmacopoeia."[18] The phenomenon of murdering women for witchcraft reflects the deepest, darkest human fear of female power.

Catherine made acceptable the seeking of wisdom from those with supernatural insight. One example was Nostradamus, who affected remarkable cures with oils during the plague in southern France. He predicted many future events as prophecies that were published under the title

Centuries in 1555. Catherine died January 5, 1589, of pneumonia. Nostradamus predicted that after her death a beautiful flower would emerge from bloodied soil. This beautiful flower could be the many gifts she gave France, the ultimate gift being an end to the French Religious Wars.

Catherine de Médicis had a strong personal relationship with divinity. For women of her time she was a worthy role model—except when fear led to things like the Saint Bartholomew's Day Massacre. She merged a robust concern for healing with essential oils, a devout faith in God, and a truth-seeking belief (some might call this a superstitious belief) in astrology and alchemy. She is the "dark aromatherapist" in our group of historical women. Like the oils she used, she seemed to continually search for balance among much conflict and during severe tests. The woman her adopted country doubted brought a dedication and creativity to the French throne that few natives ever equaled. She overcame many obstacles, upheld the power of the monarchy in spite of her children, and protected the claims of the Valois Dynasty. She was destined to scale the heights, as she had already plumbed the depths.

CHAPTER TEN

Elizabeth I, the Virgin Queen of England

When the Wise Woman wears the crown,
Marvels innumerable come to pass:
The sun rises in the East:
Seeds, well sown, swell,
Bring forth grass,
Oaks, lilies.

—ELSA GIDLOW

A s YOU ARE CROSSING a country road in England about 1575, a magnificent coach appears around the bend. As you peer inside you catch a glimpse of a noble woman who is beautifully coifed and dressed. She waves her elegantly gloved hand to you and you catch a fragrance of Lemon verbena *(Aloysia triphylla)* and Clovebud *(Syzgium aromaticum)*. Suddenly the coach stops and the incredible passenger steps out as a crowd gathers. Queen Elizabeth I smiles at her beloved people and she begins to talk. She speaks eloquently about how England and its people are God's favored company. Her satin dress has the aroma of Rose *(Rosa damascena)* on this fair summer day. She gestures to the country folk, who are delighted to see her as she offers them alms. You feel fortunate to be there to experience and whiff such a regal queen.

Of all our woman aromatherapists, Elizabeth I created the most powerful image of female authority and national pride. She was born on September 7, 1533, the extraordinary daughter of Henry VIII and Anne Boleyn, his second marriage that lasted for three years. Elizabeth's grandfather, Henry VII, had established the Tudor Dynasty and bestowed prudence and thrift on his granddaughter. She also inherited the magnificent administrative ability of her father and the charm of her mother. Elizabeth became one of England's greatest monarchs and rallied the country into a Renaissance of the arts, legislation, naval supremacy, and essential oil therapy for the average citizen. The latter half of the sixteenth century in England and Europe is called the Elizabethan Age.

Elizabeth's beginnings were painful and restrained. She was observed at the age of six to have as much gravity as a forty-year-old person. Henry VIII married Anne because after twenty years of marriage, his first wife, Catherine of Aragon, had borne him "only" a daughter, Mary, and no male heirs. The Catholic Church did not allow divorce, so Henry made himself the head of the Church of England. When Elizabeth was three, her mother was officially beheaded for adultery and treason, but really for not producing a male heir. Henry had Parliament make his marriage with Anne invalid, which made Elizabeth illegitimate. Henry married Jane Seymour. After marrying two more times, he settled on Catherine Parr, his sixth wife, who in 1537 finally gave Henry a son, Edward. Henry was more affectionate with his children than his wives. Parliament in 1544 reestablished Elizabeth in succession for the throne after Edward, her half brother, and Mary, her half sister.

Elizabeth found her new stepmother, Catherine, to be supportive and protective. She especially liked to play with her half brother, Edward. She was well-educated by a series of tutors including William Grindal and Roger Ascham. The latter said of Elizabeth: "Her mind has no womanly weakness and her perseverance and memory was equal to that of a man."[1] She learned the classics, history, sewing, and music. She spoke French, Italian, Latin, and Greek. She was quite a scholar and could talk at great length on any subject. She studied moral philosophy and theology, becoming a Protestant. As a teenager, she spent three hours a day reading just history. Her father died in 1547, when she was fourteen and Edward became King Edward VI as a boy of ten.

As a young lady, Elizabeth's plain clothes and lack of makeup showed she was a Protestant, along with her subdued, demure, and respectful manner in court. Elizabeth used the scent of Marjoram oil (*Origanum majorana*), disliking the heavy scents favored by the men and women of court such as Aloeswood, also called *Oud (Aquillaria agallocha)*, Nutmeg (*Myristica fragrans*), and Styrax (*Liquidambar styraciflua*), or her father's inventive perfume of musk, ambergris, and civet.

When Edward became ill with swollen legs and arms, doctors prescribed a stimulating medicine of Spearmint oil *(Mentha spicata)*, Fennel oil *(Foeniculum vulgare)*, liverwort, turnip, dates, raisins, an ounce of mace, and two sticks of celery. He hung on for some months but died of gangrene in his fingers and toes in July of 1553. Elizabeth's half sister, Mary, a fervent Catholic, became Queen Mary I and was married to the leading Catholic in Europe, Philip II of Spain. Elizabeth professed a desire to learn Catholicism to please her sister, who even so was advised to make Elizabeth a prisoner in the dreadful Tower of London, as her mother, Anne Boleyn, had been. Mary's fiery reign from 1553 to 1558 consisted of burning Protestants and engaging in military confrontations. These were difficult years for Elizabeth, who lived in constant fear of the scaffold. She had to swear to her unswerving loyalty, her innocence, and her pious faith. Both Protestants and Catholics thought Elizabeth lied about her true beliefs even though she conformed outwardly to Catholicism. In truth, Elizabeth died without anyone knowing—even many years later—her private, personal views on life, religion, and God.

In the face of constant hostility, Elizabeth became ill. She swelled up and was often in tears; she asked to be bled. She had no aromatics to soothe her moods, and she suffered from breathlessness and jaundice. The country was facing economic depression, poor harvests, and religious persecution. After Mary and Philip II of Spain separated, Mary relaxed the rules of Elizabeth's confinement. She was allowed to go to Hatfield, but the queen's men always watched her. After Mary died of ovarian cancer in 1558, Sir William Cecil brought Elizabeth the queen's ring and she quoted the Psalm 118: "This is the Lord's doing, and it is marvelous in our eyes."[2] She took the throne amidst public rejoicing, bells ringing, patriotic demonstrations, and bonfires.

When Elizabeth became queen, her naturally high level of energy and her strong personality emerged from the repression and difficulty of her youth. Mary Luke wrote, "To Elizabeth, the throne represented *freedom*— freedom to do as she chose as long as she remembered wherein lay her real strength: in the hearts and affections of her people."[3] The memory of her insecure childhood only stimulated Elizabeth to always responsibly give her best to the English people. "She was her father's daughter: athletic, red haired, autocratic, and vain with a stately and majestic deportment," wrote Lacey Baldwin Smith.[4] One of Elizabeth's first and most lasting acts was to appoint William Cecil (Lord Burghley) to her Privy Council. A man of learning, wisdom, and integrity, he was her most loyal, dependable councillor for forty years. She reduced the size of the Privy Council from thirty-nine to nineteen—eliminating Catholics and making the group more efficient. She appointed many talented advisors who served her well over the years. As she took the reins of government, there was religious strife, huge government debt, and failure in war with France, which brought England's fortunes to a low ebb. Upon her death forty-five years later, England had passed through one of its noblest periods in history, a period that produced Shakespeare, Francis Bacon, Walter Raleigh, and Sir Francis Drake.

Under Elizabeth's direction, England became a strong power with a great navy. Commerce and industry prospered, and colonization had begun. She had a Tudor concept of strong rule with popular support, yet at this time, in the beginning of her rule, the public mood was against a female in power. John Knox, the Calvinist, spoke vehemently about the terrors of womanly rule. However, Elizabeth's rule came to be considered an act of God. Once queen, her demure manner gave way to a dynamic energy with clear autocratic leadership. She had the heart and stomach of a king, and she would be master in her own house. She selected wise councillors but always remained in control. She was an extrovert who boxed her ministers' ears and threw slippers at them in a rage. Her temper was balanced by a sense of humor and she never held a grudge. She had strength of mind, caution, and unmatched magnetism. She worked hard at endless interviews, legislative meetings, ceaseless ceremonies, and exhausting spectacles in which the queen was always the central figure. She could sagaciously appraise people; she had a marvelous memory, handled money well, and took meticulous notes. The essential oils she surrounded herself with only served to bring more balance to her life, keeping wild impulses in check.

Mary's reign had brought disastrous results; so much reform was needed. One of Elizabeth's first acts was to reform the currency, removing the debased monetary coin put into circulation by her father, Henry VIII. She also decreed that all men who were unemployed should work the land, increasing the agricultural labor force. In foreign policy she negotiated treaties with France and Scotland to end a state of enmity. The new queen developed many aspects of the state including a standing army, a strong police force, and an efficient bureaucracy.

All of the many suitors she had throughout her life—such as Philip II of Spain; Francis, Duke of Alençon; and her favorite, Robert Dudley, Earl of Leicester—did not sway her into marriage because she always kept the interests of England first. She remarked, "I will have here but one mistress and no master. At my own time, I shall turn my mind to marriage if it be for the public's good."[5] The virgin queen concept, dreamed up by her councillors, provided her with strength, a distance, and a mystery that gave her reign its incredible Renaissance character. Painters portrayed her as a virgin in all her magnificence who brought justice and who was surrounded by the symbols of peace, virtue, truth, and majesty.

Elizabeth's love of Marjoram oil of the Lamiaceae family, with its effect of warming comfort along with encouraging a tendency toward celibacy, perhaps helped her stay true to her political values. Marjoram promoted her good health in many ways. It would ease any muscle pain during the winters spent in cold, drafty castles by dilating the arteries and capillaries, giving a feeling of warmth. It was a good tonic for her heart and lowered her blood pressure. It would relieve any headaches, menstrual cramps, or stuffy head colds due to its warming analgesic action. For Elizabeth it would steady her nerves and relieve stress at some crisis points. It would strengthen her mind, allowing her to confront issues and make weighty decisions of state. It has been used to numb the sexual drive, yet its warmth offered feelings of comfort in loneliness. After her affair with Robert Dudley, she learned that only in lonely celibacy could she ever hope to rule her jealous subjects.

Elizabeth's mother, Anne Boleyn, had been a Protestant, but religion remained mystical and personal to Elizabeth. She said, "There was only one Christ Jesus and one faith, the rest is a dispute about trifles."[6] The fiery Protestants who wanted to implement Calvinism in England and the conservative Catholics who sought the traditional course pressured her. She took the middle ground and supported the Church of England. In 1559, just one year after becoming queen, Elizabeth had Parliament reinstate Henry VIII's Act of Supremacy, which now declared the queen to be the supreme governor of the Protestant church, the Church of England. Needless to say, Elizabeth was horrified by the French royalty's involvement in the Protestant massacre of Saint Bartholomew's Day in 1572, although she maintained cordial relations with Catherine de Médicis. Elizabeth considered herself God's anointed lieutenant on earth: Lacey

Baldwin Smith said, "To God she was thankful and to men she was merciful. She believed God was on her side."[7]

Throughout Elizabeth's reign, religious conflict was a major problem. One plot to assassinate Elizabeth, called the Babington Plot, implicated Mary, Queen of Scots, as its instigator. Parliament issued a decree that Mary be executed. Elizabeth had hoped to reign amicably with her cousin and her cousin's son, James. There were many difficult skirmishes between them over the years that they had ignored or resolved. This one was too blatant a violation to look the other way. She waited three months before making a decision, but Mary was beheaded in 1587.

Elizabeth embraced the brilliant standards of the Italian Renaissance and encouraged great progress in establishing peace, and promoting culture and a flourishing social life. The Elizabethan vision was a commonwealth composed of balanced and harmonious elements, including countries and regions in which every individual would add a vital part and be content with his place. Elizabeth put through acts to encourage agriculture, commerce, and manufacturing. Under her leadership, Arnold James Cooley states, the "whole population seemed suddenly aroused and joined in the onward march of refinement and civilization. Arts, literature, science, trade, commerce, and legislation acquired new strength daily."[8]

Elizabeth established many industries in England including the perfume industry during the fifteenth year of her reign. The Earl of Oxford brought her perfumed gloves and sweet bags from Italy that totally delighted her Majesty, whose sense of smell was quite developed. Three Italians made scented gloves for her. In Shakespeare's *As You Like It*, the courtiers' hands are perfumed with civet. In London milliners who lived and worked alongside the herbalists made scented gloves in the Bucklesbury neighborhood, where the scent of Lavender *(Lavandula angustifolia)* and Rosemary *(Rosmarinus officinalis)* was ever present. Roy Genders describes the effect: "It was perhaps these delicious smells which persuaded Sir Thomas More to make plantings of lavender and rosemary in his garden when he moved to Chelsea, for rosemary was said to 'gladden the spirits' of all who inhaled its perfume. 'As for rosemarine,' wrote More, 'I let it run over my garden walls, not only because the bees love it, but because it is the herb sacred to remembrance, to love and to friendship.' In *Hamlet*, Ophelia says, 'There's Rosemary, that's for remembrance,' and every year on April 23 ... the people of Stratford-on-Avon walk in procession through the town, wearing sprigs

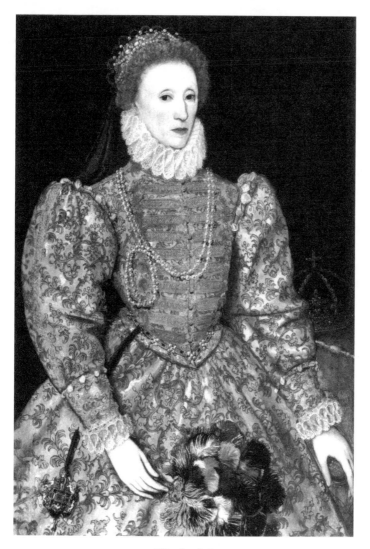

Elizabeth I

of rosemary.... They make their way to the church where Shakespeare was baptized and where he is buried, and there they place on his grave rosemary...."[9]

Not very extravagant in most ways, Elizabeth indulged her love of scent, according to Roy Genders: "Clothes were kept in coffers made of fragrant wood such as juniper, cedar or sandalwood.... Elizabeth's love of clothes and perfumes was the only feminine weakness she allowed herself for, as Queen, she had sacrificed the majority of those things a woman most enjoys so as to remain master of herself and of her kingdom...."[10] Genders also describes how Elizabeth had no alcohol-based perfumes, only perfumes derived from essential oils, as they were made during her time.

The queen's shoes and cloaks were made of leather and perfumed using a technique called Peau d'Espagne. Charles Piesse described this process in *The Art of Perfumery* (1880), according to Roy Genders: "The skins were first steeped in an otto made up of the oils of neroli, rose, sandalwood, lavender and verbena, to which was added a small quantity of the oils of clove and cinnamon All this was added to a half pint of spirit in which four ounces of gum benzoin were dissolved.... Next, a paste was made by rubbing together ... civet and ... musk, with gum tragacantha to give a spreading consistency.... the skins were then pressed with weights for several days, during which time they became so saturated with the perfume that they retained it permanently."[11]

Elizabeth inherited many palaces from her father, Henry VIII, and found it necessary to move every few months due to her sensitive nose and love of adventure. At that time there was no plumbing and the stench of the queen's entourage built up quickly. She often spent Christmas at the storybook castle of the Tudor Dynasty, Hampton Court Palace, which had hundreds of turrets and pinnacles on its whimsical roof. Its eighteen hundred inhabitable rooms were set amid formal gardens alongside the Thames. "When the queen was in residence," Carolly Erickson wrote in *The First Elizabeth*, "the palace was alive with movement and activity."[12] An army of servants repaired walls, carried firewood to the hearths (a thousand of them), and cooked feasts of roast meats, sauces, and sweets for the banquet tables. The palace had every convenience but one, indoor plumbing. "The stench of the great royal establishment must have been at least as awe-inspiring as its architecture," according to Erickson.[13] There was no sewage system for the servants' privies; that, combined with the overpowering odors from the discarded kitchen garbage, the stable sweepings, and the foul-smelling rushes on the floor, made the castle odor excruciatingly bad.

The queen didn't know how to eradicate the malodorous atmosphere, so her solution was to use fragrant oils. She and her ladies held aromatic pomanders—made in the shape of a ball composed of lavender, ambergris, and benzoin—to their noses as they passed through noxious chambers. Some "pomanders were made of gold or silver and worn as a pendant on a lady's girdle. They were constructed with a central core around which were grouped six orange-shaped segments held in place by a ring.... When the ring was lifted, the segments opened.... each one to be filled with a different perfume," wrote Roy Genders.[14] Elizabeth's favorite silver pomander can be seen today at Burghley house, sitting on a table with her thimble and notepad, next to her ancient bed with its hangings of dark green velvet.

For strewing herbs on the foul floors, Elizabeth used basil *(Ocimum basilicum)*, lemon balm *(Melissa officinalis)*, Roman chamomile *(Chamaemelum nobile)*, lavender, hyssop *(Hyssopus officinalis)*, sage *(Salvia officinalis)*, thyme *(Thymus vulgaris)*, and meadowsweet *(Filipendula ulmaria)*, her favorite. As the herbs were walked on, the essential oils were released to create a charming smell. She loved flowers and often wore them pinned to her dress. She hired a woman with a fixed salary for the sole purpose of always having fragrant plants available. She thought the scent of meadowsweet made the heart joyful and delighted the senses. Lemon balm was used to rub on furniture. Shakespeare wrote in *The Merry Wives of Windsor*:

> The several chairs of order look you scour
> With the juice of balm, and every precious flower.[15]

Rue *(Ruta graveolens)* was used for combating the fleas that multiplied on the feasting rats in these fairybook palaces. Rats were especially feared as the carriers of the plague. Dr. Turner, the author of *Herbal* written in 1551, suggests burning southernwood *(Artemisia abrotanum)* over a low flame in the fireplace, since "it will not only make the room fragrant with its pungent smoke but will drive away 'serpents' [frogs, rats, and toads] lurking in corners."[16] Elizabeth also sprinkled Rose water on the floors, or had it available in silver bowls for washing. Carolly Erickson wrote, "The Queen and those who served her walked through the raw stench and rankness of the palace in a perfumed fog...."[17]

For personal, hygienic, and political reasons, the court in summer was peripatetic. Four hundred wagons and two thousand four hundred pack-horses were used to move from palace to palace. Elizabeth's favorite was Richmond Palace, which had eighteen kitchens, lovely gardens and orchards, and towers and painted domes. She would hold balls for dancing and much musical display, both of which she delighted in participating. She was quite temperate in drink and food, but extravagant in her love of dancing. She also spent much time traveling in England to see her beloved subjects. In *The Virgin Queen*, Christopher Hibbert describes one encounter: "At Gloucester she [Elizabeth] protested to the victims of the disease who crowded around her, 'Would that I could give you help!' ... God, she told them, was the best physician of all. They must pray to him."[18]

Elizabeth extended English influence overseas. During most of her reign, the conflict between England and Spain curtailed the free movement of English ships between the North Sea and the Straits of Gibraltar. English merchants were looking for new markets of export. Elizabeth decided to establish a more comprehensive foreign trade policy. Her most famous navigator, Sir Francis Drake, made voyages to the Guineas and the West Indies and, in 1567, commanded a ship in a slave-trading expedition. In foreign policy Elizabeth sponsored privateering raids on Spanish ships and ports. Sir Francis Drake and others took valuable silver and gold from the Spanish king at the guidance of the queen. By 1585 it was clear that a war between England and Spain was imminent. In one of the most famous naval battles in the history of the world, Elizabeth's ships defeated the Spanish Armada. The Spanish fleet was destroyed by horrendous storms as they tried to sail back to Spain. This boosted English national pride.

Elizabeth gave memorable speeches. About the time of the expected invasions of Spain, she reviewed the troops even though she was advised of the danger of appearing in front of a large crowd. Elizabeth trusted her "faithful and loving people." Dressed in a white elegant gown and a silver breastplate, she began to deliver a celebrated speech. According to Christopher Hibbert, she told the troops, "I know I have the body of a weak and feeble woman, but I have the heart and stomach of a king, and a King of England too."[19] She promised to richly reward her loyal troops, but as was her custom, she broke her promise.

When the queen announced openly her pleasure in fragrance, the people of London forgot the austerity of Protestantism and delighted in perfume. To establish the perfume industry in England, Elizabeth encouraged her female subjects to cultivate gardens of fragrant plants. "The use of perfumes in every way became so popular that even the smallest country houses had their still rooms," said Eleanour Sinclair Rohde.[20] All classes used perfumes. Books from the Elizabethan period on gardening and stillrooms contain recipes for Rose water, honey of violets, Lavender oil, syrup, Lily of the Valley spirit, Rosemary oil, Jasmine water, and sugar of damask rose. The lady of the house made scented ointments, wash balls, scented waters, pomanders, and sachets for the household. Sachet powders were popular in Elizabethan times to place among clothes. Sir Hugh Platt mixed into powder for the queen's sachet: orrisroot *(Iris florentina)*, calamus *(Acorus calamus)*, clovebud, styorax *(Liquidambar orientalis)*, and rose petals *(Rosa damascena)*. This powder retained its perfume for a year or more.[21]

An Elizabethan woman presided over others or did her own distillation of scents in a "stylling house." Elizabeth I encouraged every family with land to grow aromatic plants and build a stillroom to create hydrosols and essential oils for cosmetics and medicines.[22] Sir Francis Bacon, an unofficial member of Elizabeth's learned court, wrote in his "Sylva Sylvarum" essay, "And because the breath of flowers is far sweeter in the air, where it comes and goes like the warbling of music, than in the hand, and therefore nothing is more fit for that delight, than to know what be the flowers and plants that do best perfume the air."[23]

Elizabeth had her own stillroom, as did all the ladies of the court, where she composed her own perfumes. One of her recorded compositions was a pomatum made from apples, the fat of a young dog, and fragrant oils. Ralph Rabbards was Elizabeth's perfumer. He created her famous "Water of Violets" which she used until the end of her life. Perfumes were never richer, more elaborate, more costly, or more delicate than during the reign of Elizabeth. Arnold Cooley wrote, "Her majesty's nasal organs were quite fine and sensitive and nothing offended her more than an unpleasant smell."[24] At the end of her reign, Rabbards suggested special floral waters "to cleanse and keep bright the skynne and fleshe and to preserve it in a perfect state," as disclosed by Roy Genders.[25] Perhaps this is why Elizabeth outlived everyone in her court and had an overabundance of energy even at the age of sixty-four. After applying her daily scent—compounded of Violet water, Lavender, Musk, and Rose water—she went for long walks, even up to the age of seventy. She rubbed the sweet hydrosol on her hands. The smell of her toiletries, especially the pungent smell of lemon, permeated her bedroom.

Of all the scents she used, Lemon *(Citrus x limon)* of the Rutaceae family was her preference due to its strong antibacterial quality as well as its uplifting fragrance. This was the time when plagues ravaged cities with disease and death. There was a horrible plague in London in 1603, the year of Elizabeth's death, when people intuitively used essential oils and fumigating herbs for protection. The perfumers who constantly used essential oils usually survived. In the nineteenth century research at the Pasteur Institute in Paris revealed that the microorganisms of yellow and typhoid fever were killed by essential oils of Cinnamon, Thyme, and Lemon within half an hour. This was the beginning of future European research on the anti-infectious nature of essential oils. No doubt this intelligent queen sensed that Lemon stimulated her white blood cells against infection. Lemon also offered her a heart tonic to keep her blood pressure low. If she did contract a cold, Lemon would relieve a sore throat and a cough. It made her whole digestive system more alkaline, allowing the kidneys and liver to function better. She liked Lemon since it brightened her pale complexion by cleansing away dead skin cells. She felt more alert and queenly after using lemon because it was elevating and produced clarity of thought. She chose oils that calmed her passionate nature and gave her the balance to rule with wisdom.

For thirty years Elizabeth kept the country at peace. Shortly before she died, she appointed James VI of Scotland, Mary's son, to be her successor. He became King James I of England. Her relationship with the English people, who called her "Good Queen Bess," was the core of her monarchy. In a speech to Parliament she related, "... though God hath raised me high, yet this I count the glory of my crown that I have reigned with your loves.... I do not so much rejoice that God hath made me a Queen as to be Queen over so thankful a People."[26]

Though Elizabeth has been accused of being vain, fickle, prejudiced, and miserly, she was endowed with immense personal courage and a keen awareness of her responsibility as a ruler. Throughout her reign she commanded the unwavering love and allegiance of her subjects. Her exceptional vitality and keen intelligence encouraged exploration of so many aspects of life, including foreign lands such as America and the many nuances of fragrance. She did honor to women and aromatherapy by placing a high value on the use of the essential oils of her time for enhancing her life and those of her beloved citizens.

CHAPTER ELEVEN

Marguerite Maury, the Holistic Healer

To live, to be alive, means to be in motion, to evolve, to trans-
form oneself, and transmute things according to the alchemy of
the spirit and body.

—MARGUERITE MAURY

IMAGINE YOU ARE RECEIVING a massage from an energetic woman who
seems wise about the healing of the human body and mind. You can
hear classical music quietly playing in the background. You feel her hands
firmly applying fragrant oils to your spine. As she slowly massages down
each vertebra, you detect an invigorating, life-restoring aroma seeping
through your skin into your bloodstream and energizing your body. The
blend is grounded in Cedarwood *(Cedrus atlantica)*, revivifying with Lime
(Citrus x aurantifolia), rebalancing with Geranium *(Pelargonium grave-*
olens), and regulating with Frankincense *(Boswellia carteri)*. She seems to
know you completely and to carefully choose the essential oils that will
awaken you on the deepest spiritual level. You feel restored to who you
truly are, leaving all the emotional traumas and worldly strains behind.
You emerge as a newly born person!

Marguerite Maury has been very important in the modern development of essential oil therapy by giving it a connection to the ancient healing philosophies of India, China, and Tibet while reemphasizing a personal,
holistic approach through massage. Our eleventh woman is a bridge from
the past to opportunities of the present. She was born Marguerite Konig
in Austria in 1895 and was raised in Vienna. She attended boarding school,
where she focused on music, a passion throughout her life. She sang in the
choir of Saint Stephen's Cathedral in Austria. In later years her devoted

student, Daniele Ryman, wrote about how Marguerite would play Chopin, Schubert, and Liszt under the eye of her favorite cat that sat on top of the piano. Her hands were very supple at an elderly age since she moisturized them regularly with essential oils.

Marguerite married at the age of seventeen, but within two years her husband, her child, and her father had died. After so many losses she decided to return to her studies, and subsequently received degrees in nurse and surgical assistance. She moved to France, working as a surgeon's assistant in Alsace for many years. One day she came across a fascinating book that would change her life: *Les Grandes Possibilités par les Matiéres Odoriferantes (The Great Possibilities of Odoriforous Materials)* by Dr. Chabenes published in 1838. This book became Marguerite's bible, as did studies by René-Maurice Gattefossé.

Marguerite met Dr. E. A. Maury in the early 1930s and began an exciting partnership while exploring a mutual love of art, literature, and music. Above all they shared a desire to heal through alternative, natural methods: "They explored homeopathy, naturopathy, acupuncture, osteopathy, meditation, Zen, yoga, macrobiology, and radiesthesia.... They formed a remarkable team, working, researching, and writing books together."[1]

The pivotal point in Marguerite's career was in the 1940s when she began research on the effects of essential oils on the nervous system and how they created rejuvenation. Dr. Maury became a specialist in homeopathic medicine and acupuncture treatments that were still on the fringes of established Western medicine. Marguerite borrowed two concepts from homeopathy: First, essential oils like homeopathic granules create vibration in cells of the body, even though imperceptible to human senses. And second, the prescribed remedy relates to the individual, not the illness. Marguerite invented the extremely important concept of the "individual prescription" for aromatherapy, where the blend of oils is custom-created for the individual in a holistic sense: physically, emotionally, mentally, and spiritually.

The individual prescription (IP) consists of a thorough examination of the client from observation, questions of past health history, and even what Marguerite called "blood spectrography" (the study of intracelluar hemoglobin). It is strange to discover the similarity between the impression produced by the composition of the perfume and that given by the living person. The IP blend needs to compensate for the deficiencies and reduce the excesses of the person's persona. It serves to balance the rhythms and life force of the individual.

For example, Marguerite used a blend of Elemi *(Canarium luzonicum)*, Galbanum *(Ferula gummosa)*, Violet leaves *(Viola odorata)*, and Lemongrass *(Cymbopogon citratus)* for a woman who had gray skin, gray hair, and a joyless attitude. The first two oils are reminiscent of advanced age since they were employed in impregnating the bandages of Egyptian mummies. These oils also revivify lifeless skin and bring the user more into the present moment, letting go of the past and enjoying the creativity of the now. Violet leaves dissolve rheumatic toxins and bring back an elasticity of tissues and muscles. Elemi of the Burseraceae family from the Philippine Islands is a wonderful oil for rejuvenating aged skin and relieving chronic health problems. It is very helpful for nervous exhaustion and the stress-related conditions that Marguerite's client experienced. Elemi is an expectorant for bronchial congestion and strengthens the immune system. On a psychic level it balances our spiritual practices with worldly responsibilities. Mentally it has a grounding yet joyous effect, making it good for meditation and visualization. Results: After two months of treatment with these oils, the woman's gray skin became alive and pink, and her behavior was youthful. She slept better and had even fallen in love!

Marguerite realized the significance of externally applying the oils (diluted in vegetable oil) and combining their application with massage. This concept had not been used in almost a thousand years. She sought an "alternative to oral application."[2] Perhaps she explored other methods because she was a biochemist, not a doctor, and she did not feel confident about prescribing the use of essences internally. She developed a special massage technique of applying essential oils along the nerve centers of the spine as well as to the face. Her wealthy women clients reported dramatic improvements in their complexions. Christine Wildwood writes, "To their amazement, there were also some interesting 'side-effects'; many experienced relief from rheumatic pain, deeper sleep, and a generally improved mental state."[3] The development of holistic aromatherapy massage as it is practiced in the UK today is deeply indebted to Marguerite.

These were busy years for Marguerite. She lectured and gave seminars throughout Europe, and she opened aromatherapy clinics in Switzerland, Paris, and England. At her London clinic, she taught aromatherapy to beauty therapists. She explained that she introduced her ideas to the beauty industry in England instead of the nursing field because she thought the estheticians would be most receptive to the topical applications of essential oils. Many of those students now teach too. Daniele Ryman, her most famous student, wrote a book about essential oils and her mentor, *The Aromatherapy Handbook*. Both of them felt essential oils were like drugs and should not be administered orally without a prescription. They had a profound effect on how essential oils were first used in the UK, mainly in inhalation and topical applications or massage.

Today the third generation of Marguerite's pupils includes a wide variety of medical practitioners like acupuncturists, osteopaths, nurses, reflexologists, modern herbalists, and orthodox doctors who want to avoid the overprescribing of Western medicine's drugs. The Royal College of Nursing insurance policy has helped to make essential oils used by thousands of British nurses for improved patient care. According to Shirley Price, who now has her own training schools, in between body massage treatments Marguerite used inhalations for her clients for tension, headaches, colds, sore throats, and blocked sinuses. Her clinics were established to treat both the physical symptoms and the emotional causes of disease, as well as to improve the appearance of the skin.

Marguerite wrote extensively and made a film on massage using essential oils. Her husband, Dr. Maury, said, "Marguerite was a great dynamo in my life. She would always come up with new ideas, suggestions and treatments."[4] Perhaps this is why one of her favorite oils was the lively Ginger. Ginger *(Zingiber officinale)* of the Zingiberaceae family comes from the root distilled in Britain, China, and India. Maury loved the warm, woody-spicy scent that brought balance to the digestive system for problems like indigestion, cramps, and nausea. She also found it useful for colds and coughs, and great in steams. She enjoyed how it warmed her emotions and gave her mental energy for her many projects. She appreciated how it sharpened her senses and stimulated her memory.

Marguerite Maury was awarded two international prizes in 1962 and 1967 for her research on essential oils and cosmetology. The 1962 Prix International d'Esthetique et Cosmetologie was for her contribution to the field of natural skin care. Daniele Ryman wrote, "In France, she single-handedly reestablished the reputation of aromatherapy."[5] Marguerite wrote *Le Capital Jeunesse* in 1961, which was translated and republished in 1987 by C. W. Daniel Co. under the English subtitle *The Secret of Life and Youth*.

Her work eventually led to the establishment of more than eighty aromatherapy colleges in the UK with thousands of practicing aromatherapists abiding by the decisions of a standards council for the quality of the oils and for educational certification. Patricia Davis, who established the first school, London School of Aromatherapy, was inspired by Marguerite's fine work. Patricia wrote the world's bestselling aromatherapy book, *Aromatherapy: An A–Z*, and acknowledges Marguerite in her introduction. Patricia would be included in my list of illustrious women, but she is still alive and will have to wait for another book.

Daniele Ryman, who was twenty-five years old at the time of Marguerite's death, has intently carried on her work, always giving credit to the charismatic and magnetic genius who was her mentor. She wrote, "Marguerite was a veritable whirlwind of energy and enthusiasm, working tirelessly until she quite literally died of sheer overwork of a stroke on Sept. 25th 1968."[6] She was buried in Switzerland in the mountains she loved.

Marguerite stated, "I am not trying to add years to a life, but to add life to the years."[7]

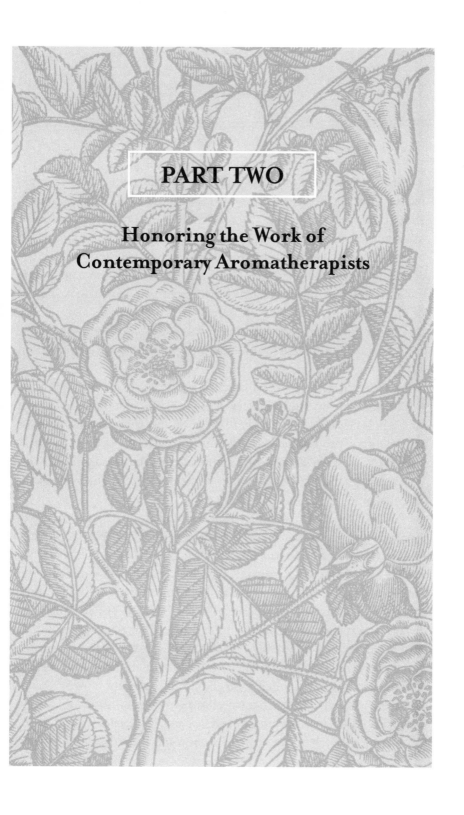

PART TWO

Honoring the Work of
Contemporary Aromatherapists

WHAT NEW ADVANCES HAVE BEEN DISCOVERED that will benefit essential oil therapists and dedicated users? We can see what science has discovered about our sense of smell and its connection to the limbic brain. Women like Zenobia and Catherine de Médicis could only use their intuition about how smell affected them. Today we have more concrete information to use as the standard of our practice. Brain research will continue to unfold more fascinating facts about smell, memory, and emotions. We can look at some of the myriad methods of applications for essential oils that have developed. Theodora's baths are still valuable, but many new external and internal ways to apply essential oils are now intriguing today's practitioners. In Part 2, some of the safety issues will be given for specific oils, as well as some of the chemical research that offers a new scientific basis to the practice of essential oils. The chemistry of oils could provide enough material for a whole new book; here I offer some GC-MS (gas chromatography–mass spectrometry) profiles and what they mean. Chapter 15 includes an examination of case studies: how to do a comprehensive study and some enlightening samples to support the modern practitioner's work in healing with essential oils.

Research has shown how effectively essential oils rid the body of infection, whether bacterial, viral, or fungal. Europeans have produced many clinical trials—often in vitro, but recently more in vivo—on the antimicrobial success of oils. Trota would have loved having this research at her fingertips. This discussion naturally leads to a glimpse of the immune system with its heroic white blood cells, which protect us from microbial invasions. Essential oils strengthen the ability of the phagocytes, B cells, and T cells to act without any side effects. Research has also shown the mind-body connection, with the immune system, the endocrine system, and the nervous system intelligently linked in a constant nonverbal conversation within us. Hildegard, who instinctively knew this truth, would be fascinated with our present-day investigation. Part 2 ends with an exploration of the search for understanding how the body, the mind, and the spirit interact.

CHAPTER TWELVE

The Sense of Smell and the Limbic Brain

Man only doth smell and take delight in the odours of flowers and sweet things.

—WILLIAM BULLEIN (1562)

IMAGINE YOUR LIFE without a sense of smell. It would be dreary, dull, and flat. Some people have anosmia or the total lack of the smell sensation, which can lead to depression and a sense of isolation. They cannot experience the ocean with its fresh, salty, surf fragrance mixed with pungent seaweed and fish. The ocean becomes more two-dimensional than three due to its bland odor. As people with anosmia walk through a forest on a hot summer day, they miss the earthy wood and balsamic dust fragrance that makes it so satisfying. Smell makes any day come alive.

I recently experienced the joy of fragrance with a group of about thirty people who were discussing some spiritual concepts and how they work in their lives. Although the conversation was interesting, everyone was in the intellectual mode and the energy felt low and stagnant. Someone asked me to share some essential oils with the group. I had with me only Bergamot (*Citrus x bergamia*) and an immune blend that contained Thyme (*Thymus vulgaris*), Lemon (*Citrus x limon*), and Eucalyptus (*Eucalyptus globulus*). I asked everyone to stand in a circle and hold out their open hands. I put two drops of bergamot in each hand and asked them to rub their hands together. Then they cupped their hands over their face and inhaled deeply. All of a sudden the energy in the room change as people began to smile and talk to each other. After each person rubbed the immune blend on the neck to boost the white blood cells, the group felt excited to be alive! The room was humming with energy. Oh, the power of scent and essential oils was demonstrated once again.

Describing various scents with words is difficult. The brain intuitively and sensually comprehends the fragrance of a rose, but grapples with trying to find the appropriate adjectives. Have you ever smelled a haunting fragrance that intrigued you and elicited a shadowy memory of a past experience? You almost did not want to find the logical explanation for it but sought to keep the secretive scent in the emotional realm, where it had depth and sacrament.

As our world moves into accepting the mysterious, feminine mode, a shift toward using our olfactory and tactile senses is taking place alongside the use of the visual and auditory. As we close the gap of our separation from nature and our emotional heart, we can use these fragrant oils to facilitate the alliance. For example, the smell of Lime oil *(Citrus x aurantifolia)* oil refreshes the mind and elicits memories of key lime pie or a cold lime soda on a hot July day.

Let us look at why a fragrance, an emotion, and a memory are bonded together. Smell is a subliminal sense, registering first in the more primitive part of the brain and eventually in the right temporal lobe of the neocortex. The right hemisphere of the brain is the more intuitive, subliminal one. An experiment with two offices painted and furnished identically showed how the room with a diffused fragrance of Lemon and Lavender *(Lavandula angustifolia)* was perceived by many observers as "brighter and cleaner." Yet no one noticed the smell. This is often how essential oils work on a subconscious level. It is difficult to consciously give an essential oil credit for the experience of feeling uplifted and less stressed. I believe this lack of olfactory awareness is due to our consciousness still being undeveloped and usually caught between the past and the future. If we live in the *now* we are more aware of how the oils are directly affecting our psyche.

Smell is more powerful than sight as it evokes an immediate response in the catacombs of the olfactory system and in the limbic brain. The process of smell begins as the molecules of an essential oil are released in the nose and then travel high up into the rear of the nasal cavity, where there is a small patch of mucous membrane called the epithelium. The fifty million receptor cells of this membrane (twenty-five million in each nostril) have millions of cilia on the other side that send neuronal information about the scent through nerves to the olfactory bulb, where the molecular information is translated into an olfactory "picture." Forty nerve cells need to be stimulated before a cell sensation can be perceived. This is the only area in the body where brain nerves contact the outside world. The translation of the molecular information into nerve language enters the brain, not the scent itself.

The millions of nerves going into the olfactory bulb coalesce into two main olfactory nerves on the other side as the smell neurons travel across the blood-brain barrier into the limbic brain system. There they are received by the many parts of the limbic brain, the mammalian evolutionary part of the brain that is sometimes called the *smell brain*. The olfactory nerves first reach a small almond-shaped subcortical nucleus lobe called the *amygdala*, which governs emotional response and presents emotional data with the smell. Immediately the amygdala decides if the incoming information is dangerous or innocuous. It is concerned with sensory input from all senses together with an emotional association. For example, if you were walking through a garden with your grandmother and together you smelled Clary sage *(Salvia sclarea)* just as she told you that she loves you, you would always associate clary sage with love.

After reaching the amygdala, the neuronal information travels to the hippocampus, which looks to me like a seahorse on its side. The hippocampus is involved in the formation and storage of short-term memories (from the previous three years). This is known because removal of the hippocampus in a man with epilepsy resulted in no short-term memory. The smell, the memory, and the emotions attached to the smell are immediately bonded together and can easily be revived by a future hit of that smell. Essential oils used to awaken the hippocampus are the mind-memory stimulating Rosemary *(Rosmarinus officinalis)* and Peppermint *(Mentha piperita)*. Gerhard Buchbauer's research found that the limbic system is responsible for feelings of harmony and peace as well as sexual desire.[1] Smell can have a psychological effect even when it is below human consciousness or when the human is asleep.[2] I know the oils can calm anxiety and panic, which was apparent with one friend who has very little sense of smell. It seems an essential oil can affect the limbic system even when the fragrance is not registered in the neocortex or the person is not consciously aware of it.

After reaching the hippocampus, the neuronal information travels on to the hypothalamus, one of the most amazing tissues in the body. The hypothalamus regulates the endocrine system via messages to the master gland, the pituitary. It also invigorates the autonomic nervous system and stores long-term memories. It essentially regulates metabolism, sex drive, stress response, respiration, growth, energy use, and the trigger of neurotransmitters such as serotonin and noradrenaline. The chemistry of hormones can be deeply affected by the smell of essential oils. Myrrh *(Commiphora myrrha)* has a stabilizing effect on thyroxine from the thyroid glands and on neurotransmitters. Ylang-ylang *(Cananga odorata)* has a calming effect on noradrenaline in the sympathetic nervous system. Essential oils that affect the hypothalamus are the chemically complex Geranium *(Pelargonium graveolens),* Rosewood *(Aniba rosaeodora),* and Frankincense *(Boswellia carteri);* both are considered regulating oils, mimicking the action of this very complicated bit of tissue.

After reaching the hypothalamus, the neurons go to the thalamus, which is a relay station for the scent to be catapulted through the cingulate gyrus to the neocortex, the human brain. When it reaches the neocortex in the temporal lobe, we become conscious of the smell and we can identify it by name. Before this last stage, though, there was a deep recognition of the smell on an unconscious emotional and memory level. Of all the senses, smell is the most immediate and the first to trigger memories due to its journey via the olfactory limbic nerve track.

To illustrate this phenomenon, a friend recently traveled to northern Italy where she visited the town of Bergamo. There grew many orchards of the citrus tree producing small green fruits from which is handpressed the oil of Bergamot. The town radiated with this delightful fragrance. The first sniff by my friend transported her back in time to a memory of her uncle, who always drank Earl Grey tea that is flavored with Bergamot oil. This uncle had been very kind and sensitive to her. The fragrance created waves of pleasure in my friend since her amygdala and hippocampus had positive feelings and memories stored with the smell of Bergamot. Of course one of the characteristics of this essential oil is its tendency to bring joy, relieve depression, and soothe tension.

I once attended a seminar called OptimaLearning during which the two hemispheres of the neocortex were described as partners in bringing the conscious and unconscious mind together in learning and life experiences. Music was used as a link between the two hemispheres. Specific classical concertos from Hayden, Chopin, and Beethoven were recommended. The left hemisphere of the brain is logical, analytical, and conscious, and keeps track of time. The right side is spontaneous, intuitive, emotional, and unconscious, and keeps track of space. Smell neurons travel through the olfactory system to the limbic brain, sojourning in the unconscious side of the brain before entering the conscious, integrating parts of the brain in the neocortex. Like classical music, smell can link both hemispheres, although it initially resonates with the right side and is more unconscious.

Odor as a bridge between the two hemispheres of the brain was shown in a 1964 Japanese study of the tracing of brain waves made on an electroencephalogram (EEG). The researchers, led by S. Torri, placed electrodes on each participant's scalp and recorded the brain-wave movement after the inhalation of over twenty different essential oils. Both hemispheres of the brain began to immediately work in greater symmetry. Oils like Geranium and Rosewood showed both an increase and a decrease in the magnitude of contingent negative variation (CNV). These two oils, as mentioned, help to regulate the autonomic nervous system and the endocrine system via the hypothalamus and the pituitary gland. Peppermint increased the brain waves and Sandalwood *(Santalum album)* decreased the activity.[3] Therefore, fragrance can deeply affect our ability to feel and think, taking us into mental alertness or into a peaceful, meditative state.

Paolo Rovesti at the University of Milan conducted important research on the emotional, mental, and psychological effects of essential oils. Rovesti treated patients who exhibited signs of depression and hysteria with the following combination of oils: Jasmine *(Jasminum grandiflorum)*, Neroli *(Citrus x aurantium l. amara)*, Lemon verbena *(Aloysia triphylla)*, Sandalwood, and Lemon. For the treatment of anxiety, he suggested Bergamot, Cypress *(Cupressus sempervirens)*, Petitgrain *(Citrus x aurantium l. amara)*, Lime, Rose *(Rosa damascena)*, Violet *(Viola odorata)*, and Marjoram *(Origanum majorana)*. He had great success with these treatments. Rovesti, who was honored for his work, came to an important conclusion regarding the use of essential oils on the mind: They bring a person into a place of "relaxed alertness." I feel this is a brilliant insight because what is more ideal than to live in a state of being relaxed yet alert.

Rovesti's lovely saying from *In Search of Perfumes Lost* speaks to our modern lack of nature's fragrant bounty: "We who are immersed in the unnaturalness of modern-day life cannot recall without nostalgia and sadness those gifts of nature at man's disposal, now neglected or in disuse.

Among those are the lost paradises of natural perfumes, of the perfumes of the past and of the spirit."[4]

Both learning and healing are optimal when all parts of the mind, soul, and personality are engaged in a creative process. Inhaling a beautiful oil stimulates an opening of the mind-body connection to the higher self that can participate in bringing balance through the parasympathetic system on the physical level to harmonizing the auric field on the energetic level. This fabulous process is discussed in more detail in Chapter 19, "Essential Oils and the Mind-Body Connection."

CHAPTER THIRTEEN

Modern Methods of Using Essential Oils

Sweet perfumes work immediately upon the spirits: for their refreshing, sweet and healthful ayres are special preserves to health, and therefore much to be praised.

—RALPH AUSTEN (1653)

M Y FIRST TECHNIQUE OF using essential oils, similar to Hatshepsut's, was to rub them directly onto my skin, like my feet or my neck, for maximum strength and effect. I loved the fragrance and the tingle I derived from this method. Putting drops of Peppermint *(Mentha piperita)* on my stomach made my skin sting a little, yet gave me great digestive benefits. I have since developed many other ways of applying essential oils, but I always come back to my original method because it works so well!

I prefer the term *essential oil therapy,* which includes all ways of using essential oils described in this book. The more specific term *aromatherapy* means personal healing via the sense of smell by inhalation. I include aromatherapy as just one of the methods used in essential oil therapy.

External Methods

INHALATION

Enjoying the sensation of smell: Just inhaling an essential oil from the bottle can bring amazing changes to the body and the mind. I recently sniffed the intriguing, smoky, husky scent of Vetiver *(Vetiveria zizanioides)* distilled in Haiti. I was transported to the grassy fields of Haiti and felt my shoulders and back relax while my mind came more into the present.

Inhaling a blend in a diffuser: Inhalation from a scent stick or diffuser is one step removed from direct contact with a plant or essential oil, but still quite effective in stimulating the odor receptors of the epithelium. In a large room such as our classrom, a nebulizing diffuser can be used to give the space a fragrance such as a blend of Lavender *(Lavandula angustifolia)*, Mandarin *(Citrus reticulata)*, and Cedarwood *(Juniperus virginiana)*. A diffuser with a timer can be set to come on every hour for thirty minutes, which seems to match the pattern of overload that the human olfactory system experiences. After a thirty-minute break, the receptors are again able to pick up the scent trail. Otherwise, a student needs to leave the classroom and return ten minutes later to smell the blend diffusing lightly in the room. The amount of oil inhaled is minimal due to the gradient concentration of oil molecules throughout many cubic feet of air.

Inhaling a blend with steam: My favorite method of dealing with an oncoming cold is the exhilarating method of steam inhalation. Using three oils in a ceramic or stainless-steel bowl of boiling water creates a powerful rush. I recommend one drop of Eucalyptus *(Eucalyptus globulus)*, one drop of Peppermint *(Mentha piperita)*, and one drop of Tea tree *(Melaleuca alternifolia)*. Sit directly in front of the bowl of water, put in the three drops of oil, and cover the head and bowl with a towel. If an infection has begun, the essential oil and steam mixture will hurt as the oils attack the bacteria or virus. Sometimes hurt is good; the steam is eliminating some of the infection. It might take three to six sessions over a couple of days to totally eliminate the infection, or only one if you catch it early.

SKIN ABSORPTION

I believe the most effective way to use essential oils is to apply them onto the skin. Rub Cypress *(Cupressus sempervirens)* on the throat when a sore throat appears. Apply Lavender to the temples and the back of the neck for a stress headache. Always test for any skin irritation. Dilute with a carrier oil (2 to 3 percent essential oil). Put Tea tree on a cut or a wound. In all three cases, immediate results are experienced. In 1992 Jager showed that linalool and linalyl acetate, two chemicals in lavender oil, in a 2 percent dilution in peanut oil, were absorbed through the abdominal skin into the blood plasma within minutes. The maximum level was reached in twenty minutes.[1] The chemicals remain in the bloodstream a short while (ninety minutes), and then—being fat-soluble compounds—they are stored in adipose tissue before being filtered out through the liver and kidneys in twenty-four hours.[2]

Below is an important chart to aid in the measurement of oil and the conversion of the amounts given in recipes.

Metric Conversion Table

30 drops (0.033814 fluid ounces)	1 milliliter
1 ounce	30 (29.57) milliliters
1 teaspoon	4.93 milliliters (147.9 drops)
1 tablespoon	17.70 milliliters
1 fluid ounce	29.57 milliliters
1.62 teaspoons (0.27 fluid ounces)	8 milliliters
0.68 tablespoons (0.338 fluid ounces)	10 milliliters
3.38 fluid ounces	100 milliliters
33.814 fluid ounces	1 liter (1000 milliliters)
1 cup (8 fluid ounces)	0.2365 liters
1 pint (16 fluid ounces)	0.473 liters (473 milliliters)
1 quart (2 pints, 32 fluid ounces)	0.95 liter
1 gallon (4 quarts, 128 fluid ounces)	3.7854 liters
1 dry ounce	28.35 grams
1 pound (16 dry ounces)	454 grams

Suggested dilution of essential oils in carrier oil:

6 to 7 drops of essential oil in 8 milliliters of carrier oil	= 2.5 percent solution
22 drops of essential oil in 30 (29.57) milliliters (1 fluid ounce) of carrier oil	= 2.5 percent solution

Here are some favorite recipes that use the direct method of application.

Salt scrub

Use equal parts of Epsom salt, sea salt, and baking soda. Add 8 drops of a blend of these essential oils per cup of salts:

3 drops Rosemary *(Rosmarinus officinalis verbenone),* a
chemotype of Rosemary

2 drops Sage *(Salvia officinalis)*

3 drops Orange *(Citrus sinensis)*

Body wrap

Into a 4-ounce bottle with a spray attachment, add 4 ounces of water and these lymphatic essential oils:

6 drops Grapefruit *(Citrus x paradisi)*

3 drops Lemon *(Citrus x limon)*

4 drops Fennel *(Foeniculum vulgare)*

3 drops Angelica *(Angelica archangelica)*

4 drops Juniper *(Juniperus communis)*

Blend in the spray bottle. Spray a large towel until it is damp. Wrap body of client in a towel, then in a plastic sheet, and then in a blanket. Play music and have the client relax for 20 minutes until the client begins to perspire and feel hot. Wait 10 more minutes before unwrapping. Have client take a shower. Leaves skin detoxified and soft.

Facial routine

First add 2 drops Lavender *(Lavandula angustifolia)* to a facial cleanser and clean skin. Then do a five-minute steam with 2 cups of boiling water by adding:

1 drop Geranium *(Pelargonium graveolens)*

1 drop Patchouli *(Pogostemon cablin)*

1 drop Sandalwood *(Santalum album)*

Make a mask with 1 teaspoon white clay, 1 teaspoon oatmeal, and 1 teaspoon cornmeal. To 1 tablespoon of the clay mixture add:

1 drop Rose *(Rosa damascena)*

1 drop Palmarosa *(Cymbopogon martini)*

Blend oils and clay with 2 drops of water. Apply and leave on for 10 minutes. Use a hydrosol (Rose or Neroli) to tone the skin as a finishing touch. Feel the velvety texture of your skin!

Compress

Compresses are valuable for painful sprains, PMS cramps, or eye irritation. You will need a bowl, 2 cups of body-temperature water, a cotton cloth or small towel, and essential oils.

For irritated, red eyes

Wet two chamomile tea bags in 1 cup of warm water. Add:

2 drops Roman chamomile *(Chamaemelum nobile)*
1 drop German chamomile *(Matricaria recutita)*

Use a dark-colored cloth due to the blue color of German chamomile. Apply tea bags to eyes and lie down. Resubmerge tea bags every 10 minutes until irritation is soothed. This is wonderful for allergies, too much champagne, and wind irritation.

For PMS cramps or heavy periods

Put 2 cups of warm water in a bowl. Add:

4 drops Clary sage *(Salvia sclarea)*
2 drops Cypress *(Cupressus sempervirens)*
3 drops Lavender *(Lavandula angustifolia)*

Dip a cloth in the water and apply it to the lower abdomen, directly on the skin. Lie down and reapply every 10 minutes until ache is relieved.

For sprained ankles or wrists

In two cups of warm water, add:

6 drops Rosemary *(Rosmarinus officinalis)*
4 drops Marjoram *(Origanum majorana)*
3 drops Cajeput *(Melaleuca cajuputi)*
7 drops Juniper *(Juniperus communis)*

Dip cloth in water, lie down, and wrap around injured limb. Reapply for half an hour three times a day. Continue this procedure for several days until the pain has subsided. RICE (rest, ice, compression, and elevation) would be valuable too.

Hair and scalp oil

Before shampooing your hair, make a blend in 2 ounces of jojoba oil. Add:

10 drops Rosemary *(Rosmarinus officinalis)*
8 drops Ylang-ylang *(Cananga odorata)*
8 drops Petitgrain *(Citrus x aurantium I. amara)*

Mix together in a 2-ounce bottle and apply to hair, beginning at the scalp and moving downward. This is great for dry hair with brittle ends. It adds luster and body. Let it sit (under a plastic cap) on hair and scalp for one hour. If you wish, shampoo afterward.

Massage

The combination of smell (essential oils) and touch (massage) triggers deep responses in the human right brain. Today massage therapists are using essential oil therapy to enhance the healing of their therapeutic touch. Massage and pure essential oils is an excellent way to treat and strengthen all the body's systems, to manage stress, and to maintain general health. You do not have to be sick to greatly benefit from these dual therapies. Massage plus the proper oils can:

• Improve circulation
• Help relieve constipation
• Reduce muscle tension
• Aid the circulation of the lymph system
• Stimulate the immune system
• Deepen sleep
• Increase physical energy

Massage Procedure Template: The are many books available that illustrate the value of adding essential oils to any massage practice. Here are some brief suggestions on how to add the oils to increase the benefit of the experience for a client:

Create a mood in the massage room with low lighting, soft music, and a diffuser with a few drops of essential oils operating softly in the background.

Interview the client for ten minutes in a Marguerite Maury individual prescription way. Ask basic information about the client's physical health.

Here are a few questions you might consider asking: What is the weakest part of your body? How is your digestion? Your sleep? Your menstrual and respiratory patterns? Do you often get a cold? Do you have good circulation? Adequate physical energy?

Then ask how your client would rate herself on a scale of one to ten on the following:

Mental fatigue	Mental alertness
Anxiety	Joy
Fear	Confidence
Stress	Peaceful
Anger	Emotional balance
Spiritual path	

As answers are given, chose the appropriate three or four oils that will bring balance and health to the client. Have the client smell the chosen oils to be sure that he enjoys these fragrances.

Mix the chosen oils with 1 ounce of vegetable oil or lotion in a small dish. Put one drop of oil on a Kleenex to place in the massage table's face cradle for enjoyment, relaxation, or respiratory stimulant.

Take some of the oil mixture out of the dish to rub between your hands and apply to the body.

The client is receiving the maximum essential oil treatment through application of the oils to the skin of the whole body and the continual inhalation of the oils on the Kleenex and in the room. This is immersion in a total-body aromatherapy envelope!

Relaxing massage oil

In a 4-ounce bottle add a mixture of vegetable oils such as:

1 ounce apricot kernel oil
1 ounce grapeseed oil
2 ounces almond oil

Add to the carrier oil the following essential oils:

10 drops American cedarwood *(Juniperus virginiana)*
12 drops Orange *(Citrus sinensis)*
6 drops Bergamot *(Citrus x bergamia)*

5 drops Geranium *(Pelargonium graveolens)*
9 drops Rosewood *(Aniba rosaeodora)*

Apply in the evening for a delicious, calming massage.

Dry brush

Before taking a shower, in a small bowl mix together:

1 ounce vegetable oil
4 drops Peppermint *(Mentha piperita)*
3 drops Lemon Eucalyptus *(Eucalyptus citriodora)*
3 drops Sage *(Salvia officinalis)*
4 drops Lemon *(Citrus x limon)*

Apply the mixture to your body using a stiff bristle brush. Experience the aromatic tingle as you help your skin to breathe.

Carrier Oils

Oils produced from nuts, vegetables, fruits, and seeds are fantastic carriers for the essential oils. They are healing agents on their own. Skin needs the vitamins and essential fatty acids that can only be found in these wonderful carrier oils.

When using vegetable oils for any blend, always use cold-pressed oils. Store oils in amber or dark-colored bottles. Keep massage oil and all blends in a cool, dark place.

The average standard for dilution is 2 to 3 percent essential oils to carrier oil. If you are using 1 ounce or more of carrier oil in hot climates (over 85ºF), keep the mixture in the refrigerator. If kept protected, vegetable oils are the perfect medium to use with essential oils. The carrier oils enrich the skin with vitamins, minerals, and emollients.

Vitamin E Oils: Some oils such as wheat germ *(Triticum spp.)* and grapeseed oil *(Vitis vinifera)* contain vitamin E, which fights free radical damage, the principal cause of premature aging. Vitamin E is an antioxidant for the collagen and elastin fibers in the dermal layers of the skin. By using foods, vegetable oils, and supplements with Vitamin E, the risk of cancer (skin and other forms) and cataract formation in the eyes can be reduced.

Vitamin A Oils: Vitamin A is another vitamin for the skin. It keeps other carrier oils from oxidizing. It soothes and diminishes rashes, acne, and dermatitis. Carotenoids, rich in vitamin A, are available in Carrot seed oil *(Daucus carota)* and rose hip seed oil *(Rosa mosqueta)*. The rich reddish-orange color of these oils reveals their carotene base. Another vegetable oil containing large amounts of vitamin A is apricot kernel oil *(Prunus armeniaca)*, which benefits mature, dry, sensitive, even inflamed skin. This vitamin is especially important in the repair of skin tissue since it helps regulate the rate at which skin cells are shed and replaced. A shortage of this vitamin makes skin sluggish and flaky; the resulting accumulated sebum makes acne more likely to form.

Gamma Linoleic Oils: Other oils like evening primrose oil *(Oenothera biennis)* and borage oil *(Borago officinalis)* provide gamma linoleic acids. Liz Earle describes this process in *New Vital Oils:* "By supplying the skin with high levels of essential fatty plant oils, they [these plant oils] are able to strengthen the fragile cellular membranes and act as antiagers."[3] Gamma linoleic oils help build the membranes that surround every cell. This process guards against moisture loss. Without essential fatty acids, we would have a dry, devitalized complexion. Evening primrose oil and borage oil are also great remedies for eczema and psoriasis; apply topically by piercing a capsule or taking a capsule internally. Other sad results of a lack of these precious fatty acids are premature aging, weak collagen fibers leading to slow wound healing, and hair loss. Besides using these oils as a base for essential oil blends, we can eat deep-water fish like salmon or supplement our diet with fish body oils that contain omega-3 and omega-6 fatty acids.

Polyunsaturated Vegetable Oils: Polyunsaturated vegetable oils such as olive oil *(Olea europaea)* and sunflower oil *(Helianthus annuus)* are also rich in linoleic acid. If these oils are overheated, the fatty acid chemical structure is changed and they become unhealthy for skin and body. It is always important to purchase cold-pressed oils.

Liquid Wax: Another important skin oil is jojoba *(Simmondsia chinensis)*, which is really a liquid wax extracted from the jojoba bean. Light and similar in texture to the skin's natural oil, sebum, it is good for body blends of essential oils. Jojoba is also a healthy base for hair blends with oils such as Rosemary and Ylang-ylang. It has a long shelf life and does not need to be refrigerated.

Aloe Vera: Another carrier that is really not an oil is aloe vera gel *(Aloe barbadensis)*. It is an incredible healing substance for burns, eczema, and wounds. I recommend growing a plant so you can always break off a frond if needed. Add some drops of essential oil directly to the gel that fills the leaves. This amazing gel helps moisturize skin, prevent bacterial and fungal infections, and reduce inflammation from conjunctivitis, gingivitis, and dermatitis. Studies show aloe vera accelerates the healing of wounds caused by full-face dermal abrasion, burns, and psoriasis. Adding essential oils such as lavender, palmarosa, tea tree, and sandalwood to the aloe vera gel for these skin conditions makes a powerful remedy. Whenever you need a carrier for essential oils that is not oily (for example, for acne), consider using aloe vera.

Care of Vegetable Oils: All of the carriers and vegetable oils described here need to be kept cool, out of the sun, and ideally in an amber bottle. Vegetable oils oxidize (except jojoba), meaning their long chains of carbon atoms and hydrogen atoms become unstable when subjected to heat. A rancid oil smells bitter and should be thrown away. Most vegetable oils have a shelf life of six months. Essential oils, if stored properly, can last for two to three years.

METHODS WITH WATER

Essential oils and water do not dissolve together due to the variance in size of molecules, water being much larger. The lipophilic quality of essential oils makes them attracted to fatty substances, not to water. Oils high in ketones such as Spearmint *(Mentha spicata)* dissolve more easily. Using essential oils in water requires an extra effort to temporarily emulsify them by stirring or shaking.

Bath

One of the most delightful ways to use essential oils is to sprinkle them on top of a freshly filled bathtub of warm water. Keep the bathroom door closed. Light a candle after turning off the lights, then lean back to enjoy the warm fragrance. The oils penetrate the skin as your body soaks. Swish them around for more body exposure. Your olfactory system picks up molecules in the air so breathe deeply. This is like a light steam for the respiratory system.

Early morning bath

3 drops Cardamom *(Elettaria cardamomum)*

4 drops of Mandarin *(Citrus reticulata)*
5 drops of Black pepper *(Piper nigrum)*
2 drops Ginger *(Zingiber officinale)*

Fill the tub to the top. Add the drops for a great way to start the day and have a stimulating morning meditation.

After a stressful day

3 drops Bay laurel *(Laurus nobilis)*
2 drops Elemi *(Canarium luzonicum)*
1 drop Spikenard *(Nardostachys grandiflora)*
5 drops Grapefruit *(Citrus x paradisi)*

Feel your nervous system unwind as your body relaxes and your mind comes back into the present moment.

Hydrosols

This delightful form of using essential oils has aroused much interest in recent years. Created during the steam-distillation process, a hydrosol is the water that lies under the essential oil after flowing through the condenser. There is always more watery substance than oil in the final product. A hydrosol contains 99 percent water that is chemically bonded to less than 1 percent essential oil. Some of the water-soluble constituents of the plant remain married to the powerful qualities of the essential oil. This creates a perfect phytotherapy wedding of the herb and the oil. In California a hydrosol is the only product of distillation that can be created and sold for a profit due to the high cost of labor and the huge quantity of plant material needed to bring about a small quantity of essential oil.

Elizabeth I encouraged noble women of her time to make hydrosols with their backyard still—for medicine, cosmetics, and fragrant pomanders. Hydrosols carry some of the chemical traces of the water-soluble plant composition to combine with the chemistry of the essential oils. For example, hydrosol of Saint John's wort contains tannins, flavonoids, and xanthones that do not exist in the essential oil. This makes the hydrosol a more complete carrier of the chemical imprint of the whole plant.

There are many magical ways to enjoy hydrosols. We offer a demonstration of the steam-distillation process three times a year at the College of Botanical Healing Arts. We focus on one plant at each open house—

lavender, rosemary, and geranium. In a glass or copper still, we get about 4 milliliters (0.81 teaspoon or 0.135 ounce) of essential oil in 4 quarts of hydrosol. The hydrosols and oils are so vital and beautiful in their fragrance and quality. Here are some ways to use them:

I always carry both Rose hydrosol and Roman Chamomile oil in my purse for any allergic reaction during the pollen time of year. They seem to inhibit the histamine reaction, calm my nasal passages, and soothe my itchy eyes. They also de-stress my emotions and bring me into my heart for more compassion in any situation. Additionally, Rose hydrosol helps my skin feel moisturized and toned. All of this with three quick sprays!

Another hydrosol I enjoy is Neroli *(Citrus x aurantium l. amara)*, which is especially delicious in warm, humid weather. Spray on your face, your temples, and the back of your neck. Its cooling, orange flower power cuts through the heat and uplifts my mind and emotions. It is helpful for headaches or nervous tension. I feel ready to connect to my higher self and handle whatever challenge might come along.

Use Rose hydrosol *(Rosa damascena)* for emotionally tense situations and skin care for all skin types.

Use Neroli hydrosol *(Citrus x aurantium l. amara)* to help a client deal with anger or insomnia, and during spiritual meditation retreats.

Use Melissa *(Melissa officinalis)* hydrosol to spray on herpes-infected skin, on people who are near death for solace, and on hyperactive children who have trouble concentrating.

Hydrosols can be the base for a blend too. Although vegetable oils provide the ideal base for these lipophilic oils, the hydrosol offers a good water base.

Healing throat spray

Add the following essential oils to a 2-ounce spray bottle filled with Lavandin hydrosol *(Lavandula x intermedia l. grosso)*. This hydrosol is more antiseptic and less relaxing than lavender due to its chemical constiuents of camphor and borneol. This would be great to use on a plane; spray on the throat or in the mouth when surrounded by coughing passengers.

5 drops Ravintsara *(Cinnamomum camphora)*
2 drops Thyme *(Thymus vulgaris)*

4 drops Fir needle *(Abies alba)*

3 drops Pine *(Pinus sylvestris)*

3 drops Bergamot *(Citrus x bergamia)*

Douche

I do not recommend douches on a regular basis. Too many can dissipate the natural bacterial flora in the vagina. They are useful for vaginal infections, either bacterial or fungal. Use the following blends twice a day until all infection disappears.

Antibacterial douche

Fill a rubber douche bag with 1 pint (2 cups) warm water. Add:

3 drops of Niaouli *(Melaleuca quinquenervia viridiflora)*

4 drops Marjoram *(Origanum majorana)*

3 drops Lemon *(Citrus x limon)*

Antifungal douche (for candida)

Fill a rubber douche bag with 1 pint (2 cups) warm water. Add:

5 drops Tea tree *(Melaleuca alternifolia)*

3 drops Lemongrass *(Cymbopogon citratus)*

2 drops Lemon eucalyptus *(Eucalyptus citriodora)*

2 drops Geranium *(Pelargonium graveolens)*

Jacuzzi (Hot Tub)

Hot tubs usually have three hundred fifty to five hundred gallons of water in them. As you drop the essential oils into the tub, much of it evaporates—especially if the jets are on. There is no need to worry about essential oils damaging the tub or its pipes if you use the following recipe.

Romantic blend

6 drops Jasmine *(Jasminum grandiflorum)*

5 drops Ylang-ylang *(Cananga odorata)*

7 drops Cardamom *(Elettaria cardamomum)*

3 drops Nutmeg *(Myristica fragrans)*

4 drops Vanilla *(Vanilla planifolia)*

Blend in a bottle (without carrier oil) and put 6 drops per person in tub every 15 minutes.

Shower

Since most people shower daily, here's a method to use essential oils in running water during an early morning shower.

Aromatic washcloth blend for an early morning shower.

3 drops Basil *(Ocimum basilicum ct linalool)*

3 drops Black pepper *(Piper nigrum)*

3 drops Mandarin *(Citrus reticulata)*

Gargle

Sore throat gargle

When a sore throat is coming on, nip it in the bud by rubbing Cypress *(Cupressus sempervirens)* on your throat and doing a gargle.

Put 3 drops of Cypress on your fingertips and rub it onto the skin on the throat.

Then put 3 drops of Cypress into a 4-ounce glass of water. Put 1 tablespoon of the mixture in mouth. Gargle for 1 minute but do not swallow.

Repeat until the glass is empty. This has arrested the infection for me many times.

Sweet breath gargle

Follow the procedure for sore throat gargle, but use 3 drops of Peppermint *(Mentha piperita)* instead of Cypress. Gargle for at least 3 minutes. Your breath will feel minty clean.

Spray Bottle

Fresh air spritzer

When the air in your house or office smells bad or stale, create a refreshing air spray. To a 4-ounce bottle filled with distilled water, add:

10 drops Lime *(Citrus x aurantifolia)*

8 drops Pine *(Pinus sylvestris)*

7 drops Tea tree *(Melaleuca alternifolia)*

12 drops Grapefruit *(Citrus x paradisi)*

6 drops Lemongrass *(Cymbopogon citratus)*

8 drops Bay laurel *(Laurus nobilis)*

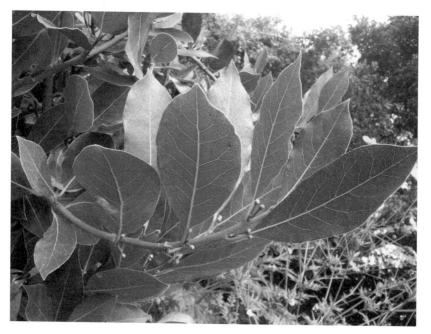

Bay laurel

Internal Methods

SAFETY ISSUES

Less is more! There are a few important safety considerations for internal use of essential oils. The only known deaths or poisoning caused by essential oils have occurred after someone (mostly children) swallowed large amounts of the oils. In *Essential Oil Safety*, Robert Tisserand and Tony Balacs wrote, "The bioavailable dose of an essential oil given orally is significantly higher than after inhalation or topical application."[4] Oral dosage is usually eight to ten times greater in its impact on the body's internal environment than massage or application to the skin. Absorption into the bloodstream after dermal application is much slower than after oral intake. Internal use is much riskier.

Concentrations on the skin will not become too high because as the oil slowly enters the body through the stratum corneum of the skin, it is continually being circulated and removed by the liver. The amount of oil absorption from inhalation or any of the above water applications will be even lower than from massage. The average amount absorbed through massage is 0.025 to 0.1 milliliters (½ to 3 drops) when it is in a 2 to 3 percent dilution.[5]

My safety guidelines are diluting the oils 1 to 5 percent for external use, depending on age and condition of client. It is best to use 12 drops diluted in 1 gallon of liquid (1 drop per 8-ounce glass) for oral use over a 24-hour period. Any more than that is dangerous and the taste is overpowering.

Only well-educated medical essential oil therapists, herbalists, or doctors should prescribe any oral use of essential oils for medicinal purposes. At College of the Botanical Healing Arts (COBHA), we recommend that Level One (beginning) students do not orally ingest oils, and in Level Two (advanced) it is used on a personal experimental basis. We do not prescribe oral use of oils when students are interviewing the public and offering treatments in our clinic. See Chapter 16, "Essential Oils for the Treatment of Infection, for more safety issues."

KEEPING RECORDS

It is wise for essential oil therapists to keep accurate records of how many drops of essential oils are used with the exact quantity of dilution in different methods of treatment (massage, bath, injury application, steam) for each client. Record on the client's chart the method suggested, the volume of carrier oil, the number of drops and the percentage of essential oils, the length of contact with body surface, and the results (for example, no irritation, fast healing, contact dermatitis, or painful reaction).

Date	Name	Phone number	Main Symptoms
04/12/09	John Roberts	(831) 462-2908	Respiratory infection, stress

Method used	Amount of carrier	# drops of each oil	Time of contact	Body results
Steam	2 cups of water	1 drop tea tree 1 drop eucalyptus 1 drop niaouli	Twice a day for 5 days in 4 days	Respiratory clear

ESSENTIAL OILS IN DRINKS

Oral doses of essential oils should be taken with large amounts of water or dissolved in water substances like fruit juice or aloe vera juice. Safe oils like Tea tree and Myrtle *(Myrtus communis)* can be taken using 1 drop per 8-ounce cup and no more than 8 to 10 drops in a 24-hour period.

A favorite drink of mine is one drop of Lemon oil *(Citrus x limon)* in an 8-ounce glass of water. It is a refreshing oil and purifies the water with its antibacterial action. If you carry some with you, you can get in the great habit of using it at a restaurant or when traveling.

We just had a distillation of Geranium *(Pelargonium graveolens)* from plant material that grows in our inner courtyard at the College of Botanical Healing Arts. The hydrosol was so fresh, so volatile in its aroma that we all felt exhilarated smelling this lovely watery substance. It brought balance to our endocrine system and a sense of community. We added 2 cups of the Geranium hydrosol to a punch drink; each person drank ¼ cup.

ESSENTIAL OILS IN FOOD

A flavorful experience! I like to add a few drops of essential oils to highlight a special flavor. Adding a drop of Rosemary *(Rosmarinus officinalis)* and a drop of Dill *(Anethum graveolens)* to a salad dressing gives it a delicious sparkle.

When baking a lemon curd tart, I like to add a drop of Lemon *(Citrus x limon)* and a drop of Lavender *(Lavandula angustifolia)* as the lemon curd is beginning to cool.

When using a blender to create a drink of strawberries, bananas, protein powder, lecithin, and 3 cups of orange juice, add 1 drop of Orange *(Citrus sinensis)* and 1 drop of Grapefruit *(Citrus x paradisi)*.

Add a drop of cardamom *(Elettaria cardamomum)* to a slice of dried, crystallized ginger to make a delicious snack or a before-dinner appetizer. It will also aid in digesting dinner. My husband loves it!

There are a multitude of delicious aromatic recipes to include in another book.

SUPPOSITORIES

Suppositories are often used in French medical aromatherapy. This method is especially effective for respiratory illnesses. Kurt Schnaubelt states in *Medical Aromatherapy* that by being absorbed into the rectal veins, the essential oils bypass the liver and reach the heart-lung circulatory system, the lower bronchial tract, and other organs without having been altered by the liver metabolism.[6]

To create a suppository, use 2 tablespoons cocoa butter, 1 teaspoon olive oil, and 1 teaspoon beeswax. Heat, cool, and add 9 to 10 drops of essential blend. For children (ages 3 to 10), use 3 drops of essential oils to 1 tablespoon cocoa butter. A study in France showed that using German chamomile *(Matricaria recutita)* for children with diarrhea in the form of a suppository proved to be quite effective.[7]

Suppositories for treating the flu

In a clinical science class at the College of Botanical Healing Arts, we create respiratory suppositories by heating 2 tablespoons cocoa butter, ½ teaspoon beeswax, and 1 teaspoon olive oil. Then add:

2 drops Oregano *(Origanum vulgare)*
1 drop Hyssop *(Hyssopus officinalis)*
1 drop spike Lavender *(Lavandula latifolia)*
2 drops Ginger *(Zingiber officinale)*
2 drops Lemon *(Citrus x limon)*

1 drop Thyme *(Thymus vulgaris ct cineol,* a chemotype of thyme*)*

Mix and cool. Then fold aluminum foil in a trough 10 to 12 inches long. Make an indentation with a pen or pencil in the center of the trough. Pour the oil mixture into the rounded pen fold. Let it cool and freeze as soon as possible. Then cut into 1-inch pieces that will be used as suppositories when needed. Use no more than once a day for adults.

PESSARIES

Make pessaries (vaginal suppositories) as described for suppositories, with olive oil, beeswax, and cocoa butter. Keep a pessary in a solid state until inserted; the body temperature will melt it.

Pessaries for vaginal infections

Niaouli is effective as a remedy for a vaginal infection. Heat 2 tablespoons cocoa butter, 2 teaspoons beeswax, and 1 teaspoon olive oil. Add:

7 drops Niaouli *(Melaleuca quinquenervia)*
2 drops Geranium *(Pelargonium graveolens)*

Freeze. Use one ovule (a 1-inch pessary) once a day until infection is gone.

The methods for making suppositories and pessaries should be used by advanced students and practitioners who have graduated from a certified essential oil college with 400 plus classroom hours. These two methods should be used with caution and with comprehensive knowledge of each individual oil involved. Oils used in this manner enter the body immediately and more completely than through the skin. This is not recommended for beginning or even intermediate students.

In Closing

Essential oils have unlimited, creative applications for treatment of the human body and spirit. You can experiment thoughtfully, always using small amounts and safe oils, especially with children under the age of ten and the elderly over the age of seventy.

CHAPTER FOURTEEN

The Importance of Chemical Makeup

All the functional groups (alcohol, ketones, esters, lactones,
acids, and aldehydes) are represented in the thousands of essen-
tial oil chemicals and almost all of them have optical isomers.
The human body's chemistry is based on receptor sites that are
optically active (enantometric). This explains why essential oils
are such effective healers with no side effects due to the chemical
binding to receptor sites on human cells so naturally.

—LAWRENCE JONES, SPECTRIX LABS

CHEMISTRY IS TO ESSENTIAL OILS as physics is to atoms. This explains why chemistry and physics do what they do. Chemistry explains the healing effect of essential oils on humans and physics explains why atoms come together to form molecules of matter that move through space-time, creating force and energy. Chemistry is a practical tool the essential oil therapist uses to explain scientifically the positive effects of the oils. Our world demands science to be the foundation of any healing modality.

In the beginning of this new century, the medical sciences are in great transition. Consumers ask for more from their medical treatments than just technologically advanced surgery or pharmaceutical drugs. They want a medical approach that is personal, preventive, and holistic. Losing clients and appointment time is forcing the medical profession to be more open to some of the alternative healing modalities. At the same time, consumers want a practitioner to be grounded in science, whether she is practicing acupuncture or essential oil and herbal therapy. They want a professional, learned attitude that offers the best of Western medicine along with the ancient wisdom of natural, even energetic systems.

The scientific method uses randomized controlled clinical trials to evaluate the effectiveness of any substance. Essential oil therapy needs to more readily adopt this method with clinical studies to show the importance of this therapy in the field of medicine. For example, a randomized clinical trial on the effect that specific essential oils have on MRSA (methicillin-resistant *Staphylococcus aureus*) is more than appropriate today. Since thousands of patients return home from a hospital with this infection, an effective and safe alternative to resistant antibiotics is vitally needed. As a starting point, this is why teachers, students, and practitioners in the field of essential oils need to know the organic chemistry of these powerful substances. Understanding the chemistry of an oil gives a common language and a verifiable makeup that can be shared globally.

Essential oils are made up of chemicals mainly based on three elements: carbon, oxygen, and hydrogen. At the College of Botanical Healing Arts, beginning students are required to take four hours of organic chemistry. A student who graduates from the 400-hour program can look at the patterns of chemical constituents in an oil and deduct the actions of that oil. Knowing the functional families and their characteristics helps an essential oil therapist see the possibilities of healing in every oil.

Cleopatra around 1 AD and Trota in 1200 AD could use essential oils with a shrewdness and uncanny intuitive adeptness. They did not need chemistry to show the effectiveness of fragrance for psychological impact. By the late 1880s perfumery was thoroughly developed in France, especially in the city of Grasse, Provence, where Catherine de Médicis encouraged the beginning of this lucrative business in the 1500s. Yet the chemical composition of essential oils was still unknown. This changed with the work of a chemist, Otto Wallach; from 1880 until 1914 he found some old essential oil bottles and discovered the benzene ring molecule, a six-sided figure with a circle inside. No doubt he was examining oils like Thyme (*Thymus vulgaris*) or Oregano (*Origanum vulgare*) due to their phenol (benzene ring) content. Then he was able to differentiate nine different terpenes that formerly had been all lumped together: fenchene, pinene, phellandrene, camphene, limonene, terpinolene, sylvestrene, dipentene, and carene.[1]

Other chemists began experimenting with terpene molecules and in 1910 F. W. Semmler found the first correct structure of a sesquiterpene, beta-santalene. Several chemists won Nobel Prizes for their essential oil research. They had to tediously separate molecules with a distillation process. Today we have chromatography to separate the chemical constituents of an essential oil on a graph and spectrometry to identify every peak. At College of the Botanical Healing Arts (COBHA), we have a gas chromatograph and a mass spectrometer analysis for every essential oil we study, thanks to my chemist husband Larry Jones. How far we have come from the days of Catherine de Médicis when analysis of scented material was done solely by prophetic visions!

Knowledge of essential oil chemistry allows the present-day therapist to explain why certain oils have special therapeutic effects. For example, an essential oil with many sesquiterpenes such as German chamomile *(Matricaria recutita)* has an anti-inflammatory effect due to the chemical constituents of 6 percent chamazulene, 36 percent farnesene, and 40 percent alpha-bisabolol.

To start at the beginning is to start with atoms and elements. Organic chemistry is the study of living organisms, which all contain carbon. Chemistry is also the study of properties, composition, and the transformation of substances. After many years of testing and experimenting with different materials, chemists decided there were one hundred plus naturally occurring basic substances called elements and eight more artificially created elements. They realized elements such as calcium are made up of indivisible particles called atoms. The atoms of each element are identical in their properties. Atoms join together to form larger groups called molecules.

In 1909 Ernest Rutherford gave a visual image to atoms: a structure amazingly similar to planets orbiting the sun in the solar system. He described an atom as mostly empty space with a nucleus of protons and an equal number of neutrons. The neutrons acted as cushions to prevent the positively charged protons from repelling each other. Neutrons and protons are the same particle held together by a superior force charge that rapidly oscillates between them to hold the nucleus together. The electrons are negatively charged and orbit the nucleus at a high speed. Since negative and positive attract, the electrons stay in orbit just as the planets do. The electrons have orbits in which to travel (two orbits for the elements involved in essential oils). The number of protons, which usually equals the number of neutrons and electrons, differentiates one element from another. For example, hydrogen has one proton and one electron (uniquely no neutron); carbon has six protons, six neutrons, and six electrons; and oxygen has eight protons, eight neutrons, and eight electrons.

These three elements (hydrogen, carbon, and oxygen) are the main building blocks of essential oils with a few nitrogens and sulfurs added in oils like Jasmine and Garlic. Carbon is the backbone of almost all molecules in essential oils. It has two electrons in the first orbit and four electrons in the second orbit. Since an atom seeks eight electrons in the second orbit for stability and satisfaction, the carbon atom has four vacancies it likes to fill by attaching to another carbon atom. This is the reason carbon atoms form chains, rings, and many, many compounds.

GC-MS: What's in a Name?

The perfect marriage of two instruments is a gas chromatograph and a mass spectrometer. Almost everything you can think of that was chemically discovered or produced was done so with the help of gas chromatography (GC) and mass spectroscopy (MS). The GC-MS is ideally suited for the analysis of essential oils, which are made up of a class of chemicals called *volatile organics*. GC-MS can identify and quantitate in a three-dimensional way that leaves little doubt as to the identification and quantization of all the chemical constituents of essential oils. Essential oils must be analyzed to understand the proper use, to identify the chemotypes, to check for adulterants and solvents, and to determine the quality of the oil and its origin. Of all the available methods of analysis, the gas chromatograph–mass spectrometer gives the most illuminating, complete, and undisputed look into the chemistry of essential oils.

The data output and interpretive nature of this instrument draws from three dimensions in its analysis output: two quantitative (the X and Y of retention time and peak area) and one qualitative (Z, the mass spectra, which has a wealth of information stored in each millisecond slice of the chromatogram). This information may be searched, calculated, analyzed, compared, and discovered by a powerful computer system operated and directed by the truth-hungry scientist. This is the most powerful and versatile instrument for chemical research and, in this case, for the scientific discovery of essential oils that is accurate and reproducible from lab to lab. GC-MS analysis combined with in vitro and clinical studies is pushing the frontier of the discovery and use of essential oils.

The basic principal of the GC-MS is that the gas chromatograph separates the chemical constituents of the essential oil and the mass spectrometer ionizes each chemical, which produces a molecular "fingerprint." This fingerprint is then identified by the computer software. The process is accomplished by injecting a very small amount of essential oil into the GC's "column," a quartz tube at least twenty-five meters in length and only about 0.25 millimeters in diameter. Globally, this equipment is made using only the metric system as its standard. The sample is forced through the column by helium pressure as the column is gradually heated within the gas chromatograph. This separates and sorts the various chemicals of an oil, depending on each oil's boiling point, molecular weight, structure, and polarity, and then resolves them in the form of "peaks" that are proportional to the percentage of each constituent.

These separated molecules then flow into the mass spectrometer where they are ionized under a high vacuum and become fragmented. The fragmented molecules are electronically filtered and patterns are detected by the data system that become the fingerprint of that chemical. A vast computer library searches to identify the molecular fingerprint.

Essential oil purity and quality is vital to essential oil therapy and should be the cornerstone of using essential oils in a therapeutic setting. GC-MS analysis of essential oils, if done properly, can reveal the purity and quality of any given sample, and hence the value, safety, and effectiveness of the analyzed oil. Without GC-MS essential oil therapists would be on their own with a label that says "pure" and a nose that is not sure. The fortuitous coming together of the healing power of essential oils and the technology of instrumental analysis is a major step forward to uplift the quality of essential oils used for alternative medicine. GC-MS provides an accurate and reproducible scientific basis of comparing and understanding essential oils.

Terpenes

Terpenes, chains of carbons and hydrogens, are the most common chemical constituents in essential oils, and they all end in *ene*. There are three main types of terpenes in essential oils: monoterpene, sesquiterpene, and diterpene.

MONOTERPENES

Monoterpenes have two isoprene units with ten carbons and at least one double bond *(C=C)*. Surrounding each carbon are one or two or three hydrogens (they are not written). A famous monoterpene in almost all citrus oils is limonene. Instead of writing the *C*s for carbons, chemists simplify limonene into the structure shown below.

Most monoterpenes are antibacterial, slightly stimulating, quite volatile, less dense than water, highly fragrant, and slightly analgesic (pain relieving). Oils with large amounts of terpenes are Orange *(Citrus sinensis),* limonene; Grapefruit *(Citrus x paradisi),* limonene; Pine *(Pinus sylvestris),* alpha pinene; and Juniper *(Juniperus communis),* myrcene. A 1991 study by Igimi et al. discovered limonene can dissolve gallstones in 48 percent of cases especially if the stones are cholesterol-based.[2] A 1988 study by Elson, Maltzman, Boston, Tanner, and Gould isolated anticarcinogenic activity in d-limonene, which was found to be effective in lowering the number of developing tumors in mammary cancer. A study by Elson et al. found that "... d-limonene may have a potential application in the chemoprevention of human cancer."[3]

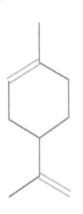

Limonene

SESQUITERPENES

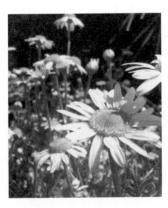

German chamomile

Sesquiterpenes have three isoprene units or fifteen carbons and a varying number of hydrogens. Some of the characteristics of sesquiterpenes are anti-inflammatory, sedative, choleretic (aids secretion of bile by liver), hypotensive (lowers blood pressure), and hormonal effects. They have more complex actions than monoterpenes in essential oils such as Rose *(Rosa damascena),* farnesene; and American cedarwood *(Juniperus virginiana),* thujopsene.

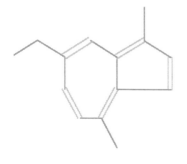

Chamazulene

Chamazulene in German chamomile (*Matricaria recutita*) was studied by Safyh, Sabieraj, Sailer, and Ammon in 1994 and showed great anti-inflammatory action by inhibiting leukotriene formation, which normally produces and sustains inflammatory diseases. The study concludes that in vivo, chamazulene furthers anti-inflammatory effects due to its antioxidative properties.[4]

DITERPENES

Diterpenes have four isoprene units or twenty carbons. They are rarely found in essential oils due to their large molecular structure. An example is cembrene in Frankincense *(Boswellia carteri)* or curcumene in Helichrysum *(Helichrysum italicum)*.

Curcumene

Functional Groups

The definition of a functional group is the addition of oxygen in some form to the carbon and hydrogen structure. There are approximately ten different functional groups: alcohols, esters, lactones, phenols, aldehydes, ketones, ethers, oxides, acids, and coumarins. They all have oxygen added in different arrangements to the carbons and hydrogens. These varying forms change the action of the molecule, giving each functional group certain actions.

All three terpene groups can modify the functional families. When a terpene has a functional group added to it, it is called a *terpenoid*. Some examples are linalool in lavender *(Lavandula angustifolia)*, which is a monterpenol. The functional family of alcohols has added OH (oxygen hydrogen) to the basic structure of a monoterpene. Clary sage *(Salvia sclaria)* has a diterpenol of sclareol, which is OH added to the basic structure of a diterpene. This diterpenol is so large a molecule that it begins to resemble a steroid in its structure and action. It gives *Salvia sclaria* an ability to balance human hormones (estrogen and progesterone) as during a woman's PMS episode.

PHENOLS

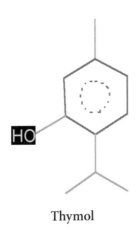

Thymol

A group that is stimulating and aggressive in its effects, especially against infection, the phenol molecule contains a benzene ring. The figure shows the way electrons are shared in the ring. Thymol has an OH attached to the ring and creates hot and fiery effects for an oil that contains a phenol.

This group can be quite irritating to skin and mucous membranes. Phenols need to be used in small doses and for short periods of time. Examples are Cinnamon *(Cinnamomum verum)* and Thyme. Phenols end in *ol* since they are connected to the alcohol functional group (phenols and alcohols are chemical cousins). One of their basic effects is pain relief. For example, eugenol in Clovebud *(Syzgium aromaticum)* helps relieve tooth pain. Carvacrol in Thyme has been shown in studies to kill bacteria and viruses by making cell membranes more permeable to hydrogen and potassium molecules, leading to death of the microorganism.[5] In 1987 studies at the Arch Institute of Pasteur found Thyme to have great antibacterial strength against *Staphylococcus aureus* and *E. coli.*[6]

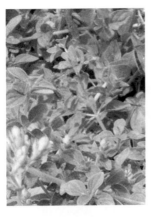

Oregano

An essential oil rich in phenols is Oregano. The following figures show a shortened version of an essential oil profile with its main medicinal effects and then the GC-MS. I will show the correlation between the healing qualities and the chemical constituents.

Essential Oil	**Oregano *(Origanum vulgare)***
Country of origin	Greece, Russia, Bulgaria
Botanical family	Lamiaceae
Extraction	Steam distillation of the dried flowering herb
Plant description	Bushy, hardy perennial herb up to 35 inches high with a hairy stem, dark green ovate leaves, and pink, purple flowers
Key	Stimulating anti-infectious oil
Medicinal	Good for extreme infections on the skin, respiratory, or digestive system.
	Antiviral against flu, polio, and herpes virus.[7]
	Antifungal property; in a study the high carvacrol effectively inhibited three strains of *Candida albicans.*[8]
	Antiparasitical property; in a study oregano at 1 percent inhibited the growth of *Aspergillus parasiticus.*[9]
	As a pain reliever, showed its analgesic quality for patients with osteoarthritis.
	Aids digestive system to help an acid liver, spleen, or stomach.[10]
	Works as a laxative.
Mind	Stimulating nerve tonic.
	Warming and gives a feeling of well-being.
Precautions	Avoid in pregnancy.
	Do not use on babies, children, or the elderly.
	Skin irritant.
	Hepatotoxic when used in large doses or longer than 7 to 10 days.
How to use	Mix 10 drops in 4 ounces of massage oil or put 1 drop in a quart of water to drink.

The main constituent in Oregano is about 80 percent carvacrol, a phenol. Carvacrol is a similar molecule to thymol but more bioactively aggressive against some bacteria and viruses. Oregano contains other antimicrobial chemicals like para cymene and thymol. Oregano is produced by steam distillation.

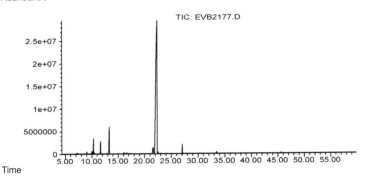

GC-MS CHROMATOGRAM OF OREGANO ESSENTIAL OIL
Abundance

TIC: EVB2177.D

GC-MS IDENTIFACATION OF THE MAIN CHEMICAL CONSTITUENTS AND THIER PERCENTAGES

OPERATOR: SPECTRIX LAB, INC.
SAMPLE NAME: OREGANO E03-30-09 089CB

Pk#	RT	Area%	Library/ID	Pk#	RT	Area%	Library/ID
1	7.04	0.13	Thujene<Alpha->	23	27.06	1.31	Caryophyllene(E-)
2	7.26	0.29	Pinene<Alpha->				
3	7.73	0.13	Camphene	24	27.85	0.12	Carvone Oxide
4A	8.60	0.08	Octen-3-Ol<1->	25	28.43	0.08	Humulene<Alpha->
4B	8.60	0.10	Pinene<Beta->				
5	9.05	0.42	Myrcene	26	30.11	0.08	Viridiflorene
6	9.56	0.09	Phellandrene<Alpha->	27	30.58	0.09	Bisabolene<Beta->
7	10.01	0.48	Carene<Delta-2->				
8	10.29	2.63	Cymene<Para->	28	31.19	0.07	Cadinene<Delta->
9A	10.47	0.03	Limonene				
9B	10.47	0.20	Phellandrene<Beta->	29	33.26	0.07	Spathulenol
9C	10.47	0.06	Cineole<1,8->	30	33.48	0.31	Caryophyllene Oxide
10	11.63	2.02	Terpinene<Gamma->				
11	11.92	0.09	Sabinene Hydrate<Cis->				
12	12.82	0.11	Terpinolene				
13	13.28	5.40	Linalool				
14	16.08	0.42	Borneol				
15	16.60	0.31	Terpinen-4-Ol				
16	17.12	0.07	Terpineol<Alpha->				
17	17.31	0.07	Terpineol<Gamma->				

Gas chromatograph–mass spectrometer analysis of Oregano (*Origanum vulgare*)

The chemistry of *Origanum vulgare* clearly shows why it acts as it does. The collection of six monoterpenes—tricyclene, alpha pinene, beta-myrcene, alpha-terpenene, para cymene, and gamma-terpinene—gives this oil a stimulating, antibacterial shine. These components also increase the speed of absorption of the oil into the human body via the respiratory or dermal routes.

The three monoterpenols—linalool, borneol, and terpin-4-ol—provide oregano oil with a tonifying, analgesic, and anti-infectious quality. A 1995 study by Carson and Riley showed terpin-4-ol and linalool were effective against *E. coli, Staphylococcus aureus,* and *Candida albicans.*[11]

The large percentage of phenols—thymol (5 percent) and carvacrol (71 percent)—makes oregano oil an irritation to skin, a low state of volatility, a strong smell, and an extremely effective antibacterial, antifungal, and antiviral agent. A 1996 study by Sivropoulou et al. showed *Origanum vulgare* to be the most effective antibacterial oil at dilution of 1 to 4,000. It was also shown to be cytotoxic against Hep 2 (human epidermoid larynx carcinoma) and HeLa (human epithelial cervix carcinoma), causing cell death at dilutions up to 10,000.[12]

Another group of researchers, Ultee et al., found that carvacrol causes bacteria cell membranes to increase permeability to hydrogen and potassium ions, eventually leading to cell death.[13]

Caryophyllene is a sesquiterpene with anti-spasmolytic activity that helps the oil to work as a laxative in the digestive system.[14]

ESTERS

A functional family with an opposite effect to the flaming phenols is soothing esters. Acids found in plants, carboxylic acids, easily combine with alcohols to form esters. Esters are usually created or broken down during steam distillation. Linalyl acetate, an ester, is formed from linalool and acetic acid. Water (H_2O) is created with the ester. This action is always changing. It is a functional group in motion, often changing chemically due to heat, pressure, or *pH*.

Esters always end in *ate*. They rarely have toxicity involved, perhaps only a little skin irritation on people with very sensitive skin. The only exceptions are sabinyl acetate, which causes birth defects, and methyl salicylate (98 percent in Birch, *Betula benta*), which is so irritating it can become pain relieving. Esters make an essential oil relaxing to the central nervous system[15] and help to regulate the sympathetic nervous system as well as parts of the endocrine system. For example, esters in Lavender like linalyl acetate and geranyl acetate help soothe the nerves and maintain the progesterone-estrogen balance during PMS and menopause.

Buchbauer et al. found that esters in Lavender created a sedative effect on mice and decreased their motor ability.[16] For people esters were found to produce a calm state of mind and reduced stress. This is what makes Lavender the most popular essential oil in our stressful world. Esters are also hypotensive with a sedative action on the heart and lowering cholesterol in the blood.[17]

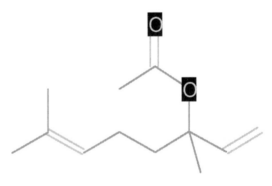

Linalool acetate

To illuminate the effects of esters, The figures on the next pages show a profile of Bergamot, an essential oil that contains 31 percent esters.

Essential Oil	Bergamot *(Citrus x bergamia)*
Country of origin	Italy
Botanical family	Rutaceae
Extraction	Cold expression of fruit peel, then steam distillation
Plant description	Small tree up to 15 feet high with smooth, oval leaves and small round fruit that turns from green to yellow
Key	Refreshing
Medicinal	Valuable antiseptic for the urinary tract.
	Relaxes the cardiovascular system; significantly reduces coronary dilator action.[18]
	An immune stimulant.[19]
	Good remedy for cold sores, chicken pox, shingles, eczema, psoriasis, and herpes.
Mind	Sedative medicine for the central nervous system.[20]
	Helps balance the emotional mood swings of PMS.[21]
Precautions	Phototoxic when used before going in sunlight.[22]
How to use	In the evening bath, directly on the skin, or in a massage oil. Wait at least two hours before entering sunlight.

Bergamot is very safe and soothing containing about 44 percent total esters, mainly linalool acetate. The whole oil does contain the sun sensitizers dimethoxy-coumarin and bergaptene. Other relaxing constituents are limonene, linalool, and many others in smaller quantities.

GC-MS CHROMATOGRAM OF BERGAMOT ESSENTIAL OIL

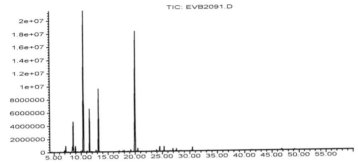

Abundance

TIC: EVB2091.D

Time

GC-MS IDENTIFACATION OF THE MAIN CHEMICAL CONSTITUENTS AND THIER PERCENTAGE

OPERATOR: SPECTRIX LAB, INC.
SAMPLE NAME: BERGAMOT ITALY C9-23-08 267BA

PK#	RT	AREA%	LIBRARY/ID
1	6.98	0.29	Thujene<Alpha->
2	7.20	1.16	Pinene<Alpha->
3	8.43	0.98	Sabinene
4	8.57	6.02	Pinene<Beta->
5	8.98	1.00	Myrcene
6	9.93	0.17	Terpinene<Alpha->
7	10.20	0.34	Cymene<Para->
8	10.47	33.63	Limonene
9	10.69	0.04	Ocimene<(Z)-Beta->
10	11.10	0.16	Ocimene<(E)-Beta->
11	11.57	6.55	Terpinene<Gamma->
12	12.74	0.34	Terpinolene
13	13.24	13.33	Linalool
14	17.04	0.11	Terpineol<Alpha->
15	17.95	0.19	Octanol Acetate
16	19.18	0.27	Neral
17	20.03	32.01	Linalool Acetate
18	20.47	0.45	Geranial
19	23.90	0.23	Terpinyl Acetate<Alpha->
20	24.51	0.70	Neryl Acetate
21	25.30	0.61	Geranyl Acetate
22	26.92	0.35	Caryophyllene(E-)
23	27.55	0.33	Bergamotene<Alpha-Trans->
24	30.47	0.55	Bisabolene<Beta->
25	46.79	0.15	5,7-Dimethoxycoumarin
26	49.17	0.09	Bergaptene

Gas chromatograph–mass spectrometer analysis of bergamot (*Citrus x bergamia*)

Here is a quick look at the chemistry of *Citrus x bergamia:*

This oil has a large group of ten monoterpenes: thujene, alpha-pinene, sabinene, beta-pinene, myrcene, para cymene, limonene (32 percent), beta ocimene, gamma-terpinene, and terpinolene. This group of ten carbon molecules makes the oil stimulating, even somewhat irritating, and drying on the skin. Plus it has antimicrobial effects. Research shows that the monoterpene limonene has an antitumor effect.[23]

Bergamot has been shown to be effective in preventing mammary cancer.[24]

Bergamot has a fairly large amount (13 percent) of linalool, the monoterpenol. It has an anti-infectious and sedative effect found by Elizabetsk et al. on examining the effect of linalool on the central nervous system as it modifies the neuronal response to L-(H3)-glutamate.[25]

This oil has a large amount of esters: octanol acetate, linalyl acetate (32 percent), neryl acetate, and geranyl acetate. Esters are known to relax, soothe, and calm emotions and nerves. They provide the famous antidepressant effect in Bergamot. The anti-inflammatory and antispasmodic effect of esters was shown in a study on the cardiovascular properties of *Citrus x bergamia.* F. Occhiuto et al. found this oil to have a "protective effect against vasopressin-induced coronary spasm and arrhythmias . . . [and to] prevent ventricular tachyarrhythmias by suppressing the digitalis-induced ectopic pacemaker."[26]

KETONES

Another important functional group is ketones. They have a carbon atom and an oxygen atom double-bonded on a carbon atom that is bonded to two other carbon atoms. They are derived from secondary alcohols by oxidation in the plant. Ketones and alcohols are rapid penetrators of the skin. An example is methone in Peppermint *(Mentha piperita).*

Ketones end in *one.* There is a problem of toxicity with ketones. Joy Bowles, an Australian chemist, wrote, "Ketones are relatively stable and may pose problems in the body because they are resistant to metabolism by the liver."[27] According to Tisserand and Balacs, ketones can produce liver and central nervous system damage that can lead to convulsions and a coma.[28]

The ketone thujone is found in most of the plants of the Artemisia family, including wormwood *(Artemisia absinthium),* tarragon *(Artemisia dracunculus),* mugwort *(Artemisia vulgaris),* tansy *(Tanacetum vulgare),* thuja *(Thuja occidentalis),* and western red cedar *(Thuja plicata).* Other ketones are pulegone in pennyroyal *(Mentha pulegium);* carvone in spearmint *(Mentha spicata);* and camphor in camphor *(Cinnamomum camphora),* rosemary *(Rosmarinus officinalis),* and yarrow *(Achillea mille-folium).* Any oral intake of the oils with ketones (except rosemary and yarrow) is not recommended in more than 0.2 milliliter doses in an essential oil practice.

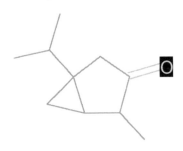

Thujone

Taken orally, 14 grams (½ ounce) of any of the ketones listed here can be lethal. Anything over 2 grams can create unpleasant effects such as hallucinations, nausea, and lack of coordination. These effects were experienced by many of the French impressionist painters when they drank "the green fairy" or absinthe from Wormwood *(Artemisia absinthium),* which was popular among French soldiers in Algeria in the 1830s as a remedy against dysentery. The drink rapidly became fashionable back home in Paris. The painter Toulouse-Lautrec carried a small shot of what he called "earthquake" in the hollow top of his walking stick. By 1910 the French government banned the drink. Today distillers are beginning to produce a diluted, low-proof copy.

One of the positive effects of ketones is as an antimucosal for urinary and respiratory infections.[29] Peppermint has close to 30 percent of menthone and 1 drop is very effective in a steam to clear the sinuses and throat of mucous. Another effective use of ketones is wound healing. Hyssop *(Hyssopus officinalis),* for example, will help to form scars and disperse bruises when a cold compress is applied soon after injury. It contains 31 percent pinocamphone.

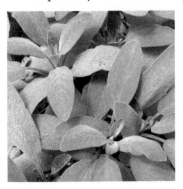

Sage

The figures on the next pages show an example of a ketone oil, Sage, that must be used with caution.

Essential Oil	**Sage** *(Salvia officinalis)*
Country of origin	Croatia, Indonesia
Botanical family	Lamiaceae
Extraction	Distillation of whole plant
Plant description	Evergreen, perennial shrub up to 32 inches high with a woody base, soft, silvery, long leaves, and deep blue flowers.
Key	Regenerative
Medicinal	As a stimulant for the adrenocortical glands.
	A general stimulant for metabolism and the central nervous system.
	Highly regenerative; tonic for low blood pressure.
	Cleansing action on the circulatory and lymphatic system.
	Aids in ridding the body's skin of cellulite.
	Phytoestrogen so regulates the menstrual cycle.
	Tonic for digestive system and constipation.
Mind	To calm the parasympathetic system, use 1 to 2 drops.
	Good to combat fatigue, memory loss, and Alzheimer's disease.
	Use 1 drop to develop visualization in meditation.
Precautions	Never use on pregnant women or epileptics.
	Do not use on babies or children.
	Less is better.
How to use	Use 1 percent in massage oil or bath.
	To cleanse the skin and lymph system, add 6 drops of Sage, 5 drops of Geranium, and 7 drops of Grapefruit to 1 ounce of lotion. Rub on the face, neck, chest, and underarms.

Sage has many chemotypes but the dalmatian is the most widely known and used. This chemotype has more than 44 percent total ketone with alpha- and beta-thujone comprising the largest percentage. This oil can be toxic to the nervous system. Essential oils generally have no or low toxicity, but some—like sage dalmatia—should not be used internally or in large amounts on the skin (only 1 percent dilution). Thujone is very trans-dermal.

GC-MS CHROMATOGRAM OF SAGE DALMATIAN ESSENTIAL OIL

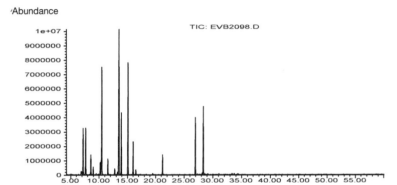

GC-MS IDENTIFACATION OF THE MAIN CHEMICAL CONSTITUENTS AND THIER PERCENTAGES

OPERATOR: SPECTIRIX LABS, INC.
SAMPLE NAME: SAGE DALMATIAN C9-29-08 273BA

PK#	RT	AREA%	LIBRARY/ID
1	6.86	0.47	Tricyclene
2	6.98	0.35	Thujene<Alpha->
3	7.20	5.55	Pinene<Alpha->
4	7.66	5.84	Camphene
5	8.56	2.25	Pinene<Beta->
6	8.98	0.85	Myrcene
7	9.49	0.16	Phellandrene<Beta->
8	10.21	1.44	Cymene<Para->
9	10.50	13.94	Cineole<1,8->
10	11.55	1.65	Terpinene<Gamma->
11	12.75	0.73	Terpinolene
12	13.23	0.42	Linalool
13	13.51	22.11	Thujone<Cis->
14	13.92	6.88	Thujone<Trans->
15	15.11	14.84	Camphor
16	16.01	3.65	Borneol
17	16.49	0.57	Terpinen-4-Ol
18	19.48	0.12	Carvotanacetone
19	21.22	2.12	Bornyl Acetate
20	26.96	6.68	Caryophyllene(E-)
21	27.27	0.14	Ylangene<Beta->
22	28.16	0.23	Aromadendrene
23	28.35	8.11	Humulene<Alpha->
24	28.62	0.13	Aromadendrene<Allo->
25	29.11	0.09	Cadina-1(6),4-Diene<Trans->
26	31.06	0.13	Cadinene<Delta->
27	34.35	0.12	Humulene Epoxide Ii

Gas chromatograph–mass spectrometer analysis Sage *(Salvia officinalis)*

The chemical constituents of *Salvia officinalis* reveal these patterns: The monoterpenes in Sage, such as tricyclene, alpha-pinene (5 percent), camphene (5 percent), beta-pinene, beta-myrcene (1.7 percent), beta-thujene, menthadiene, para cymene, limonene, gamma-terpeniene, and 4-carene, all have a stimulating, antibacterial, antiviral effect. They help relieve fatigue and activate the mind.

Sage has eucalyptol (also known as 1,8-cineol), a powerful anti-infectious and expectorant agent at 12 percent.

The ketone thujone comes out in two parts: alpha-thujone (23 percent) and beta-thujone (6 percent), which is dangerous as a central nervous system depressant. On the other hand, thujone reduces mucous and fat, giving Sage the cleansing action on the circulatory and lymphatic systems. Because thujone is cell regenerative, it aids the body's regeneration.

In Sage there are seven monoterpene alcohols, all in low amounts of less than 1 percent, such as linalool, pinocarveol, thujanol, borneol (4 percent), terpin-4-ol, alpha terpineol, and pinocampheol. These tonics with zero toxicity would add to the stimulating effect on the glands and metabolism. They are warming and would be effective tonics for anemia and debility.

Sage is made up of 15 percent camphor, a type of ketone that can have carcinogenic effects on the liver. Camphor adds to the highly regenerative quality of Sage. It helps to dissolve lipids such as cellulite on skin. Mixed with the other chemicals in Sage, it is mild on the skin.

Three esters in Sage—bornyl acetate (3 percent), thujyl acetate, and terpinyl acetate—help to calm the parasympathetic nervous system. These esters act as hormonal calming agents for PMS and menopause.

The two sesquiterpenes in sage—beta-caryophyllene (6 percent) and alpha-caryophyllene (4 percent)—give the oil an anti-inflammatory and antiallergenic quality. They also make this oil a tonic for the digestive system. One study showed beta-caryophyllene, when administered orally, reduced stomach cell damage from alcohol poisoning in rats. It worked better than standard anti-inflammatory preparations since it did not harm the stomach mucosa.[30]

Two oxides also known as cyclic ethers, caryophyllene oxide and humulene oxide, contribute to the strong fragrance of this essential oil. They also have an anti-inflammatory effect.

The sesquiterpenol ledol gives sage oil a mild antispasmodic and anti-inflammatory effect. This would help calm the cramps of the menstrual cycle.

Overall, even with the ketone thujone, this oil is more beneficial than toxic for many human conditions.

ALDEHYDES

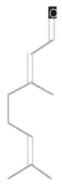

Another functional group is aldehydes, which have an oxygen atom double bonded to a carbon atom with a hydrogen bond next to it. They too are derived from alcohols due to oxidation. A good example is citronellal derived from citronellol in an oil such as Lemon Eucalyptus *(Eucalyptus citriodora).* They end in *al.*

All essential oils with aldehydes have the same lemony fragrance. Geranial and neral usually occur together in essential oils such as Lemongrass *(Cymbopogon citratus)* and Melissa *(Melissa officinalis).*

Geranial

Aldehydes are antiviral. For example, Lemon Eucalyptus *(Eucalyptus citriodora),* which has 82 percent of citronellal, can be used to strengthen the immune system during flus or diseases such as chicken pox. It is also very effective with shingles, a viral nervous disorder, along with the oil of Ravintsara *(Cinnamomum camphora),* which has several toxic constituents. Aldehydes are also antifungal. Lemongrass can be used as a vaginal douche for *Candida albicans.* Aldehydes also are sedatives and analgesic. A massage oil of Rosemary, Juniper, and Lemongrass creates a powerful analgesic tonic for arthritis, rheumatoid arthritis, and muscle aches.

Examine the profile of Lemongrass shown in the following figures.

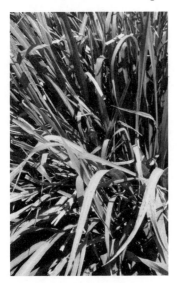

Lemongrass

Essential Oil	**Lemongrass *(Cymbopogan citratus)***
Country of origin	Guatemala, Brazil
Botanical family	Poaceae
Extraction	Steam distillation of grass
Plant description	A fast-growing, tall, aromatic perennial grass that produces a network of rootlets
Key	Restorative tonic
Medicinal	Boasts the parasympathetic nervous system.
	Aids in recovery from illness.
	Reduces pain in aching muscles.
	Acts as a vasodilator.
	Great for athlete's foot and *Candida albicans*.
	Anti-inflammatory effect.
	Calming to headaches
Mind	Good for fatigue and exhaustion.
	Calms the nervous system while energizing the mind.
	Encourages optimism and courage.
Precautions	Can irritate the skin so use in low doses.
How to use	Mix 5 drops of Lemongrass with 4 drops of Peppermint and 8 milliliters (1.62 teaspoons) of safflower vegetable oil. Rub on aching muscles and temples for headaches.

Lemongrass essential oil is rich in aldehydes (almost 80 percent), which accounts for its aggressive antimicrobial action. It can be sensitizing to the skin. The two aldehydes in lemongrass, neral and geranial (commonly called *citral*), are found in other essential oils in similar quantities and with similar qualities. Lemongrass is produced by steam distillation.

GC-MS CHROMATOGRAM OF LEMONGRASS ESSENTIAL OIL

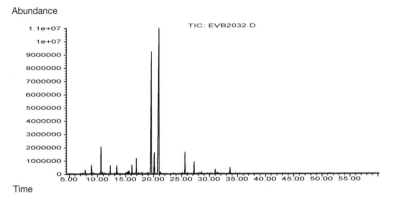

GC-MS IDENTIFACATION OF THE MAIN CHEMICAL CONSTITUENTS AND THIER PERCENTAGES
OPERATOR: SPECTRIX LABS, INC.
SAMPLE NAME: LEMONGRASS L5-8-08 129BB

PK#	RT	AREA%	LIBRARY/ID
1	7.84	0.55	Pinene<Beta->
2	8.94	1.23	Hepten-2-One<6-Methyl-5->
3A	9.17	0.07	Myrcene
3B	9.17	0.10	Cineole<Dehydro-1,8->
4	10.60	3.67	Limonene
5	10.90	0.21	Ocimene<(Z)-Beta->
6	11.31	0.17	Ocimene<(E)-Beta->
7	12.24	1.10	4-Nonanone
8	13.38	1.07	Linalool
9	15.28	0.29	Isocitral<Exo->
10	15.51	0.37	Trans-Chrysanthemal
11	15.63	0.40	Citronellal
12	16.14	1.20	Isocitral<Z->
13	16.92	1.97	Isocitral<E->
14	17.30	0.17	Terpineol<Alpha->
15	17.92	0.26	Decanal<N->
16	18.96	0.31	Linalool Formate
17	19.61	31.62	Neral
18	20.11	4.24	Geraniol
19	20.94	43.62	Geranial
20	21.19	0.19	Carvone Oxide
21	25.60	2.86	Neryl Acetate
22	27.23	1.66	Caryophyllene(E-)
23	28.26	0.18	Isoeugenol<E->
24	28.61	0.29	Humulene<Alpha->
25	31.02	0.68	Cadinene<Gamma->
26	31.37	0.31	Cadinene<Delta->
27	33.67	1.00	Caryophyllene Oxide

Gas chromatograph–mass spectrometer analysis of Lemongrass (*Cymbopogon citratus*)

The chemistry of Lemongrass oil weaves a path with several functional families, but mostly alcohols and aldehydes.

A chemical analysis of Lemongrass begins with two ketones: hepton-2-one (3 percent) and 4-nonanone (1.5 percent). This makes the oil great for bathing or to use diluted in water as a cleanser. Ketones are quite hydrophilic (easily dissolved in water).

Lemongrass oil contains limonene (5 percent), ocimene, and perillene, the monoterpenes that have a stimulating, antibacterial, and antitumoral effect.

The alcohol family is represented in this oil by linalool (1 percent), verbenol trans (1.5 percent,) verbenol cis, alpha-terpineol, carveol, 7-octen-2-ol, and geraniol (3 percent). These chemicals make the oil tonifying and an aid in recovering from illness.

The strong suit of Lemongrass is the aldehyde family. It has beta-citronellal, decanal, dimethylocta-3, 4-dienal, neral (33 percent), and geranial (43 percent). With over 78 percent aldehydes, the antifungal, antibacterial, and immune-strengthening effect is potent. In a 1984 study by Onawunmiet et al., the antibacterial activity of neral and geranial was found to be strong against *Staphylococcus aureus, E. coli,* and *Bacillus subtilis.*[31]

In another interesting study on the aldehydes in Lemongrass, the concentration of citral required to achieve a 50 percent reduction in viable P388 leukemia cells was 7.1 micrograms per milliliter. The mixture contained the two geometric isomers, neral and geranial, in the ratio of 2.5 to 7.5 respectively. The conclusion was that citral may have potential as a chemotherapeutic agent and more clinical trials are necessary.[32]

If a small amount is used, the aldehydes make the oil relaxing but mentally uplifting. In a larger or undiluted dose, they make the oil irritating to the skin.

The last family represented in this oil is the esters: citronellyl formate, neryl acetate, and geranyl acetate (1.5 percent). Their action, along with that of the alcohols, contributes to the calming of the central nervous system and the reduction of headaches.

Two sesquiterpenes, caryophyllene (2 percent) and bergamotene, support lemongrass's anti-inflammatory effects and the activities of the parasympathetic system.

ALCOHOLS

Alcohols end in *ol*. They are usually considered the most beneficial chemical constituents in essential oils. They have a hydroxyl group or OH group attached to one of their carbon atoms. Phenols are actually a type of alcohol but have a structure consisting of an aromatic or benzene ring. Monoterpenols are alcohols with the structure of monoterpenes and the OH group attached.

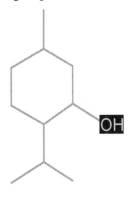

Menthol

Alcohols are mostly soluble in ethanol and other vegetable oils but only slightly in water. They are often middle notes in perfumery. When exposed to air, alcohols slowly oxidize to aldehydes. For example, geranium oil will become harsh with a lemon odor as it ages (geraniol becomes geranial). Alcohols have little toxicity on the skin and require imbibing more than one or two gallons to cause internal toxicity according to Tisserand and Balacs.[33]

One of the most important alcohols for its antibacterial action is terpinen-4-ol in Tea tree *(Melaleuca alternifolia)*. Terpinen-4-ol is a large peak in the oil and needs to be 40 percent or more to be effective as an anti-infectious agent. It is active against *E. coli*, *Staphylococcus aureus*, and *Candida albicans*, according to many studies including the 1995 study by Carson and Riley.[34] They found that terpinen-4-ol was also effective against *Pseudomonas aeruginosa*.

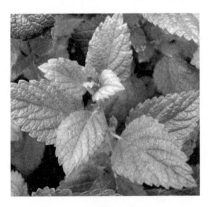

Peppermint

Alcohol also has an analgesic property. Examples are menthol in Peppermint and linalool in Lavender. H. Gobel in 1995 found menthol reduces pain caused by headaches and strained muscles.[35] The oil of Rosewood *(Aniba roseaodora)* has 85 percent linalool, which makes it helpful as a remedy for nervous headaches. This analgesic effect is partly due to the anti-inflammatory effect of menthol and linalool.

Monoterpene alcohols have a modulating and balancing action on the immune system. This action occurs by their ability to lower the increased levels of gamma globulins.

Let's focus on the profile of Peppermint as shown in the following figures.

Essential oil	Peppermint *(Mentha piperita)*
Country of origin	United States (Oregon, Washington), England
Botanical family	Lamiaceae
Extraction	Distillation of leaves and flowers
Plant description	Perennial herb up to 3 feet high with underground runners, green serrated leaves, and violet flowers
Key	Energizing
Medicinal	Has dual action: cooling when hot (menthol) and warming when cold (menthone).
	Important digestive for even acute problems like vomiting, diarrhea, constipation, travel sickness.
	Analgesic for muscle aches, colds, flus, headaches, and rheumatism.
	Induces sweating in a fever.
	Helps varicose veins with an astringent action.
	Antispasmodic on smooth muscle.
	Antibacterial for stomach and respiratory infections.
Mind	Has a cooling action on anger and hysteria.
	Cephalic action brings clear thinking; a mental stimulant.
Precautions	Can irritate sensitive skin and eyes.
How to use	Dilute in vegetable oil 1 percent for children and the elderly.
	Avoid in pregnancy and nursing mothers.
	Put 1 drop of Peppermint, 1 drop of *Eucalyptus globulus,* and 1 drop of Tea tree in a bowl of boiling water. Cover head and inhale the steam.
	For upset stomach, dilute 1 part essential oil and 1 part vegetable oil to rub directly on stomach and intestinal area.

Peppermint oil is easily absorbed through the skin due to the large percentage of very polar constituents comprising functional groups like ketones (alcohols and others including cineole and menthofuran). The acetates and sesquiterpenoids, being larger and less polar, take much longer to be transported through the skin. Peppermint essential oil is produced by steam distillation.

GC-MS CHROMATOGRAM OF PEPPERMINT ESSENTIAL OIL

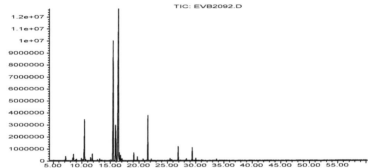

GC-MS IDENTIFACATION OF THE MAIN CHEMICAL CONSTITUENTS AND THIER PERCENTAGES

OPERATOR: SPECTRIX LABS, INC.
SAMPLE NAME: PEPPERMINT C10-2-08 LOT MO7314

PK#	RT	AREA%	LIBRARY/ID	PK#	RT	AREA%	LIBRARY/ID
1	7.18	0.65	Pinene<Alpha->				
2	8.41	0.44	Sabinene	27	25.48	0.27	Bourbonene<Beta->
3	8.54	1.01	Pinene<Beta->	28	26.91	1.92	Caryophyllene(E-)
4	8.94	0.17	Myrcene	29	28.36	0.23	Farnesene<(E)-Beta->
5	9.05	0.26	Octanol<3->	30	29.40	1.79	Germacrene D
6	9.92	0.37	Terpinene<Alpha->	31	30.03	0.31	Bicyclogermacrene
7	10.18	0.22	Cymene<Para->	32	33.68	0.23	Viridiflorol
8	10.46	7.06	Cineole<1,8->				
9	10.66	0.20	Ocimene<(Z)-Beta->				
10	11.53	0.41	Terpinene<Gamma->				
11	11.83	0.96	Sabinene Hydrate<Cis->				
12	12.72	0.17	Terpinolene				
13	13.13	0.29	Linalool				
14	15.10	0.19	Isopulegol				
15	15.52	22.81	Menthone				
16A	15.91	4.00	Menthone<Iso->				
16B	15.91	4.91	Menthofuran				
17	16.44	41.12	Menthol				
18	16.55	0.97	Terpinen-4-Ol				
19	16.77	0.69	Menthol<Iso->				
20	16.98	0.18	Menthol<Neoiso->				
21	17.04	0.23	Terpineol<Alpha->				
22	19.11	0.96	Pulegone				
23	19.73	0.57	Piperitone				
24	20.73	0.26	Menthyl Acetate<Neo->				
25	21.56	5.94	Menthyl Acetate				
26	22.16	0.21	Menthyl Acetate<Iso->				

Gas chromatograph–mass spectrometer analysis of peppermint (*Mentha piperita*)

The Importance of Chemical Makeup

Let's examine the chemical constituents of *Mentha piperita* to understand its actions:

There are many small peaks of monoterpenes: alpha-pinene, sabinene, beta-pinene, terpinene, benzene, limonene (1 percent), alpha-terpinene, and gamma-terpinene. These give a stimulating, antibacterial effect to the oil. One study examined ten essential oils against twenty-two bacteria (including *Staphylococcus aureus, E. coli, Pseudomonas aeruginosa,* and *Klebsiella* species). Petitgrain *(Citrus x aurantium l. amara),* Lemon Eucalyptus *(Eucalyptus citriodora),* and Peppermint affected all of the bacteria. The other oils varied in their activity.[36]

Peppermint has an abundance of alcohols such as 3-cyclohexen-1-ol, linalool, menthol (45 percent), terpin-4-ol, isomenthol, dihydro terpineol, and alpha-terpineol. Some researchers think monoterpene alcohols have a positive electrical charge that can change the acidity or alkalinity of any medium. The seven alcohols in *Mentha piperita* give the oil an ability to deal with digestive upsets. Making the stomach more alkaline would help alleviate food poisoning, constipation, and travel sickness.

Menthol in peppermint was found to have the greatest spasmolytic activity in a study done on the contractile electro-induced response of guinea pig ileum. The oil inhibited muscle contraction by antagonizing acetylcholine.[37]

To prevent colonic spasm discomfort and physical hindrance during sigmoidoscopy, twenty patients received peppermint oil injected along the biopsy channel of the colonoscope; in every case colonic spasm was relieved in thirty seconds. A diluted suspension of the oil had the same effect.[38] The oil would be a great aid to controlling vomiting and diarrhea for these reasons.

There are three esters in *Mentha piperita,* including menthyl acetate (6 percent), that balance the fast energy of the monoterpenes and alcohols. They would help induce sweating in a fever and calm anger and hysteria. The five sesquiterpenes—bourbonene, caryophyllene (1 percent), farnesene, germacrene, and bicyclogermacrene—bring a strong anti-inflammatory effect to this oil. The oil is known for its pain-relieving action.

A study on the neurophysiological and psychological parameters of headache mechanisms investigated thirty-two healthy subjects in a double-blind placebo controlled trial. Four preparations of varying amounts of Eucalyptus and Peppermint were used. Peppermint alone had a significant analgesic effect with reduction in sensitivity to headache.[39]

SESQUITERPENOIDS

Sesquiterpenoids are sesquiterpenes with a functional group added like an alcohol (OH). Oils with these alcohols are thicker and slower to move. Examples are farnesol in Jasmine *(Jasminum grandiflorum)* and alpha- or beta-santalol in Sandalwood *(Santalum album).* They are considered base notes in perfumery. They are often anti-inflammatory such as bisabolol in German chamomile. A calming sesquiterpenol for brain nerve cells, alpha-eudesmol, has been studied in Cedarwood *(Juniperus virginiana)* by Asakura et al.[40]

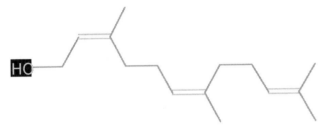

Farnesol

Sesquiterpenols also act as immune stimulants, such as the small amount of zingiberol in ginger *(Zingiber officinalis)* and patchouli alcohol (40 percent) in patchouli *(Pogostemon cablin).* These sesquiterpenol molecules also have been studied in relation to reducing cancer tumors.

A 1999 study by Luft et al. researched the way farnesol works on the smooth muscle of a rat's aorta. The results showed that farnesol greatly reduced the hypertensive rats' blood pressure for up to forty-eight hours. Farnesol prevents heart contraction by blocking L-type calcium ion ($Ca2+$) channels. Farnesol exists at a level of 92 percent in Rose *(Rosa damascena)* and 4.6 percent in Ylang-ylang *(Cananga odorata).* Both of these oils are known for their relaxing effects on the heart. The alcohol group is extremely valuable for many complex, intricate human problems.[41]

As shown in the following figures, Ylang-ylang has many sesquiterpenoids.

Essential oil	Ylang-ylang *(Cananga odorata)*
Country of origin	Philippines, Java, Madagascar
Botanical family	Annonaceae
Extraction	Distillation of flowers from trees
Plant description	Tall, tropical tree up to 65 feet high with long folded leaves and large yellow flowers
Key	Euphoric and calming
Medicinal	Has ability to slow down overly rapid breathing and heartbeat.
	As a nervine, has a calming effect; use for shock, fear, and anger.
	A tonic to the womb after a cesarean section birth.
	Has aphrodisiac qualities; helps alleviate impotence and frigidity.
	Antiseptic action on intestinal infections.
Mind	Regulates adrenaline flow; relaxes nervous system.
	Brings feelings of joy; eases anxiety, panic, and anger.
	Is an antidepressant.
	"It will open our hearts to the pleasures that God has given us. ..." (Valerie Worwood).[42]
Precaution	If used in too high a concentration for too long a time, ylang-ylang can cause nausea or headache.
How to use	Create a blend with two other oils and 7 drops in 8 milli liters (1.62 teaspoons) of vegetable oil like jojoba oil. Wear on the neck and wrists. For emotional upsets, put on a Kleenex and smell every few minutes. Rub oil on heart area.

Ylang-ylang essential oil is very diverse in its chemical makeup with very light and powerful top notes of esters, alcohols, and phenylpropanoids. The esters and sesquiterpenes make up a very dominate middle note. The base note is comprised of sesquiterpenols plus phenyl esters. Ylang-ylang is produced from steam distillation of the flowers.

GC-MS CHROMATOGRAM OF YLANG YLANG COMPLETE ESSENTIAL OIL

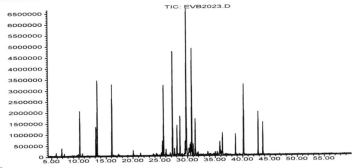

GC-MS IDENTIFACATION OF THE MAIN CHEMICAL CONSTITUENTS AND THIER PERCENTAGES

OPERATOR: SPECTRIX LABS, INC.
SAMPLE NAME: YLANG YLANG COMPLETE 1-25-08

PK#	RT	AREA%	LIBRARY/ID	PK#	RT	AREA%	LIBRARY/I
1	5.86	0.33	Buten-1-Ol Acetate<3-Methyl-3				
2	6.88	0.61	Buten-1-Ol Acetate<3-Methyl-2	31	30.35	0.83	Bicyclogermacrene
3	7.36	0.22	Pinene<Alpha->	32	30.47	0.90	Muurolene<Alpha->
4	9.89	0.16	Hexyl Acetate	33	30.62	0.96	(Z,E)-.Alpha.-Farnesene
5	10.20	3.62	Anisole<Para-Methyl->	34	30.78	9.68	Farnesene<(E,E)-Alpha->
6	10.67	0.26	Cineole<1,8->	35	31.02	0.92	Cadinene<Gamma->
7	13.15	2.26	Methyl Benzoate	36	31.39	3.21	Cadinene<Delta->
8	13.41	5.55	Linalool	37	31.73	0.20	Cadina-1,4-Diene<Trans
9	16.11	5.89	Benzyl Acetate	38	31.92	0.25	Cadinene<Alpha->
10	17.29	0.13	Terpineol<Alpha->	39	33.67	0.45	Caryophyllene Oxide
11	20.04	0.52	Geraniol	40	35.01	0.35	Junenol
12	21.39	0.26	Anethole<E->	41	35.36	0.29	Cubenol<1-Epi->
13	23.75	0.25	Elemene<Delta->	42	35.86	1.62	Cadinol<Epi-Alpha->
14	24.28	0.16	Cubebene<Alpha->	43	36.00	0.44	Muurolol<Alpha->
15	25.21	0.28	Ylangene<Alpha->	44	36.32	2.03	Cadinol<Alpha->
16	25.40	1.17	Copaene<Alpha->	45	38.70	1.56	Farnesol<Z,E->
17	25.62	5.46	Geranyl Acetate	46	40.19	6.82	Benzyl Benzoate
18A	26.06	0.20	Cubebene<Beta->	47	42.84	3.30	Farnesyl Acetate <2z,6e
18B	26.06	0.44	Elemene<Beta->	48	43.70	2.62	Benzyl Salicylate
19	26.83	0.21	Gurjunene<Alpha->				
20	27.27	10.11	Caryophyllene(E-)				
21	27.61	0.59	Copaene<Beta->				
22	28.07	2.43	Cinnamyl Acetate<E->				
24	28.62	3.38	Humulene<Alpha->				
25	29.00	0.26	Muurola-4(14),5-Diene<Cis->				
26	29.41	0.25	Cadina-1(6),4-Diene<Trans->				
27	29.57	1.43	Muurolene<Gamma->				
28	29.79	15.44	Germacrene D				
29	29.88	0.57	Prenyl Benzoate				
30	30.24	0.89	Amorphene<Gamma->				

Gas chromatograph–mass spectrometer analysis of Ylang-ylang (*Cananga odorata*)

Observing the chemistry of *Cananga odorata,* we can see why it affects us as it does. This is an essential oil rich in esters, alcohols, and sesquiterpenes.

An analysis begins with esters such as 3-methyl acetate, hexyl acetate, methyl benzoate (3 percent), benzyl acetate (9 percent), geranyl acetate (4 percent), and cinnamyl acetate (4 percent). There are three main esters: farnesyl acetate (3 percent), benzyl benzoate (7 percent), and benzyl salicylate (3.5 percent). The last two are phenyl esters. All of these esters are quite stable and safe, and offer sedative and antispasmodic effects to the oil. This would explain why *Cananga odorata* is a tonic to the womb after a cesarean birth.

Esters re-equilibriate and regulate the sympathetic autonomic nervous system and, Pierre Franchomme and Daniel Pénoël suggest, the neuroendocrine nervous system.[43] This is why *Cananga odorata* regulates adrenaline flow and relaxes the central nervous system. These esters make this oil effective for reducing panic, shock, fear, and anger. With all of the above esters, this oil truly is a nervine. The alcohols are numerous too: cresol, methyl ether (4.6 percent), linalool (5.6 percent), geraniol, and the sesquiterpenols cubenol, alpha-muurolol (1.5 percent), alpha-cadinol (0.9 percent), and farnesol (1 percent). As stated previously, the alcohols, especially farnesol, have a relaxing and tonic effect on the heart, slowing down a rapid heartbeat and relieving hypertension. A study on epilepsy patients at the Neuropsychiatry and Seizure Clinic of Birmingham Hospital used Bergamot, Lemongrass, Chamomile, Lavender, and Ylang-ylang for stress. Of the first ten patients treated (followed up over two years), six became seizure-free and three withdrew from anticonvulsive medication.[44]

Another important quality of farnesol is its ability to kill leukemia cells. A study done in vitro on affected acute leukemia blood cells showed farnesol selectively killed leukemia cells in preference to normal hemopoietic cells. More research needs to be done in vivo. *Cananga odorata* also contains large quantities of sesquiterpenes such a copaene (1.6 percent), bourbonene, elemene, caryophyllene (6.7 percent), humulene (3.3 percent), farnesene, alpha-farnesene (9.6 percent), humulene (2.5 percent), muurolene (1.4 percent), amorphene (1.1 percent), germacrene D (17 percent), and delta-cadinene (2.5 percent). These sesquiterpenes make the oil very anti-inflammatory, increasing the positive effect on the heart for high blood pressure. They also have a sedative characteristic, which is the main mental-emotional effect of this oil.[45]

The sesquiterpenes in *Cananga odorata* accentuate the antifungal action as seen in a study of twenty-six essential oils and cultures of *Trichomonas vaginalis* compared to metronidazole (a standard pharmaceutical antimicrobial agent). Of the oils, *Cinnamomum cassia* was the most effective, followed by *Vetiveria zizanioides* and *Santalum album,* and then *Cananga odorata.* None of the oils had activity comparable to that of metronidazole.[46]

Another study of some Philippine plants revealed that ylang-ylang gave good results against *Staphylococcus aureus.*[47]

Because of the antifungal quality of the sesquiterpenes, Ylang-ylang oil is effective for intestinal infections, whether fungal or bacterial.

Overall, the chemistry of Ylang-ylang backs up the claims in the profile shown on pages 173 and 174. This oil is euphoric due to all the esters and alcohols and calming due to the large amount of sesquiterpenes. It is an amazing phenomenon that the science of essential oil chemistry today is proving the assertions of people in the time of Zenobia when they received the oils from the spice trade.

In Closing

Chemistry gives us more answers and deeper insights! Mastering some basic organic chemistry gives the practicing essential oil therapist and consumer some vital tools based on scientific data for choosing the right oil for the right person.

CHAPTER FIFTEEN

Case Studies

Work is love made visible.

—Kahlil Gibran

E SSENTIAL OIL THERAPY offers many scintillating avenues for creating healthy lives. Let us look at where we are now in our evolutionary path toward preventive medicine with essential oils. We will examine some methods of use and real applications in the field. Interspersed in the discussion are amazingly rich personal and student case studies. This method, which originated with Marguerite Maury's individual prescription, looks at the whole person instead of the disease or illness.

Today the essential oil therapist shows the physician how to produce holistic medicine with compounds or blends from nature's cornucopia of fragrant oils and herbs. The subject of modern doctors is addressed in Chapter 21, "Integrative Medicine." The modern aromatherapist realizes how many diseases can be eliminated by creating a healthy lifestyle and using the gentle power of essential oils to create balance.

All students at the College of Botanical Healing Arts do about thirty case studies, making this practice the heart of the program. As students learn to look objectively and compassionately at family members and friends during the interview and to create an individualized prescription blend, as initiated by Marguerite Maury, they grow in the wisdom of healing. These case studies are based on women and men dealing with the stresses of modern life. Some are classically timeless in their approach to tension and to healing these imbalances. Some will seem achingly familiar. We sense the spirit of Trota in the directions and plant medicines chosen for healing by many of the students.

How to Do a Great Case Study

Begin with a short interview that looks at the whole person—physically, emotionally, mentally, and spiritually (PEMS). Find a quiet, private place to conduct your interview, whether in person or on the phone. In the presence of your client, initially ask to work for the highest good and benefit.

Respect the answers of the person you are interviewing, even if you know the client may not be completely honest with you or himself. Imbalances in a person's health often entail some denial, especially in the emotional area. Looking at his situation and discussing his problems can be a healing process in and of itself. Record the answers faithfully and give a copy of the interview form to the client. Let him know that his identity will remain anonymous and only you will know the true source.

Then work on a form that only you will see. Begin with a description of how you see the person may be out of balance and show a clear picture of his life's situation, including family, social relationships, job reality, lifestyle habits, and spiritual growth. Use all of your knowledge about essential oils: traditional uses, scientific experiments, therapeutic actions, chemical makeup, and energetic effects. Choose four to seven essential oils that will stimulate and tonify the different levels of healing needed. Ask for higher guidance in these choices. Perhaps you can write down essential oils that intuitively come to you during the interview process.

Create a blend with great care. Make it a very sacred, conscious process that is not hurried. Write down the oils you have chosen for this person. Put one drop of each oil in a bottle. With each drop, rub the bottle horizontally between your fingers, thoroughly mixing the fragrant elixir. Smell the blend after each drop is added. Then put one drop more of the oils you want to emphasize therapeutically. Add some extra drops to create a smooth fragrance, not letting one oil dominate. As a less important, secondary practice, put a top, middle, and base note in the blend for balance. Write down each drop you add with a hatch mark, crossing it if you reach five. Depending on the person's size, age, and condition, use 2 to 5 percent essential oils in a carrier oil. Keep this record with all the forms you accumulate for this person with his initials and the date. A therapeutic blend can be a beautiful aromatic blend too!

Write down the chosen oils with the reasons for each choice. On the same form describe how your client is to use this blend—massage, bath, neat (without dilution), lotion, mist—the number of times each day, and for how many days. Be sure to give your client the information in writing on how to use each oil or each blend. Offer any lifestyle suggestions at this time such as nutritional focus or elimination, herbal supplements, special exercise or yoga, meditation time, and any other healing modalities you think would be beneficial.

Check in with your client in two days, five days, and ten days. Check his progress and stress the importance of using the oils daily. Commend him for all his effort.

During a clinic for graduating students, done as the last two classes (clinical practice and clinical theory), students conduct ninety-minute sessions with a client. These are more comprehensive case studies that offer graduating students a chance to work with the public and apply all they have learned in the entire program. Here the work with nutrition, herbs, and lifestyle changes is extended, yet the integrity of the basic case study and the creation of an individual prescription blend is maintained. Other factors such as herbal teas, essential oil footbaths, and reflexology on the feet are added for the enhanced experience of both the attending client and the budding practitioner.

Here I will share some examples of the multitude of case studies that I have done and that I have received from my students. All student case studies are included with the permission of the student. These case studies show the breadth and depth of healing possible with the beautiful, mighty power of essential oils along with a healthy lifestyle.

These case studies will be generally classified into four categories: physical, emotional, mental, and spiritual. My experience is that there are always correlations between physical symptoms, emotional traumas, negative thinking, and spiritual imbalances. This will be more thoroughly discussed in Chapter 19, "Essential Oils and the Mind-Body Connection."

Physical Level Case Studies

CASE STUDY #1 PHYSICAL LEVEL

My first personal experience with how essential oils work on the feet was at a health spa in Calistoga, California, where I had just received a mud bath. It was spring and my allergies blossomed into inflamed, painful sinuses. A massage therapist began rubbing my feet. She applied eucalyptus *(Eucalyptus globulus)* to the tips of my toes. I suddenly experienced a complete release of my impacted sinuses. The oil and massage totally drained my sinus area and I left the spa breathing deeply with no pain! This was a major revelation to me in how well touch and essential oils can relieve suffering.

CASE STUDY #2 PHYSICAL LEVEL

This is a touching story shared by C.L., a registered nurse working for a hospice and doing outreach work on dying patients. C.L.'s client suffered from severe cancer of the respiratory and digestive systems. She had a tumor mass inside the right cheek of the buttocks on the anus and in the lungs. The anus tumor had a cauliflower-like growth 6.5 centimeters (2½ inches) in diameter and caused 90 percent of her pain. She had swollen legs from knees to toes. Emotionally she expressed fear of the unknown and of how she would die. Mentally she was alert and in control, very outgoing. She expressed anger and hatred toward her family members and some of her friends. She worked at living each day to the fullest.

Three oils were chosen for their holistic actions and specifically to help her edema:

- Grapefruit *(Citrus x paradisi),* a draining and a lymphatic stimulant that can increase appetite. It has a balancing effect on the central nervous system with an uplifting, euphoric effect.
- Fennel *(Foeniculum vulgare),* a cleanser to help the body remove toxins from the blood. It is a tonic for digestion and good for the relief of constipation. For the mind, it can release suppressed emotions and build courage.
- Geranium *(Pelargonium graveolens),* which balances and regulates the endocrine system through the hypothalamus and the adrenal cortex. It can alleviate inflammation and has diuretic properties to reduce swelling. It brings emotional balance, alleviating anxiety and depression. It brings happiness and a positive outlook.

C.L. instructed the caregiver how to do a lymphatic massage on the client's legs. She recommended a bedtime massage when the patient was able to stay off her feet.

Results

After three days the patient stated that her swelling is almost completely gone. Her spirits are good and she wonders why. Never having used essential oils before, she attributes her positive outlook to not seeing her negative friend in the last few days. She has become quick to laugh and finds herself telling stories of her past to the hospice caregivers, something she never did before. Also, her bowels started working well.

There is more to this case study, but C.L. was very happy with the immediate results.

CASE STUDY #3 PHYSICAL LEVEL

One of my early students, P.W., did a case study on her hairstylist, who had chronic tendonitis on the right anterior lateral side of her foot. The tendonitis was constantly aching due to her job of standing on her feet all day, every day. She also had referral pain up the tendon of her calf behind her knee. She was emotionally very stressed and tired due to a difficult family situation and the pain in her foot. She was overweight.

P.W. chose the following oils:

- Roman chamomile *(Chamaemelum nobile)*, which is good for chronic aches and inflamed joints and tendons. It has a calming action on emotions and is an antidepressant.
- Lavender *(Lavandula angustifolia)*, which relieves the pain of sprained tendons and ligaments. It relieves stress and exhaustion in the central nervous system.
- Juniper *(Juniperus communis)*, a detoxifying oil that helps regulate appetite and obesity. It relieves pain in the feet and legs.
- Rosemary *(Rosmarinus officinalis)*, a brain stimulant that strengthens the mind when a person feels weak and fatigued. It is definitely pain relieving and brings warmth to muscles. It also is a diuretic for cellulite and obesity.

P.W. suggested blending these four essential oils in 2 ounces of carrier oil. She recommended massaging the affected areas of the foot and the tendons by the knee.

Results

The client was amazed at the results! She went on vacation and used the massage oil the morning and evening after she arrived. She said her foot was swollen and painful. The next day she had no pain. She was very surprised and continued to use it while on vacation. When she returned to work, her foot still got a little swollen, but not nearly as bad as before. She wanted a refill on the blend and planned to use it indefinitely. She experienced less emotional tension and more peace.

As P.W.'s teacher, I pointed out that recommending some nutrition and herbs would have been beneficial too.

CASE STUDY #4 PHYSICAL LEVEL

This is an in-depth case study by V.M., a thoughtful, enthusiastic healer. The client interview revealed a person with indigestion, constipation, acid reflux, physical fatigue, depression, fear, mood swings, PMS, and mental fatigue. She is overweight and finds it hard to get out of bed in the morning due to lack of physical vitality. She had a doctor prescribe an acid-reflux medication. She appears healthy and has an open mind. She does worry a lot.

V.M. decided to begin with nervines. "The healing strategy here will be to calm the nervous system, redirect focus, acknowledge needs, and make simpler, healthier food choices," V.M. wrote on the patient's form. "Essential oils will play many roles in healing including sedating the nervous system, helping damaged esophageal tissue, soothing the digestive tract, and aiding digestion." V.M. asked the client to keep a journal, noting each day her emotional and eating habits.

V.M. began with lavender hydrosol for her client to rub on her neck and belly. The following blend was to be rubbed on her abdomen before each meal:

- Dill *(Anethum graveolens)*, a soothing digestive aid that promotes healing of damaged tissues. It helps with constipation and brings awareness to a situation.
- Spearmint *(Mentha spicata)*, a tonic to the digestive system that stimulates healthy liver bile production. It releases urine retention;

helps alleviate mental fatigue, headaches, nervous strain, and stress; and develops greater self-trust.

- Peppermint *(Mentha piperita)*, which relaxes stomach muscles and removes toxic congestion. It helps relieve nervous tension and pain, and promotes concentration.

V.M. felt this blend would bring an awareness of health to her client's present moment. While inhaling the aroma, she was instructed to think "I am feeding my body what it needs to burn brightly." V.M. said to use the blend several times throughout the day, applying it with downward strokes from the center of the chest toward the lower intestines. She also recommended drinking a cup of calendula *(Calendula officinalis)* and licorice *(Glycyrrhiza glabra)* tea plus tinctures of calendula and licorice, 25 drops each four times a day after meals. V.M. asked her client to choose a variety of whole foods for five days and to write in her journal what she ate. She was instructed to wait several hours after eating before napping or sleeping. Here are V.M.'s written instructions:

Daily:
Do eat raw or simply prepared foods.
Do eat "live" sauerkraut before meals.
Do eat small meals instead of large meals.
Do eat meats first in a meal.
Do reach for a hydrosol mist instead of a snack.
Do add cold-pressed oils to food after it has been prepared.
Do drink fresh vegetable juice.

For five days:
Avoid carbohydrates.
Avoid sugar.
Avoid coffee, tea, fruit juice, alcohol, and caffeine.
Avoid processed prepared foods.
Avoid snacking.
Avoid the bakery aisle like the plague.

Results

It was a struggle for the client to make such big changes. She felt a big change from using the blend and changing her eating habits. She no longer felt the burning pain in her esophagus. She loved the hydrosol and took it with her everywhere. After five days she decided to make most of the changes permanent and continued using the blend before meals. She began to lose weight and she had more peace of mind.

CASE STUDY #5 PHYSICAL LEVEL

This is an interesting case study by an intelligent student, N.S. She describes the client as a hard-working, capable woman who is worn out. She is fifty-three years old and has raised four children mostly by herself (divorced). She worked in a law firm for many years and then worked as an investigator of police misconduct, only to leave this stressful environment to take classes in healing therapies, one of which was the study of essential oils. By this time she had developed high blood pressure, high cholesterol, asthma, mouth sores, and low back pain.

N.S. chose three oils:

- Frankincense *(Boswellia carteri)* to relieve her asthma, regulate secretions, break the emotional ties to her former employment, and elevate her mind to her higher self.
- Lavender *(Lavandula angustifolia)* to reduce high blood pressure, relieve exhaustion, improve asthma and bronchitis, help with bile and digestion of fats, and energize all the chakras.
- Orange *(Citrus sinensis)* to improve her digestion and lymphatic flow, to gain control of her weight, and to uplift the emotions for warmth and joy from the heart.

N.S. instructed her client to rub the Frankincense on her chest and throat, morning and night, and to use it in a diffuser in her bedroom when sleeping. She was also told to rub the oil lightly over her tongue, gums, and cheeks prior to going to bed for mouth sores.

She took nightly baths with Lavender oil.

She massaged the Orange oil onto her stomach and hips before lunch and dinner.

Results

The client found the Frankincense more effective in relieving coughing fits than prescribed inhalers. Her stress level began to drop, knowing help was there if coughing fits occurred. She began to sleep better and the exhaustion dropped away. After two nights of application in her mouth, the inflammation of the tongue, gums, and cheeks almost totally disappeared. As her stress level decreased, so did her high blood pressure and cholesterol. She continued using these oils for several months, adding a few more as her knowledge increased. Bringing balance to the body, mind, and spirit was a reality for this woman.

As N.S.'s teacher, I recommended that the treatment of the client could have continued with more essential oil blends plus nutritional and herbal remedies for at least six months.

CASE STUDY #6 PHYSICAL LEVEL

A graduate, D.M., does this case study on an elderly person eighty years of age. Her health problems are multiple, including poor heart circulation, high blood pressure, diabetes, joint pain, neuralgia, arthritis, and obesity. She had both wrists operated on for carpal tunnel syndrome. Both hands and arms are swollen, the right worse than the left. The swelling gives her almost constant pain and she is unable to wear jewelry.

The main focus of this case study is to reduce the inflammation in the forearms and hands. The edema is probably from the heart problems, lymphatic build-up, arthritis, or diabetes. The goal is to reduce the inflammation so the pain will subside significantly.

On an emotional level, the client experiences mood swings with bouts of anger, depression, anxiety, poor judgment, and negativity. As in the case of multiple system problems in the body, the emotions tend to be unstable too. She was on antidepressants for a couple of years and has anxiety attacks when she is away from home for too long. These attacks usually manifest in either constipation or diarrhea.

D.M. felt her client exhibited a general feeling of being unloved and is in need of nurturing and touch. D.M. had done a previous study on this woman, who had cried and said she was so touched that someone would take the time to care for her. The woman's husband shows love and affection in certain ways, yet as the primary caretaker of her household she does all the cleaning, cooking, and financial management. She has some money issues, feeling everyone is after hers. She has a distrust of people, even those in her closest circle.

Based on the conditions described, D.M. chose oils for the whole person, but specifically to eliminate accumulated fluids and reduce the inflammation. In addition oils were chosen to tonify the heart, help circulation, reduce pain, balance the emotions, control the diabetes, reduce anger, and transform pessimism into optimism. D.M. chose these essential oils and herbs:

- Ginseng *(Panax quinquefolius)*, selected for its documented results to help alleviate edema, diabetes, arteriosclerosis, depression, hypertension, and stress, and to increase the immune system. A ginseng drink is to be consumed two to five times per week as a tea. Ginseng has eighteen saponins or plant hormones called *ginsenosides* that fight stress and fatigue, protect the liver, and guard against memory loss.
- Cypress *(Cupressus sempervirens)*, an astringent to reduce excess fluids and edema, and to help stay balanced in the middle of emotional storms. It is also good for aches and pains and reduces anger and irritability.
- Orange *(Citrus sinensis)*, which benefits edema, digestion of fats, lymphatic movement, circulation, and heart palpitations; brings down high cholesterol; calms stomach and nervous states; and balances diarrhea and constipation. It spreads sunshine on gloomy thoughts and depression. It helps develop patience during life's challenges.
- Nutmeg *(Myristica fragrans)*, which breaks down fats, is good for relieving rheumatic pain, and acts as a warming balm to chronic muscular pain. It lessens the stabbing pain of neuralgia and is a stimulant to the heart and circulation.
- Lemon *(Citrus x limon)*, which stimulates white blood cells (phagocytes and lymphocytes). It is a tonic to the circulatory system and an effective heart tonic, and it brings down high blood pressure. It is used to treat diabetes and benefits arteriosclerosis, arthritis, and inflamed joints. Lemon is refreshing and cooling when feeling hot. It increases inner joy while transforming pessimism into optimism.
- Geranium *(Pelargonium graveolens)*, which balances and regulates. It helps sluggish circulation and edema, and has diuretic properties when the system is congested and elimination is poor. It

guards against fluid retention and swollen ankles. It is a tonic to the nervous system and regulates mood swings. It produces a joyful heart and promotes self-love.

- Castor oil *(Ricinus communis)*, the yellowish fluid expressed from the seed of the castor bean. Applied topically, it can stimulate the lymph system to drain in problem spots along the spinal cord, the abdomen, or areas of lymph node concentration.

Castor oil has been used for centuries, both internally and externally. Hatshepsut probably used it during her reign since it is discussed in the pharmacopoeia of the Ebers papyrus, one of six Egyptian medical papyrii from the Eighteenth Dynasty. Dated about 1534 BC during the reign of Amenhotep I, the document was purchased in 1972 by Georg Ebers and first published in 1875 in an Egyptian-Latin vocabulary. An English translation was first published in 1937. The original scroll is 110 pages long and was written by an Egyptian scribe about the structure of the body, diseases, and remedies. The products of the castor oil plant are systematically described in the Ebers papyrus:

Knowledge of what is made from (or done with) the Ricinus plant, as that which was found in ancient writings and as that which is useful to mankind.

a) One crushes its roots in water, to place on a head which is sick: he will then become well immediately, like one who is not ill.

b) A little of its fruit (beans) is chewed with beer by a man with *wehi*-condition in his faeces. This is an elimination of disease from the belly of a man.

c) The hair of a woman is also caused to grow by its fruit (beans); it is ground and made into one thing and added to oil; then the woman should anoint her head with it.

d) Its oil *(merhet)* is also prepared from its fruit (beans); to anoint [a man] with *wehau*-skin disease ... which is painful.... Really excellent, a million times.[1]

It is difficult to translate the exact name of the disease mentioned in the ancient writing.

Castor oil is native to Africa and grows as a tree in tropical and temperate regions like Egypt. Medicinal castor oil is prepared from the yield of the first pressing and is used as a purgative and laxative.

D.M. says making a castor oil pack is a simple procedure that can produce good effects. For the maximum effect, use a hot oil pack. Physiological effects of the castor oil pack include stimulating the liver, increasing elimination, relieving pain, increasing lymphatic circulation, improving gastrointestinal function, increasing relaxation, and reducing inflammation.

Castor oil pack

> 3 layers of natural, uncolored wool or flannel cotton to cover the area being treated
>
> Castor oil (½ to 1 cup)
>
> Plastic wrap to cover the cloth
>
> Hot water bottle or electric blanket

Soak cotton with castor oil. It should be saturated but not dripping.

Place the pack on the area being treated.

Cover the pack with plastic wrap and place a hot water bottle over the pack.

Leave the pack on for 30 to 60 minutes. Use the castor oil pack 3 to 7 days per week.

Same pack can be used for months; refresh with additional oil if necessary.

Precautions: Avoid use close to meal times. Do not use during heavy menses. Avoid contact with fabric that could become stained.

Treatment Administered

D.M. mixed the essential oil blend of Cypress, Orange, Nutmeg, Lemon, and Geranium with the castor oil and with a light touch massaged it into the skin, moving toward the lymph nodes under the arms. She finished by rubbing the oil onto one hand and the lower part of the arm, using the long, light, smooth strokes recommended in lymph massage. After the massage, D.M. wrapped unbleached cotton muslin around her client's arm and hand. A towel was wrapped around the muslin and then surrounded by a heating pad. This was left on for one hour, and then the other arm and hand were given the same treatment. While the arms were being treated, D.M. served her client a cup of ginseng tea and they watched *Gone with the Wind*.

In addition to being treated with a hot castor oil pack, the woman was advised to drink water with freshly squeezed lemon juice and a drop of lemon essential oil. This was designed to help with cleansing the liver, digesting the fats and cholesterol, and suppressing the appetite. D.M. also recommended the client walk, starting with fifteen minutes per day and working up to one hour. The walk is to take place along the ocean or country scenic areas around her house. This will help with her weight and blood circulation, and act as a meditation to reduce stress.

Results

The client noticed a throbbing feeling (not painful), but said the arms felt really good. The client and D.M. both noticed a reduction in fluid around the arms and hands immediately after the cloth was removed. The swollen arm was less puffed out and resembled the other arm that typically does not swell up as much. She commented how nice the treatment felt and how she would like to continue them. She was so relaxed that she actually dosed off a couple of times. The treatment was not only a physical relief, but also provided stress relief and relaxation for a person who rarely takes time to care for herself.

Emotional and Mental Level Case Studies

CASE STUDY #7 EMOTIONAL LEVEL

This is a case study done by S.S., a student committed to healing. She chose a client who was in her thirties and had been abused by an ex-husband. The woman had endured many beatings and at the time of her case study had damaged thumbs. She is described as a warm, loving, outgoing, caring person.

S.S. chose the following leaf oils:

- Hyssop (*Hyssopus officinalis*), which releases the deep emotions hidden beneath the surface. It releases emotional pain and helps clear grief. It expands perceptive abilities and fortifies your resolve to walk your path. It also protects the aura.
- Vetiver (*Vetiveria zizanioides*), which balances the central nervous system. It is calming for stress and tension. It promotes sleep and relaxes nightmares. It stimulates the root chakra for grounding.

- Lavender *(Lavandula angustifolia)*, which relieves anger, exhaustion, and fear; creates calm; and heals the passions that create turmoil. It promotes patience and inspires feelings of security.
- Cypress *(Cupressus sempervirens)*, which promotes balance in the middle of emotional storms. It transforms old grief into inner strength. Good for transitions.
- Eucalyptus smithii *(Eucalyptus smithii)*, a milder oil than *Eucalyptus globulus* that relieves pain, arthritis, and inflammation. It clears heat.

Almond oil is the carrier. A good massage oil for slip and glide, it contains vitamin A, B, and C to reduce itching and swelling. S.S. asked her client to massage the mixture on her feet, hands, and belly twice a day.

Results

In two days the client felt better. The oils made her feel pampered and increased her life force. In five days she felt great, grounded with a sense of clarification and vision regarding her goals in life. She became very enthusiastic and passionate about her goals of becoming a massage therapist and actress. She loved the blend. It seemed to work powerfully on both the emotional and the mental level. She continued using the blend for some time.

CASE STUDY #8 EMOTIONAL LEVEL

This study by a student, B.B., reveals a common malady of today. B.B.'s client was doing way too much. She was operating totally in her head, out of touch with her body, and very stressed out. She acknowledged she had a body when the pain became severe. She had frequent headaches, lower back pain, menstrual pain, flaky skin on legs and feet, acne on her face, PMS cramps, and a sensitive stomach. Emotionally, she was letting go and ending a romantic friendship of ten years. She wanted to give her mind a rest and focus more on spiritual intuition and inner guidance. She also sought to connect with her artistic side.

B.B. chose these oils:

- Roman chamomile *(Chamaemelum nobile)*, which is good for sensitive skin, PMS cramps since it is antispasmodic and soothing for

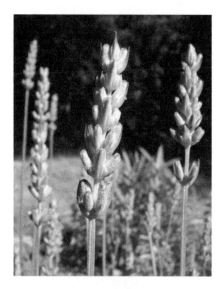

Lavender

the stomach. It will help to calm the mind and keep it positive. It aids in truthful spiritual communication even when it is difficult.

- Lavender *(Lavandula angustifolia)*, which will help with acne and promote new skin growth. Emotionally it will soothe and calm. It relieves painful stress headaches. It can reduce the anger she feels toward her ex-friend. It will energize her chakras.
- Jasmine *(Jasminum grandiflorum)*, which offers relief for menstrual cramps and helps to balance hormones like estrogen and progesterone. It can boast confidence and as an antidepressant help maintain a positive attitude.

Individual Prescription

Massage the mixture of oils into the base of the neck and shoulders twice a day. Take daily baths with 10 drops in water; make this a beautiful experience with candlelight and music. S.S. advised her client to put the oil on her temples whenever she felt the need to be more balanced.

Results

In two days B.B.'s client felt calmer and was sleeping better. There were no more emotional mood swings.

In five days she was recovering much more quickly from stressful situations. She felt more positive despite many challenging issues. She found the blend helped her stay grounded.

CASE STUDY #9 EMOTIONAL LEVEL

This student, S.T., did a study on a Taiwanese woman who obeyed rules and was very disciplined. She devoted her life to her family and barely thought of herself. According to tradition, she lived with her husband's parents for many years of her marriage. They treated her badly and she suffered from frustration and pressures due to this situation. She felt "tortured" by her parents-in-law. She is usually unhappy and quite depressed on rainy days.

S.T. chose these oils for this client:

- Spikenard *(Nardostachys grandiflora)*, an oil for emotional distress since it reduces nervous tension and balances the sympathetic with the parasympathetic system. It helps a person let go of old pain and ancient emotional blocks while opening the spirit of generosity.
- Geranium *(Pelargonium graveolens)*, an oil to alleviate anxiety and depression. It regulates the hormonal system via the pituitary gland. An oil for emotional balance, it brings self-esteem, happiness, and a positive outlook.
- Bergamot *(Citrus x bergamia)*, an uplifting antidepressant that is cooling and refreshing, helping control frustration and anger. It opens the heart and creates calm and clarity for the mind.

Suggested Uses

Since the client had an electric diffuser at home, she was advised to let the diffuser run fifteen minutes every two hours. She also used the essential oil mixture in the bath, but diluted the blend with 2 tablespoons of vodka, so the geranium and bergamot would not irritate the skin.

Results

The client loved the fragrance of the blend. She followed directions very carefully and paid close attention to her feelings. Sitting in the aromatic living room with her, my student began talking to her client, who relaxed enough to talk about something interesting in her childhood and some sweet memories of her husband. She had never shared these things before. Always before she could only complain about how her parents-in-law ill-treated her.

After two weeks, she looked much happier and even wanted to learn something new and fascinating like speaking English! She started to watch English TV programs instead of only Chinese ones. She still diffused the blend every day since she loved the delightful fragrance!

CASE STUDY #10 EMOTIONAL AND PHYSICAL LEVEL

This is a case study done by a student, K.E., on a woman who is fifty-three years old. She is generally healthy but at least sixty pounds overweight with hypertension, obesity with prediabetes, chronic bronchitis, stiff knees, and irregular heart beat. She is on several medications such as Maxide (diuretic), Toprol-XL (hypertension), baby aspirin (anticoagulant), Furacin (hives), Glucophage (prediabetes), and Provera (menstrual cycle). With all of these physical problems and medications, she has a long-standing history of chronic anxiety and depression. She says that the Toprol-XL has relieved some of her agitation as well as decreased her blood pressure and palpitations. She has extra anxiety at work where there is a new manager. She has experienced occasional panic disorders, for which her physician prescribed Klonopin. However, she is not interested in being dependent on medications and wants to try the benefits of essential oils.

As K.E.'s teacher and as an essential oil therapist, I usually recommend that people with multiple physical conditions first begin treatment with essential oils for the emotional situation. Often some of the physical problems disappear when there is an emotional uplift and clarity.

K.E. chose these oils:

- Orange *(Citrus sinensis),* an oil that relaxes and helps with insomnia. It stimulates bile for digestion, calms the stomach, and calms nervous states and anxiety. It is good for treating obesity.
- Lavender *(Lavandula angustifolia),* an oil with a sedative action on the heart and on high blood pressure. It relieves insomnia and nerve pain, and reduces stress in the central nervous system. It

promotes patience and inspires feelings of security.

- Frankincense *(Boswellia carteri)*, which slows breathing and produces calm. It elevates the mind to a more spiritual perspective, and is helpful for anxious and obsessive states linked to the past.
- Elemi *(Canarium luzonicum)*, which has a grounding yet joyous effect. A good nerve sedative for stress and exhaustion, it brings feelings of deep peace.

Methods of Use

K.E. advised her client to diffuse lavender during the night to promote rest and relaxation. The blend of the four oils she used as an inhalation from a ¼-ounce (8-milliliter) bottle instead of direct application for fear of skin irritation. The woman also wanted to begin an exercise program encouraged by her physician as part of a stress reduction program.

Results

K.E.'s client became more profoundly relaxed, and she could sleep quite soundly without interruption due to the infused lavender. She found the inhaled blend uplifting. Due to the chronic nature of the symptoms, she will need to use the oils for at least a month.

As K.E.'s teacher, I advised that a more powerful effect would come from a topical application of the blend. In subsequent use of the oils, the woman began steaming daily due to flu symptoms. It seemed to bring on a healing crisis and detoxification of her body. She recovered and began losing some weight and feeling her immune system was stronger. I recommended that she continue daily use of the oils, change her nutritional routine, and get more exercise.

Spiritual Level Case Studies

CASE STUDY #11 SPIRITUAL LEVEL
(BODY-MIND-SPIRIT INTEGRATION)

This student, R.B., loved to create blends for spiritual edification. This essential oil blend, which he named *Ba-Ka-Ra*, he made for himself and used when he needed more focus on his whole self. Here's the creative process he went through.

R.B. decided to meditate the night before putting this blend together to receive inspirational transmissions to guide him. Before going to sleep, he placed selected essential oils near two crystals (rose quartz and clear quartz) and wrapped everything in a special cloth. In a prayer ritual he offered selected essential oils to the sending and receiving energies of the two crystal objects. That night during his deep sleep phases, he experienced wonderful guided messages in colorful plant-human time-space communications. He remembered getting advice on his present life's body-mind-spirit journey, which was very helpful.

R.B. felt the rituals and dreams energized the following oils:

- Melissa *(Melissa officinalis)* of the Lamiaceae family. The energy quality is cool and dry. Being an adaptogenic that works on many systems of the body, Melissa is balancing. It works on the liver and gall bladder as well as the heart. It is both parasympathetic and sympathetic in action. "Gentle strength" is what it provides in this blend (spiritual focus).
- Spikenard *(Nardostachys grandiflora)* of the Valerianaceae family. The energy quality is neutral, the temperature is cold and dry. It is adaptogenic, balancing, and works on the liver, gall bladder, and heart. It is a parasympathetic regulator. "Surrender and faith" are what it provides in this blend (spiritual focus).
- Neroli *(Citrus x aurantium l. amara)* of the Rutaceae family. The energy quality is cool with neutral moisture. It is adaptogenic and a parasympathetic regulator, and it triggers the release of corticosteroids if needed. It also works on the liver and heart areas. "Renewal" is what it provides in this blend (spiritual focus).
- Frankincense *(Boswellia carteri)* of the Burseraceae family. The energy quality is cool and dry and it works on the parasympathetic system, the lungs, and the large intestine. It is wonderful at deepening the breath (opening up the chest). "Liberation" is what it provides in this blend (spiritual focus).
- Jasmine *(Jasminum grandiflorum)* of the Oleaceae family. The energy quality is neutral temperature and neutral moisture, and it works on the sympathetic system and the heart area. It provides "creativity" for this blend (mind focus).
- Ginger *(Zingiber officinale)* of the Zingiberaceae family. The energy quality is hot and dry, and it works on the parasympathetic

system, the kidneys, and the bladder. It is excellent at increasing the oxygen, lymph, and blood flow throughout the body and mind. It provides "confidence and will power" conviction for this blend (body focus).

- Myrrh *(Commiphora myrrha)* of the Burseraceae family. The energy quality is warm and dry. An adaptogenic, it is a balancer. It works on the spleen, pancreas, and stomach areas. It provides "peace and solitude" for this blend (body focus).

Methods of Use

R.B. used the blend nightly in his spiritual rituals by placing the oils on the crystals, which subtly diffused the fragrance all night.

Results

This blend of higher spirit essential oils brought R.B. more clairvoyance and energy to pursue his spiritual journey. He used it frequently and received the guidance he was looking for.

In Closing

The case study or individual prescription is the way forward for essential oil therapists to become vital and significant in their contributions to the health field. It allows them to offer individual treatment in a deep, holistic, meaningful way.

CHAPTER SIXTEEN

Essential Oils for the Treatment of Infection

Nature is but another name for health.

—HENRY DAVID THOREAU

TODAY WE ARE FORTUNATE to have the powerful alternative of essential oils to fight infections. This is an area where essential oils shine. Research in Europe (especially France, England, and Germany) and Australia reveals the antimicrobial potency of essential oil therapy. In fact every oil is antibacterial, some more than others. Investigation shows that using the antibacterial, antiviral, antifungal, and mind-uplifting oils gives the immune system a sustaining boost. Even when pandemic viral diseases such as bird flu and AIDS sweep the planet, the essential oils are effective tools to help ameliorate the crisis and provide holistic, systemic, long-term health.

Here is some French history on the development of essential oil therapy as clinical medicine. Catherine de Médicis might have prevented the death of her dear husband and children if she had this knowledge available to her in the sixteenth century. In 1937 René-Maurice Gattefossé introduced the discipline of essential oil therapy in *Aromatherapie: Les Huiles Essentielles, Hormones Végétales (Essential Oils, Vegetable Hormones)*. The English translation, called *Gattefossé's Aromatherapy,* edited by Robert Tisserand, was published in 1993. This book was based on scientific thought. The "new" field was considered a medical modality based on pharmacological properties. According to Gattefossé, essential oils contained active ingredients that treat disease the way pharmaceutical drugs do. According to Kurt Schnaubelt, Gattefossé was also "aware of the psychological and neurological effects of essential oils . . . that foreshadowed the holistic approach to aromatherapy that has become dominant today."[1]

In 1980 French doctor Jean Valnet followed in the philosophical-medical approach of Gattefossé in *The Practice of Aromatherapy*. Valnet wrote, "Essential oils' aggression towards microbial germs is matched by their total harmlessness to healthy tissue."[2] From 1948 until 1959 Valnet, an army surgeon during the Indochina War, did research on soldiers wounded in battle whose infections responded as well to essential oils with no side effects as to synthetic antibiotics. In fact we now know that overuse of antibiotics can deplete the white blood-cell count while certain essential oils can greatly strengthen and invigorate the immune system. When Dr. Valnet returned to France, he began teaching other doctors about the healing benefits of essential oils and herbs, which became known as *phytotherapy*.

Paul Belaiche, a student of Dr. Jean Valnet, discovered in 1979 that a mixture of essential oils was a powerful treatment against bacteria especially after it has become resistant to synthetic antibiotics. His work, *Traite de Phytotherapie et d'Aromatherapie (Treatise of Phytotherapy and Aromatherapy)*, combined extensive in vitro research on the antibacterial effects of forty-two essential oils with the clinical application of using an "aromatogram" for patients to evaluate which oils worked best for their infection in a typical Western medicinal way.[3]

The aromatogram consists of the medium of agar agar in a petri dish with the addition of some infected human tissue placed in the center. The bacterium naturally grows and increases in the agar. Three or four essential oils are placed in the dish surrounding the human tissue and left to incubate overnight. Within twelve to twenty-four hours, it is clear which essential oils stop the spread of this particular microorganism's growth by how large the circle of resistance is around each essential oil in the dish. The most effective oils are then used to treat the patient. The results of the aromatogram are repeatable and similar to the antibiogram test of allopathic medicine. Besides proving the effectiveness of the oils against twelve of the most common pathogens, Belaiche showed how the oils improve the ability of the human body to ward off disease by creating balance in the central, autonomic, and endocrine systems.

Two more-recent Frenchmen, Pierre Franchomme, a scientist, and Daniel Pénoël, a medical doctor, together wrote *L'Aromatherapie Exactement (Exact Aromatherapy)* in 1990, an important book on the scientific discovery of how valuable essential oils are for healing.[4] They explore some of the actions of oils via their chemistry and the functional families. Their book elevates the scientific basis for how essential oils work in the body and the mind. They both continue their research and medical practice, bringing more evidence to the world's table.

Essential Oils for Curing or Eliminating Microorganisms

The antiseptic power of essential oils is due to their surface activity,[5] their lipid solubility or ability to penetrate the cell membrane,[6] and their ability to influence cell metabolism (cutting off the breathing or oxygen absorption of bacteria). With all their antiseptic power, there are few side effects from using the oils. Mostly due to inappropriate, accidental oral ingestion of oils by children, there have only been a small number of deaths in the last two hundred years. Compared to the huge number of deaths from pharmaceutical drugs, this is a miniscule number. The key factor is dosage with children and adults.

An oil with camphor as one of its constituents (such as Rosemary, 10 to 20 percent camphor) could be dangerous if 8 milliliters (1.62 teaspoons) were ingested or a large quantity were used externally (8 to 10 milliliters) on someone who has epilepsy or is pregnant. Safety is dependent on dosage and methods used (oral intake being the most precarious). An aromatherapy massage with less than 10 drops in a 1 to 3 percent dilution in carrier oil is almost always safe unless skin-irritating oils are used. Some of the unsafe exceptions in the essential oil field are phenol oils such as Clovebud *(Syzygium aromaticum)* and Oregano *(Origanum vulgare),* which can irritate skin and mucous membranes with possible liver toxicity over certain periods of use (one to two weeks for adults). Also in the cautionary group are some ketone oils such as Wormwood *(Artemisia vulgaris),* Pennyroyal *(Mentha piperita),* and Thuja *(Thuja occidentalis).* When taken internally (over 10 drops for adults with no dilution), these oils can shut down the central nervous system. Aldehyde oils such as Lemongrass *(Cymbopogon citratus)* also require careful monitoring for skin irritation. Small doses are best (1 to 3 percent in a vegetable-oil dilution). For more safety information, read *Essential Oil Safety* by Robert Tisserand and Tony Balacs.[7]

Most pure oils (especially those GC-MS analyzed) are ecologically sound. There is never a built-up resistance to microbes with essential oils as there is with antibiotics. The oils are antimicrobial every time they are used. This makes the oils important additions to our pharmacopoeia of medicines for the twenty-first century.

The Antibacterial and Antiviral Effects of Essential Oils

The knowledge of the effectiveness of essential oils goes back to the Black Death (Plague) in Europe. It began with Trota and the School of Salerno, where many botanicals were used for healing illnesses of their time. During the fourteenth-century bubonic plague, doctors often wore long bird-beak masks with essential oils in them to keep them safe from the disease. Many of the following studies and trials were found in Jane Buckle's thoroughly researched *Clinical Aromatherapy: Essential Oils in Practice* (2003) and Bob and Rhiannon Harris's *The Essential Oil Resources Database,* an online database of worldwide essential oil clinical trials. Today researchers Bob and Rhiannon Harris have concluded that "the primary effect of essential oils on bacteria and viruses appears to be on the cell membrane."[8] There, according to Savino et al., "... they seem to alter the osmotic regulatory function"[9] or the absorption of fluids. Modern pharmaceutical medicines such as penicillin and other antibiotics destroy the surrounding tissue as well as the infection. They destroy bacteria by puncturing their cell walls, which allows all the toxins to spill out onto healthy and unhealthy tissue.

The powerful, synergistic effect of using three or four oils together has been shown in many studies. The synergy is usually more effective than using a single oil. Research shows Tea tree *(Melaleuca alternifolia)* with its main terpene alcohol peak, terpinen-4-ol, is powerful against flu viruses, especially in conjunction with Eucalyptus *(Eucalyptus globulus),* and Ravintsara *(Cinnamomum camphora)* which both have large peaks of 1,8-cineol. When flu virus symptoms like sore throats, congestion, and stomach upset rear their ugly heads, doing a steam with these three oils will effectively stop the infection. I have used them successfully many times for family, friends, and myself. *Melaleuca alternifolia* should be in every medicine chest on the planet.

Philippe Goeb, a French medical doctor and essential oil therapist, believes the "anti-infectious action of essential oils is indisputable, as is their strengthening action on a weakened organism."[10] He gives a 5 percent blend of the following oils to a patient with a painful, persistent cough:

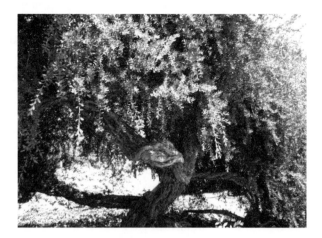

Tea tree

Rosemary *(Rosmarinus officinalis)*	25 percent
Eucalyptus *(Eucalyptus globulus)*	20 percent
Niaouli *(Melaleuca quinquenervia viridiflora)*	20 percent
Ravintsara *(Cinnamomum camphora)*	20 percent
Spike lavender *(Lavandula latifolia)*	10 percent
Peppermint *(Mentha piperita)*	5 percent

The oils are diluted in 95 percent vegetable oil in a 15-milliliter (½-ounce) bottle. Dr. Goeb suggests rubbing the blend on the chest and the back three times a day, which should greatly reduce a cough and infection in five days. As a doctor he finds essential oils are a significant part of his medicine today. They address his needs for a holistic, natural, and effective therapy.

A significant way to begin to use the essential oils in the medical community would be in the air in sickrooms, in burn and pain units, and in medical office and hospital waiting rooms. A study done in 1954 with a synergy of essential oils like Pine *(Pinus sylvestris)*, Thyme *(Thymus vulgaris)*, Peppermint *(Mentha piperita)*, Lavender *(Lavandula angustifolia)*, Rosemary *(Rosmarinus officinalis)*, Clove, and Cinnamon almost completely eliminated pre-existing microorganisms in an enclosed area.[11] A very pleasant smell was created too, something few hospitals can presently claim. This would be like the burning of the herbs rosemary and juniper in European hospitals to prevent the spread of infection during the times of Trota and Hildegard.

Since the billions of dollars spent today on studies of pharmaceutical drugs have not been allocated for clinical research of essential oils, there is a dismissal and mistrust of essential oil therapy in the American medical community. Corporations do not want to spend millions testing the oils since they would compete with pharmaceuticals. Also, the oils are difficult to patent. This is due to the myriad variations in chemotypes of plants worldwide that make it difficult to exactly duplicate any given oil's chemical constituents. With careful planting of like organic genus and species plants in similar environmental conditions and gas chromatography–mass spectrometry analysis, this problem could be mitigated.

Yet research has found some significant effects of essential oils that can't be overlooked. One is their antifungal effects. In 1936 Schmidt successfully used Cinnamon, Clovebud, Fennel *(Foeniculum vulgare)*, and Thyme against *Candida albicans*.[12] Herman and Kucera revealed their antiviral effects in 1967 when a study used Melissa *(Melissa officinalis)* and *Eucalyptus smithii* to relieve shingles (herpes zoster).[13] Plus many, many other clinical trials have been transacted worldwide. A few are outlined below.

Pure essential oils are pro-life and eubiotic as opposed to synthetic antibiotics, which are anti-life. The oils support the development and activities of the white blood cells. It is best to prescribe a blend of three powerful essential oils, tested in an aromatogram, for the synergistic effect. Immune-strengthening oils are Eucalyptus, Thyme, Niaouli *(Melaleuca quinquenervia viridiflora)*, Oregano, Tea tree, and the most powerful one, Garlic *(Allium sativum)*.

On the following pages are discussions of three general categories of microorganisms (fungal infections, bacterial infections, and viral infections) and some essential oils found to be effective in clinical studies. To begin, microbes are mindless creatures that only seek to stay alive and reproduce. To fulfill this destiny, they love human bodies, which are full of nutritious carbohydrates and other nutrients on which to munch. Humans are warm and moist. These are ideal conditions for habitation. Microbes can make humans sick and even kill them if the immune system is weak.

FUNGAL INFECTIONS

These primitive organisms have lost their chlorophyll-making behavior and are parasitic. They can cause some of the most deadly infections but do not usually occur unless the immune system is weakened. They are caught from airborne fungus spores such as aspergillosis, a disease of the lungs, or direct infection such as athlete's foot.

Candida albicans is a fungus that begins an invasion of mucous membranes when the pH of the body's tissues become too alkaline. It can spread throughout the digestive and reproductive systems of the body. "Essential oils appear to have a . . . respiration-inhibitory effect on fungi."[14] Candida is effectively treated with these essential oils:

Petitgrain *(Citrus x aurantium l. amara)*[15]
Tea tree *(Melaleuca alternifolia)*[16]
Cajeput *(Melaleuca cajuputi)*[17]
Melissa *(Melissa officinalis)*[18]

The above clinical trails are described in *Clinical Aromatherapy* by Jane Buckle.[19]

BACTERIAL INFECTIONS

Bacteria are single-celled organisms with no nucleus. They are simple, vegetable organisms with thousands of species that are little changed from the dawn of life. They do not need a host, yet they eat and divide every twenty minutes in ideal conditions such as human mucous membranes. Any human disturbances such as diet change, emotional stress, antibiotics, and certain drugs can increase susceptibility to bacterial infection. Many strains have developed resistance to antibiotics. We are surrounded by millions of these microorganisms.

Some examples of how effective essential oils are with specific types of bacteria come from studies by Paul Belaiche, Pierre Franchomme and Daniel Pénoël (1990), Valnet (1980), Deans and Ritchie (1987), and Deans and Svoboda (1988, 1989).[20]

Pneumococcus is a coccus bacterium that causes human respiratory passages to be clogged with mucous or fluid that makes breathing difficult. It can be effectively treated by Eucalyptus *(Eucalyptus globulus)*.[21]

Staphylococcus aureus is a bacterium in the shape of grapes that causes serious skin infections, often acquired during a hospital stay. It is effectively treated by Tea tree[22] and German chamomile *(Matricaria recutita)*.[23]

VIRAL INFECTIONS

Michael Roberts defines virus in *Biology: A Functional Approach:* "A virus is ... a coiled strand of nucleic acid protected by a protein coat, which can only survive and reproduce in a host cell."[24] Viruses are tiny, viscous organisms that can be classified by DNA types, either single or double strand. One of hundreds of viruses can cause a human cold, measles, hepatitis, or the flu. The flu virus doesn't make you feel tired, achy with a fever; the chemicals released by the immune system to fight the flu makes you feel sick. These symptoms reveal the lymphocytes are alive and kicking. The RNA virus (ribonucleic acid) includes the single strand retrovirus AIDS that is creating a twenty-first century plague on our planet. Most virus infections can be treated with one of these oils:

> Garlic *(Allium sativum)*[25]
> Cinnamon *(Cinnamomum verum)*[26]
> Bay laurel *(Laurus nobilis)*[27]
> Thyme *(Thymus vulgaris, Thymus vulgaris ct thymol, Thymus geraniol,* and *Thymus linalool)*[28]

Franchomme and Pénoël have found that essential oils with large peaks of 1,8-cineol are antiviral. This includes such oils as Ravintsara *(Cinnamomum camphora)*, Bay laurel, Rosemary, Eucalyptus, and Cardamom *(Elletaria cardamomum)*.[29]

Case Study: Abscessed Tooth

We can emphasize how essential oils act as important enhancements to the work of medical doctors and dentists, but they cannot replace the developments in technology and chemistry. This case study is an example.

R.T. is my student and a hypnotherapist who regularly sees clients. Her client, P.H., had an abscessed tooth that required extraction. R.T. spoke with P.H. three days before the extraction was to take place. At that time P.H. was experiencing a lot of pain and swelling around the infected tooth area. R.T. suggested that P.H. use a blend of these oils:

> 4 drops Tea tree *(Melaleuca alternifolia)*
> 2 drops Thyme *(Thymus vulgaris)*
> 1 drop Clovebud *(Syzygium aromaticum)*

R.T. mixed the above oils in 20 milliliters (1.36 teaspoons) of olive oil. She told her client that because these three oils are very antibacterial and immune-system boosters, they would be especially good for gum disease.

Three times a day P.H. applied the blend next to the area surrounding the tooth by placing a drop on her finger and spreading it around. She also gargled twice a day (morning and evening) with a solution of Tea tree and Thyme, one drop of each in four ounces of distilled water. After one day of following this procedure, P.H. experienced a great reduction in the pain and swelling. She noticed that her tooth was much less sensitive to heat and cold and she was feeling more comfortable. She continued this procedure right up to the time the tooth was extracted.

When the tooth was extracted, a cyst was found and also removed. Instead of taking the tetracycline the dentist prescribed, P.H. decided to continue her routine with the essential oils. She went back to the dentist ten days later. The first thing the dentist said was that he was amazed at how fast the gum and surrounding area were healing. The gum was healing beautifully and there was no sign of infection. P.H. told the dentist and his assistant what she had been doing, and that if her gums had not healed within a few days, she would have taken the antibiotic. The assistant said that she had heard of Tea tree. The dentist seemed a little surprised but commented, "Well, anything that will work."

P.H. continues to gargle with Tea tree and Thyme several times a week as a preventive treatment and to keep her gums healthy. This is the indirect, preventive action of essential oils in eliminating disease.

Case Study: An Alcoholic

Here is a case study from Shirley and Len Price's *Aromatherapy for Health Professionals* showing how addressing the whole person, both physically and emotionally, with essential oils can prevent death in a seriously diseased person. A male fifty-eight years of age was admitted to an Australian hospital in a semicomatose state after years of excessive drinking. He had extreme jaundice (yellow eyes), a puffy face and belly, and uncontrollable tremors. Tests showed he had impaired liver function and enzyme activity sixty times the norm. His family was informed of his imminent death.

The patient's daughter sought a local aromatherapist. She began essential oil treatments with Roman chamomile, Frankincense (*Boswellia carteri)*, Lavender, Rosemary, and Clary sage *(Salvia sclarea)* in an almond and avocado oil base. In two days he began to sleep well because his itchy skin and emotions were soothed. After ten days tests revealed the liver enzymes were decreasing. His mental attitude was improved and he loved the daily massage. He was discharged from the hospital one month from entering and a test showed his liver function to be normal. He looked and felt well. His appetite was improved and he began to enjoy life again.[30]

Marguerite Maury realized that essential oils have multiple effects when she had her massage clients do a steam with the oils. Her clients not only improved the quality of their skin and their mind, but they also eliminated sore throats, blocked sinuses, and incipient colds.

Christian Duraffourd, another student of Jean Valnet, found in his research that Marjoram *(Origanum majorana)* and Cedarwood *(Cedrus Atlantica)* affect the respiratory system with several actions at once: mucolytic, antiseptic, and anti-inflammatory.[31] Marguerite also noticed a profusion of effects when she applied the oils to the skin of her client as they promoted local circulation, vasodilation of the blood vessels, anti-inflammatory results on swollen skin, and the rubefacient glow as such oils as Eucalyptus, Rosemary, and Black pepper *(Piper nigrum)* increased the blood and lymph circulation. She was also profoundly aware of how the oils strongly influenced the digestive system of her patients as she massaged them.

Research done in 1985 by a German, Schilcher, on Fennel, Peppermint, Basil *(Ocimum basilicum)*, Roman chamomile *(Chamaemelum nobile)*, and German chamomile revealed how these oils are carminatives to settle the system and relieve gas, stimulants for the secretory activity of digestion, antispasmodic, and beneficial to gall bladder and liver function.[32] All of these actions take place when a blend of these oils is massaged on the skin. No wonder Marguerite chose aromatherapy as her favorite complementary medicine for healing.

In Closing

The evidence is conclusive that essential oils are extremely effective in eliminating infections without the side effects and resistance that antibiotics generate. Today we have MRSA, a methicillin-resistant *Staphylococcus aureus* that has patients return home from a hospital with a serious infection. This is an area where essential oils can triumph if used diligently. We need more American research with double-blind studies in vitro and in vivo to show hospital administrators that essential oils are a convincing solution.

CHAPTER SEVENTEEN

Immune Stimulating Effect of Essential Oils

It is through those encounters [with germs] that the immune system learns to protect us from serious infections.

—ANDREW WEIL

FOR WOMEN AND MEN who are healers, this is an exciting time to live. There is so much dissatisfaction with the heavy-handed, expensive, and often toxic allopathic system that many people are returning to their herbal roots and rediscovering healing arts like essential oil therapy. Since the days of Elizabeth I, improvements in social sanitation systems—garbage disposal, water filtration, and hygiene standards—have prolonged the life span of humanity. Western medicine has made incredible gains in eliminating many diseases through drugs, inoculation, surgery, and radiation. However, the terminator approach of seeking the enemy (bacteria) and destroying it with drugs kills healthy cells and beneficial bacteria as well. These drugs are often toxic to the homeostasis of the human metabolism and create many side effects. They do not deal with the real cause of disease, which often originates as a mental and emotional imbalance. For example, there is an epidemic of Americans taking pharmaceutical pain-killers to numb physical and emotional malaise. (More on pain in Chapter 19.) In addition, many tests of allopathic drugs are done on animals with positive results, and later these drugs are discovered to have horrible side effects on humans. People are realizing that we need the Western medical approach for emergencies and interceptive operations, but we also require the preventive and the building-from-within approach of nutrition, herbs, and essential oils.

There is a worldwide antibiotic crisis. According to Michael Schmidt, "The discovery of penicillin in 1928 ushered in one of the greatest changes in modern medical history—the antibiotic era."[1] Most of the medical community celebrated, thinking that infectious diseases would be totally eliminated. But eighty years later, we know now that a danger has been hidden in the overuse of these drugs. One effect of overprescribing antibiotics by doctors throughout the Western world is the disruption of the normal ecology of the millions of bacteria in a delicately balanced system in the human body. This makes the body more susceptible to yeast (fungal) and viral infections. Other effects are the suppression of the immune system, the creation of food allergies, and the nutrient loss of the C and B vitamins. A major problem that we face today is bacterial resistance to antibiotics. The microbial world reinvents itself every moment with new strains that antibiotics can't touch.

The Immune System

John Muir wrote, "Contemplating the lace-like fabric of streams outspread over the mountains, we are reminded that everything is flowing—going somewhere. The snow flows fast or slow in grand beauty making glaciers and avalanches; the air in majestic floods carrying minerals, plant leaves, seeds, spores, with streams of music and fragrance; water streams carrying rocks both in solution and in the form of mud particles, sand, pebbles, and boulders. Animals flock together and flow in currents modified by stepping, leaping, gliding, flying, swimming. The stars go streaming through space pulsed on and on forever like blood globules in Nature's warm heart."[2]

In examining the circulatory, the lymph, and the immune systems of humans, we see how many of these inner systems mimic the flows of nature occurring outside of us. The blood is like a major river with minor tributaries to connect to every particle of earth and the lymph is the smaller streams that pool in the rocky areas of the lymph nodes to filter the impurities. The immune system is the sun, rain, and earth that affect the watery tributaries and travel like minerals or white blood cells to bring the greatest balance and protection to the flow of liquid. These three bodily systems are indissolubly linked, the circulatory system bringing every cell more oxygen and eliminating carbon dioxide, the lymph system eliminating toxic waste material from the cells and blood, and the immune system preventing growth of foreign invaders that can bring disease.

Many factors can build or debilitate the human immune system. The system exists in the bloodstream as white blood cells, which are about one-sixteenth as numerous as red blood cells. Examining your blood under a powerful microscope is a fascinating experience. I once had my blood analyzed. The medical technologist put my blood between two glass plates; a TV monitor showed the activity between the plates. She exclaimed that my white blood cells were unusually active. She moved the microscope to another end of the plates and revealed an ugly, rectangular, fuzzy free radical. I was horrified at the sight but was amazed to see two white blood cells, one above and one below the strange rectangle, gobbling up the free radical right before our eyes. This was living proof that the white blood cells—the phagocytes, T cells, and B cells—are there to defend the body from infection. It was one of my proudest moments! The medical technologist asked what I did in my life to have such an active immune system. I told her I try to eat well, exercise regularly, and use essential oils. She began using essential oils the next day and recommending them to her clients.

Humans have sophisticated immune systems that can deal with specific microorganisms. They have memory immune cells that recognize bacteria invaders and they distinguish between self and nonself cells. The immune system mostly functions incredibly well on our behalf, but we also have many autoimmune diseases (such as chronic fatigue, rheumatoid arthritis, and lupus) in which the immune system mistakenly attacks normal tissues. The amazing drama of this system is one of my favorites.

The immune system consists of the following:

Skin: The first line of the body's defense is the acid pH of skin and sebum from the sebaceous glands. Microorganisms must enter the body. The skin is a strong physical barrier against them. When skin is broken, they can easily get through to the bloodstream.

Mucous membranes: The second line of defense is all the mucous membranes, for example, in the throat, the windpipe, and the bronchial tubes. They help trap viruses that manage to get past the mouth or nose. They can be expelled through sneezing or coughing. The mucous membranes of the digestive system, such as the esophagus, snare bacteria embedded in food or water. The stomach mucosa and hydrochloric acids attack infectious microbes. The intestines contain permanent colonies of helpful bacteria that kill invading harmful microorganisms. Some of these tiny destructive creatures enter our bodies during sexual intercourse, where they meet their demise due to the acidic environment of the vaginal mucous.

Lymph nodes: These are throughout the entire body, especially under the arms, in the groin, and under the collarbone. When the white blood cells are fighting off bacteria invaders, the lymph nodes become enlarged due to the proliferation and dying of white blood cells. The nodes are the home of the B and T cells, waiting to be called to action.

Bone marrow: In the center of large, flat bones like the pelvis is a soft, spongy tissue, the bone marrow. Large white blood cells called *phagocytes* are born here alongside mature red blood cells and platelets. The B and T cells originate in the bone marrow as immature lymphocytes. The T cells then move to the thymus gland and the B cells migrate to the lymph nodes.

Thymus gland: Located behind the breastbone, the thymus gland shrinks with age. Ann Percival, an English aromatherapist and nurse, writes, "Stem cells are chemically attracted to the thymus, where they are modified to become T-cells."[3] When the T cells become immunocompetent, they migrate via the blood to the lymph nodes.

Spleen: An organ lying under the lower left ribcage, the spleen functions as a filter for tired red and white blood cells. It can be a site for B cell antibody production.

Phagocytes: These large white blood cells were discovered by Elie Metchinoff in 1888 in Russia when he looked at blood through a crude microscope. These nonspecific members of the immune system (they attack any invaders) are formed in bone marrow. They literally wrap their tentacles around foreign bacteria to bring them into their central body, where they store enzymes (lysozymes) to kill them. Mature and large phagocytes are called macrophages. Phagocytes can travel freely throughout the entire body, keeping it clean of unwanted bacteria, kind of like a traveling vacuum cleaner. If they can't recognize a foreign antigen, they take it to the T cells for proper identification. Their true home is the lymph nodes, where they detoxify the liquid lymph of all impurities that flow through.

B cells: Originating in lymph tissue and bone marrow, these white blood cells identify and destroy nonself antigens. When a foreign invader such as a virus binds to the surface receptors on a B cell, it becomes activated to undergo clonal selection. This B cell multiplies to form an army of daughter duplicate cells bearing the same antigen-specific receptors. Most of these clone cells become plasma cells that manufacture antibodies from complex proteins at a rate of 2,000 per second. This flurry of activity lasts about four to five days and then the plasma cells begin to die. Some plasma memory B cells stay alive in the bloodstream after the battle. Once antibodies are produced against a certain bacteria, lifetime immunity to that particular microorganism has been established. Ann Percival states, "If an antibody has already been prepared through a previous invasion in the body, then the B-cells can react very quickly by releasing the specific antibody to help bring a new invasion quickly under control."[4] The antibodies are in five groups named IgM, IgA, IgD, IgG, and IgE (MADGE).

Immunity is actively acquired during a battle against infection or when we receive a vaccine, and passively acquired when a fetus obtains the mother's antibodies through the placenta or when an antitoxin serum is injected to fight rabies and poisonous snakebites. As stated in the *Harvard Medical School Family Health Guide*, "One of the many wonders of the immune system is its ability to produce a vast variety of very specific antibodies that are able to lock onto a huge variety of germs."[5]

Essential oils boast antibody immunity both active and passive. Studies have shown how German chamomile *(Matricaria recutita)* increases the number of B-lymphocytes.[6] Daniel Pénoël believes IgG, an antibody secreted for long-term defense, is similar to the actions of essential oils with monoterpene alcohols such as Tea tree *(Melaleuca alternifolia)* and Peppermint *(Mentha piperita)*.[7]

T cells: Activated by the thymus gland, T cells coordinate the activities of all the other types of white blood cells. This gland transforms and graduates four functionally different T cells:

- Natural killer T cells: These T cells are called *leukocytes* because they can directly kill cancer and virus cells before the B cell and other T cells, both of which are lymphocytes, are enlisted. The natural killer cells are not antigen specific like the lymphocytes. The natural T cells secrete a toxic chemical called *perforin* into the invader's plasma membrane to kill it. Elaine Marieb in *Essentials of Human Anatomy and Physiology* wrote, "They can act spontaneously by recognizing certain sugars on the intruder's surface.... They attack the cell's membrane and release several chemicals [perforin]. Thereafter the target cell's membrane and nucleus disintegrate."[8]

- Helper T cells: As the intelligent directors of the immune system, helper T cells are like soldiers on patrol, traveling through the bloodstream to every cell in the body. They are always on the lookout for any invading bacteria or virus. The macrophage acts as an antigen presenter when it is overwhelmed and has ingested an antigen to display parts of it on its surface membranes. This unique antigen is recognized by a helper T cell that bears receptors for the same antigen. Also the macrophage releases monokines that enhance T cell activation. T cells return to a lymph node and find B cells that carry the right antigen receptors for this invading bacteria scourge. T cells release chemicals called *lymphokines* that stimulate proliferation and the activity of other helper T cells, phagocytes, enhancing the B cells and killer T cells to rid the body of antigens. These amazing cells have real intelligence and the ability to communicate.
- Suppressor T cells: These cells release chemicals to suppress the activity of T and B cells after an antigen has been effectively destroyed. They help wind down the immune system response.
- Memory T cells: After a battle memory T cells stay alive to provide the immunological memory for subsequent invasions.

What an astounding community of protective molecules we all have within us!

Today we have an epidemic surrounding the immune system because HIV (human immunodeficiency virus) kills the helper T cells and thus immobilizes the rest of the white blood cells to resist invading bacteria. The immune system needs the leadership ability of the helper T cells (also called *CD4 cells*). The macrophage presenters and the helper T cells that create the "double handshake" are vital to the effectiveness of the immune system. When their number is reduced by HIV to 200, a person is considered to have AIDS (autoimmune deficiency syndrome) and is very susceptible to secondary infections, which the essential oils can help combat.

Other inhibitors of the immune system are our lifestyle of *stress*. Too many stressors, both physical and mental, cause the white blood cells to shut down or multiply too rapidly, creating a whole spectrum of modern autoimmune diseases like lupus, chronic fatigue, rheumatoid arthritis, and even lymphoma. Essential oil therapy and stress are discussed in Chapter 19, "Essential Oils and the Mind-Body Connection." Other disrupters of the immune system are chemotherapy, toxic drugs like steroids, tobacco smoke, pesticides, or petroleum-derived ingredients in our food and medicine. We have created an environment of poisonous air, water, and soil, which affects all of the plants we ingest from lettuce to peppermint.

Our immune system struggles to maintain our health by fighting off all of the free radicals created by man-made toxins. This was not a factor during the lives of Esther and the women who lived at the time of Jesus. Essential oils are vital to empowering the immune system. See the "Blend for Immune Deficiency" at the end of this chapter.

The Lymph System

The lymph system provides a means of detoxifying the body through a large series of capillaries or channels similar to the circulatory system of arteries and veins. The osmotic pressure on capillary beds forces fluid out of the blood at the arterial (artery) end of capillary beds ("upstream") so it is reabsorbed at the venous (vein) end ("downstream"). The fluid that remains behind can accumulate in the tissues and cause edema. This impairs the ability of the body's cells to make proper exchanges of oxygen and carbon dioxide with the blood. The main purpose of the lymphatic vessels is to absorb this excess fluid or *lymph* ("clear water"), filter it, and return it to the bloodstream.

Lymph flows only toward the heart. The lymph capillaries spiderweb their way through connective tissues in the body. Proteins, cell debris, bacteria, and even viruses easily enter the lymphatic capillaries, especially in inflamed areas. The lymph vessels flow through many lymph nodes where they are cleansed of toxic waste by macrophages (phagocytes) and lymphocytes with their active vacuum-cleaner enzymes to keep infection at a minimum. When large numbers of bacteria and viruses are trapped in the nodes, they become inflamed and tender to the touch. If cancerous cells overwhelm the nodes, as in lymphoma, they are swollen but not painful.

Generally, the lymph system promotes the movement of all the white blood cells around the body to fight infection. This is another fantastic system that works below consciousness to keep us healthy.

Essential oils like Rosemary (*Rosmarinus officinalis*), Grapefruit (*Citrus x paradisi*), and Fennel (*Foeniculum vulgare*) empower the lymph system to be more active in its waste management. These oils can be used in a massage on the lymph-node areas or in a bath. A lymphatic drainage massage would begin with the hands or feet and bring the strokes inward toward the clavicle bone in the upper chest. The lymph drains under the clavicle collarbone into the subclavian veins. The benefit of a massage with Rosemary, Grapefruit, and Fennel is increased by bathing in them and applying them using a dry brush with oils applied. The brush can follow the same strokes as the lymphatic drainage massage.

Elizabeth I needed an external lymph system in the castles of her time to remove the garbage and toxic human by-products that built up when so many people in her entourage lived in one building for a long period of time. With her sensitive nose we can understand why she craved using essential oils. Her love of Lemon *(Citrus x limon)* with all its antiseptic, antitoxic, depurative qualities helped to keep her lymphatic system strong under such stinky circumstances.

Case Study: Lymphatic-Stimulating Blend

A student, C.R., realized that her mother's lymph and digestive system was way out of balance when she asked her mother if she had any physical symptoms she would like to alleviate. Her response was that she had been constipated for thirty years. She had tried various drugs and over-the-counter remedies to no avail. So C.R. created a blend for her and received her mother's agreement to apply it to her abdominal area at least once a day. Here are the ingredients of the blend:

11 drops Marjoram *(Origanum majorana)*
10 drops sweet Orange *(Citrus sinensis)*
6 drops Fennel *(Foeniculum vulgare)*
6 drops Thyme *(Thymus vulgaris)*
6 drops Grapefruit *(Citrus paradisi)*
2 ounces olive oil *(Olea europaea)*

C.R. reported that the "constipation blend" was a huge success. Her mother reported that after two days of use she began going to the bathroom at a tremendous rate. She claimed not to have had such bowel movements for thirty years. She said, "I feel like I have been clearing out my body. It's like a miracle." Later C.R. needed to make an anxiety-reducing blend for her mother because the continual clearing out made her uneasy.

C.R. reported that in the following months her mother's overall health was greatly improved due to this lymphatic-stimulating blend that boosted her immune system.

The Adrenal Glands

The next incredible line of defense is the adrenal glands, which sit like little mountain peaks atop the kidneys. They have glandular (cortex) and neural (medulla) tissue. They produce three major groups of steroid hormones: mineralocorticoids, glucocorticoids (which include cortisone and cortisol), and the sex hormones. The glucocorticoids help the body resist long-term stressors by increasing blood glucose levels. They are released from the adrenal cortex in response to rising blood levels of ACTH (adrenocorticotropic hormone) from the pituitary. The ACTH loop is discussed in Chapter 19, "Essential Oils and the Mind-Body Connection."

The state of our adrenals determines how well we handle stress. They are activated by the pituitary gland, the master gland, to produce more adrenaline and cortisol hormones when the body needs to aid and bolster the white blood cells. The adrenals also control the amount of the hormone DHEA (dehydroepiandrosterone) in our system. When the adrenals become exhausted or "whipped" by too much mental stress and too many cycles of having to produce more hormones, we experience a lower resistance to infection.

The essential oils of Geranium *(Pelargonium graveolens)*, Spruce *(Picea mariana)*, and Pine *(Pinus sylvestris)* have a beneficial effect on the adrenals and other glands too. Using a diluted blend, rub the oils over the lower back area when feeling stressed or fatigued. Drinking a cup of licorice tea *(Glycyrrhiza glabra)* can help heal stressed adrenal glands.

Mental Thoughts

The next line of defense—or perhaps the first and foremost line of defense—is our mental thoughts. This is where the mind-body connection comes into play. The ability to think positive thoughts is key to having a strong immune system. Our general health is intrinsically connected to the quality of our mental life. Michael Schmidt comments, "Optimists have more

T-helper cells in their immune systems than pessimists. Optimists also suffer only half the number of infections and make fewer trips to the doctor."[9] This is discussed further in Chapter 19, "Essential Oils and the Mind-Body Connection," which focuses on pyschoneuroimmunology and essential oils. Using essential oils such as Ylang-ylang *(Cananga Odorata)*, Roman chamomile *(Chamaemelum nobile)*, Bay laurel *(Laurus nobilis)*, and Elemi *(Canarium luzonicum)* create an uplifted mental state.

The Colon

Another vital line of defense is the colon. If the colon is kept clean and clear, it allows millions of friendly bacteria to suppress and control invaders. Its major functions are to dry out the indigestible food residue by absorbing water and to eliminate this dried-out mass from the body as feces. The essential oils of Fennel, Angelica *(Angelica archangelica)*, and Juniper *(Juniperus communis)* can aid the removal of waste material and support the work of the colon. The whole immune system is thus able to more effectively resist invading viruses and bacteria. Hildegard intuitively knew this in the eleventh century. She wrote, "Most patients with gastritis, which mainly causes stomach pains in elderly persons, have a deficiency of gastric digestive juices. They ... can be helped by taking one tablespoon of Clary sage *(Salvia sclaria)* stomach tonic after each meal. Good digestion is very important to good health."[10]

Case Study: Pain and Constipation

A student, C.C., had a client, K.J., who had been in a serious car accident. Six months later, after lengthy physical therapy, K.J. was in serious physical and emotional decline. Due to much pain and continual cold infections, doctors performed a laminectomy (a spine operation to remove the portion of the vertebral bone called the *lamina*). They cleaned her vertebrae through an incision on the anterior neck and took a piece of bone from her hip to repair the neck. Postoperatively, she was taking a lot of pain medication and was confined to her home with many cold and flu bugs plaguing her.

C.C. made this blend for K.J.:

12 drops Cypress *(Cupressus sempervirens)* for balancing body
fluids and to help with constipation

7 drops Lemongrass *(Cymbopogan citratus)* to tone the muscles and
eliminate lactic acid

10 drops Juniper *(Juniperus communis)* for pain relief and to purify
body and mind

4 drops Mandarin *(Citrus reticulata)* to cheer her mind and balance
constipation

2 ounces almond oil *(Prunus amygdalus)*

K.J. applied the oil to her incision and all around her neck and hip. First
she reported that she no longer had constipation and she felt her ability
to fight off colds was improved. Also her pain subsided from twice daily
use of the blend. Here is another example of how clearing the colon provides the immune system with more strength to ward off infection.

Strengthening the Immune System

An example of the differences between traditional and integrative medicine is shown in a person with the HIV virus. When this pernicious virus
invades the body, it begins to reproduce itself in a host cell, the helper T
cells of the immune system. The HIV virus destroys the T cells, which leaves
the body at the mercy of invading bacteria, other viruses, and fungi. The
Western medical approach is to prescribe drugs that attack the virus.
However, within a short time the virus can develop drug-resistant strains.
The essential oil approach would be to administer oils that strengthen the
lymphocyte immune system specifically and provide a tonic for both physical and emotional heath generally.

Here's an example: Thyme, Tea tree, and Roman chamomile are all
immune-stimulant oils. They could be massaged over the chest, which
includes the area of the thymus gland, to stimulate production of killer
T cells and to strengthen helper T cells. Other oils such as Lavender
(Lavandula angustifolia), Orange *(Citrus sinensis)*, and Bergamot *(Citrus
x bergamia)* would be good to help the patient relax, and to feel emotionally uplifted and able to boast the immune system through mind fitness.
A potent oil, Garlic *(Allium sativum)* could best be used on the bottom
of the feet, diluted 4 percent in carrier oil for a seriously depleted person

with constant infections. The odor and effects of garlic oil are so strong it would be best to apply to the feet. This approach would build mind-body health instead of just attempting to destroy disease.

A 1995 double-blind study by Komori, Fujiwara, Tanida, Nomura, and Yokoyama is described in *Neuroimmunomodulation*.[11] Previous animal experiments showed citrus fragrance could restore stress-induced immuno-suppression. A new citrus fragrance was created using a blend of Lemon, Orange, and Bergamot oils with cis-4-hexenol. Twenty depressed male inpatients were divided into two groups. One (AD group) was given pharmaceutical antidepressants alone and the other (CF group) was exposed to the citrus fragrance while having their medication reduced weekly until their depression was in remission. By the end of the eleventh week, the CF group reduced their antidepressant drug intake to zero. The AD group still needed the medication at twelve weeks. Cortisol and dopamine levels were significantly lower in the CF group. The natural killer cell activity was significantly higher when compared to the AD group. The results support the concept that human depression is based on homeostatic dysregulation and citrus oils improve the homeostatic balance more than antidepressant drugs. The researchers concluded with the suggestion that the use of citrus oils could be of psychoneuroimmunological benefit for the treatment of emotions and the immune system.

Oil blend for immune deficiency

Blend the following:

> 6 drops Thyme *(Thymus vulgaris)*
> 7 drops Lemon *(Citrus x limon)*
> 6 drops Tea tree *(Melaleuca alternifolia)*
> 3 drops Roman Chamomile *(Chamaemelum nobile)*
> 4 drops Niaouli *(Melaleuca quinquenervia viridiflora)*
> 3 drops Ravintsara *(Cinnamomum camphora)*
> 2 ounces sesame oil *(Sesamun inidicum)*

Use twice a day for one week on neck and chest. Take a break for ten days and begin again for another two weeks. Also use this blend in a bath. Eat greens and unprocessed foods and drink lots of water. Use this blend regularly, even when you are feeling healthy. You will experience great improvement in your immune system.

Herbs for the immune system are echinacea *(Echinacea angustifolia)*, goldenseal *(Hydrastis canadensis)*, and astragalus *(Radix astragali membranaceus)*. Take 4 drops of each in tincture form every day. Echinacea is best to use in capsules or tincture when a cold, flu, or infections is coming on, then discontinue after five or six days. Astragalus is best to use long term, taking the capsules daily for three or four weeks in the fall, strengthening the immune system for the coming winter colds.

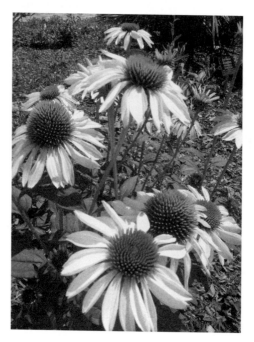

Echinacea

In Closing

Essential oils work two ways to support the immune system: They directly kill bacteria or viruses when doing a steam, applying them to the skin, or taking a bath with seven to ten drops. They also fortify certain members of the immune system, for example the way Thyme *(Thymus vulgaris)* boosts the phagocytes' actions in the body. Medicine of the future will certainly chose to include the path of preventive immune-stimulating oils and herbs when more knowledge is available. This book is intended to elicit such a response.

CHAPTER EIGHTEEN

Optimal Health with Essential Oil, Nutritional, and Herbal Therapy

What a person wants and enjoys is apt to be just what is good for him.

—ABRAHAM MASLOW

IN MY YEARS OF TEACHING, researching, reading, and living, I have come to realize that essential oils alone will not bring someone who is in a state of disease back to healthy homeostasis. As powerful as the oils are in their effects on human beings, they can work only in a limited manner over a period of time unless a healthy lifestyle of good nutrition, energetic exercise, and positive thinking is not practiced simultaneously. The oils can offer outstandingly affirmative effects when a healthy lifestyle exists. The case studies in this book show striking examples of how the oils fortified the immune system against a physical malaise or uplifted the mind to overcome an emotional imbalance. In our present-day world, in which people tend toward stress, obesity, and degenerative diseases, it takes a mighty desire and a strong will to bring a totally healthy lifestyle into being. It requires using organic, living, or lightly cooked foods, slowly replacing pharmaceuticals with herbal extracts and essential oils, and a commitment to exercising for thirty minutes five days a week. Practicing meditation on a daily basis offers the mind and the emotions a way to be grounded, inspired, and guided to spiritual health.

In my life I have found that good health depends on how many good habits I practice. Deepak Chopra writes in *Creating Health,* "Every habit is a cooperative venture between body and mind. Generally speaking, the mind leads the venture and the body follows as a silent partner...."[1] A habit such as drinking a glass of pure water with the juice of half a lemon and one drop of lemon essential oil *(Citrus x limon)* in it every morning should be acquired effortlessly over a period of time guided by positive thoughts on how the lemon cleanses the blood and liver.

In my pursuit of healthy vitality, I seek to stay close to nature. There are so many temptations in our modern world to veer off the track with fast foods, synthetic chemicals, and man-made environments. Sometimes it's the quantity that counts. Drinking a rich, melodious bottle of wine, which originates in the vineyard and nourishes the body and spirit, is healthy if imbibed in small amounts. As we all know, drinking daily in large quantities leads to a toxic body and diseases like Parkinson's, chronic heart failure, and cancer. When I eat unprocessed food that is organically grown, such as green leafy vegetables, yellow squash, and peppers, I feel on track with my body's vitamin and mineral needs. When I eat too many sweets, such as pecan pie or chocolate cookies, I begin to feel achy joints and stomach indigestion that leads to arthritis, colitis, diabetes, and colon cancer. If I replace the sweets with kiwi fruit, tangerines, and pears, I feel light and able to easily digest my nourishment. Daily taking vitamins A through E and digestive enzymes, since our food supply is not always reliable, helps to nourish my cells. When I drink pure water from a reliable source, I feel refreshed and detoxified. When I spend some time each day in the sun and fresh air, I know my skin receives some vitamin D and my lungs are replenished with unpolluted oxygen. How fortunate are those who can walk in the woods or garden to receive the oxygen directly from the plants. City parks are good too. Better yet, walking or running on the beach gives you delicious air to breathe and a chance to be in close vicinity with sea plants, which provide over 70 percent of the oxygen generated on our planet.

When I acquire essential oils from the most excellent distillers all over the globe and have them GC-MS analyzed for purity, I know I'm offering my body, emotions, and spirit the finest the plant world has to offer. I then apply the oils in my body care, using Rose *(Rosa damascena)* from Bulgaria with a facial lotion, and in first aid, using an oil like Tea tree *(Melaleuca alternifolia)* from Australia. When I use herbal extracts such as Saint John's wort *(Hypericum perforatum)* for mild depression and burdock root *(Arctium lappa)* for blood cleansing instead of pharmaceutical drugs, I know I am respecting the natural way without chemical side effects for my

ADULTHOOD, MALE AND FEMALE

These oils can be employed in perfume, baths, massage, shampoo, steam, gargle, and Jacuzzi:

Pine *(Pinus sylvestris)*
Rosemary *(Rosmarinus officinalis)*
Lemon *(Citrus x limon)*
Thyme *(Thymus vulgaris)*
Peppermint *(Mentha piperita)*
Carrot seed *(Daucus carota)*
Helichrysum *(Helichrysum italicum)*
Elemi *(Canarium luzonicum)*
Orange *(Citrus sinensis)*
Cardamom *(Elettaria cardamomum)*
Cajeput *(Melaleuca cajuputi)*
Bay laurel *(Laurus nobilis)*
Black pepper *(Piper nigrum)*

MENOPAUSE

Apply these oils to the neck and lower abdomen (4 drops each in 1 ounce carrier oil):

Cypress *(Cupressus sempervirens)*
Geranium *(Pelargonium graveolens)*
Sage *(Salvia officinalis)*
Fennel *(Foeniculum vulgare)*
Rose *(Rosa damascena)*

Use these oils to balance the adrenals and erratic emotions:

Spruce *(Picea mariana)*
German chamomile *(Matricaria recutita)*
Ylang-ylang *(Cananga odorata)*

ELDERLY YEARS, MALE AND FEMALE

Treat yourself to a foot or hand massage with carrier oil or lotion plus 2 drops each of the following:

Marjoram *(Origanum majorana)*
Spruce *(Picea mariana)*
Ravensara *(Ravensara aromaticum)*
Violet *(Viola odorata)*
Sandalwood *(Santalum album)*

Include 4 to 6 drops total (depending on skin sensitivity) of three of the following oils to 1 ounce lotion for body massage:

Juniper *(Juniperus communis)*
Melissa *(Melissa officinalis)*
Angelica *(Angelica archangelica)*
Neroli *(Citrus x aurantium l. amara)*
Eucalyptus radiata *(Eucalyptus radiata)*
Spikenard *(Nardostachys grandiflora)*
Lavender *(Lavandula angustifolia)*
Galbanum *(Ferula gummosa)*
Rosewood *(Aniba rosaeodora)*

In Closing

Enjoy the delightful scents and effects of the above oils as your life unfolds through all its myriad stages. The oils will rejuvenate your body, mind, and spirit, especially if you keep your lifestyle in balance, eating fresh local foods, sleeping seven to eight hours each night, and exercising regularly, ideally out in nature.

CHAPTER NINETEEN

Essential Oils and the Mind-Body Connection

Fragrance is a conduit for our earliest memories, on the one hand; on the other, it may accompany us as we enter the next life. In between, it creates mood, stimulates fantasy, shapes thought, and modifies behavior. It is our strongest link to the past, our closest fellow traveler to the future. Prehistory, history, and the afterworld, all are its domain. Fragrance may well be the signature of eternity.

—TOM ROBBINS

ONE OF THE MOST IMPORTANT developments in research on human health in the twentieth century was the discovery that the mind and body are indissolubly linked together on a physical, cellular level as well as an emotional or energetic level. The mind and body were separated in the beliefs of Western culture by the influence of the rationalistic ideas and writings of French philosopher René Descartes in the seventeenth century (1596–1650). His famous saying, "I think therefore I am," lingers on today. He believed in dualism: the body works like a machine and the mind as a nonmaterial entity.

Today we realize that treating just physical symptoms such as back or joint pain with a pharmaceutical drug is inadequate to heal the disease. This truth points to observing mental thoughts as being vital in helping a client find symptom relief. About 75 to 80 percent of all doctor visits are for stress-related problems, according to Bill Moyers in *Healing and the Mind*.[1] Emotional stress can cause or influence major medical problems such as high blood pressure, ulcers, and migraine headaches. Some of the pathways that the mind uses to affect the immune system, the digestive system, the endocrine system, and the nervous system are examined in this chapter. Looking at patterns of usually negative thoughts and substituting self- and life-affirming ideas can often make a paradigm shift from physical illness to health. This is a truth that Hildegard de Bingen recognized during her life about 1140 AD (see Chapter 8). She many times struggled with painful headaches and serious illness before her faith reemerged to bring her illuminating insights into the meaning of life.

Here is my understanding of the real goal we seek as human beings. Mind-body health is achieved when our thoughts, our emotions, and our physical bodies are in harmony, inspired by our inner spirit. Essential oils that work simultaneously on all levels are the perfect instruments to bring this about. They are the gifts from God in the plant world that magnetize us toward this optimum state of balance.

A friend of mine developed migraine headaches whenever she came in contact with Tom, her ex-husband and father of her ten-year-old son. She felt Tom did not see who she really was, and he had many negative judgments and unrealistic expectations that boxed her in. She sought help from her doctor, who prescribed pain medication with no understanding of her emotional and mental situation. The pain medicine made her feel more enclosed, imprisoned with only momentary relief. She described her life as if she were locked in a cage with electrical shocks painfully zapping her head through the bars. When she tried to call out, her voice was muted and she became invisible. This is a vivid example of a mind-body imbalance that requires more than a prescription drug to remedy. When she came to see me, I interviewed her looking first at all the complex relationships and emotional entanglements. I offered her an essential oil blend, an herbal tincture, and lifestyle changes that addressed the emotional stress. Later, when the migraines subsided, I offered her a pain relief blend that she could use for emergency symptoms. Thanks to the blend, meditation, some diet changes, and increased self-esteem, she now rarely experiences migraines. She and I had to address the deeper emotional issues to resolve the pain.

In the twenty-first century, we live in a much faster paced life than most of our heroines of the past. We have new kinds of struggles that many of these women did not experience. As we deal with a world of jet lag, freeway speed and road rage, pesticides in our food, bombardment from the media with murders, wars, and terrorism, and chemical overload in our environment, we feel great stress in our mind-body systems. Instead of going to war with the Romans or dealing with animosity between the Protestants and Catholics, we feel global tensions from the media's ability to immediately bring yesterday and today's happenings into our homes. Due to the emphasis on negative news, we daily absorb an unhealthy physical and emotional environment. These bombardments have brought imbalances to our endocrine, nervous, and immune systems. Together these systems make up the field of study called *pyschoneuroimmunology*. Essential oils are potent tools to help ameliorate some of the problems for modern women and men.

As we explore this new field of pyschoneuroimmunology, we must acknowledge the originator, Candace B. Pert. Her revolutionary research as a neurophysicist showed the dynamic network of peptides that link the body and the mind and establish the biochemical basis for emotions and consciousness. Deepak Chopra has written of her, "Her pioneering research has demonstrated how our internal chemicals, the neuropeptides and their receptors, are the actual biological underpinnings of our awareness, manifesting themselves as our emotions, beliefs, and expectations, and profoundly influencing how we respond to and experience our world.... There is a revolution taking form that is significantly influencing how the Western medical community views health and disease."[2]

While working at John Hopkins University as a graduate student in 1972, Pert's discovery of the opiate receptors in the limbic brain led to a mad scientific dash to find the natural substances in the body that use the receptors. Her research showed neural receptors present on almost all of the body's cells. This took her to the amazing realization that the neurotransmitters in the neurons and protein peptides, which are a string of amino acids, join together like beads in a necklace and travel in our bloodstream. This is the chemical brain that allows us to have a mobile mindbrain throughout the whole body. According to her research, a capacity for decision making, remembering, and feeling is stored in the digestive, the immune, the endocrine, and the neurological systems. Essential oils also travel in the bloodstream and find receptors, acting as catalysts for homeostasis and balance along with the hormones and wandering peptide emotions.

As the neuropeptides flow in the bloodstream, looking for the right receptors on cells, the mind-body becomes interconnected when the peptide key links with the lock of the cell's receptor. This dynamic key-lock action gives the body a communication network to inform every system and cell of the emotions and thoughts you are experiencing. There are no secrets between the mind and the body. Western medicine is beginning to acknowledge this bridge.

The mind can be subdivided into the conscious and the subconscious. The subconscious is a place of memory tapes derived from instincts and learned experience, mostly programmed during childhood. These tapes play constantly, especially when the conscious mind is distracted. If your conscious mind wants to affirm your self-worth, it can be easily undermined by the subconscious mind's program of how inadequate you are from parents' or teachers' attitudes toward you in early childhood.

As we know now, when someone experiences emotional trauma as a child or even as an adult, the emotions need recognition and release. Of course, it is important not to dump your raw emotions on another person as you process and express them. Candace Pert wrote, "... I believe that repressed emotions are stored in the body—the unconscious mind—via the release of neuropeptide ligands, and that memories are held in their receptors."[3] These unexpressed emotions eventually lead to dis-ease or disease later in life.

Expressing positive, honest thoughts can bring health to an ailing body. Unexplored unconscious emotions can make a body diseased. Sometimes transformations occur through the emotional catharsis of mind-body therapies such as visualization, Rolfing massage, essential oil therapy, sound healing, acupuncture, and many others.

Birth

One of the most poignant examples of emotions stored in the body is birth trauma. The energy and conditions of a birth set the tone for a person's whole life. During its life as a fetus, the unborn child absorbs nutrients, emotions, and hormones from its mother. A healthy birth of conscious, loving parents, who are physically and psychologically prepared, using natural means, can bring immense benefits to all. Each birth is unique. A birth that requires many hours of labor (due to blockages, such as a plugged cervix, a uterus that can't contract, or a breech baby) can leave emotional scars on the baby. The mother's and father's mental state and mood have an impact on how easy or difficult a birth can be. The baby can experience these emotions as a growing fetus or as a newly born baby. Sometimes these emotions will surface later as an adult due to energetic therapies or events.

Once labor has really started—the cervix is dilating and the uterus is contracting every ten minutes—an essential oil blend can be applied to invigorate the birth process. The oils of Frankincense *(Boswellia carteri),* Lavender *(Lavandula angustifolia),* and Jasmine *(Jasminum grandiflorum)* can be applied to the sacrum (lower) area of the spine and on the bottom of the feet. These oils help to calm the mother yet revitalize the energy of the baby moving down the birth canal. It makes labor more effective, so it usually is no longer than four hours for many of my students. The mother is activating her emotional, intuitive limbic brain consciousness during this process, not the logical neocortex. Frankincense is a strong regulator of the hypothalamus, which during childbirth directs the release of hormones via the pituitary and the autonomic nervous system. Lavender relaxes the central nervous system and the stressed uterine muscles in the mother to provide an easier passage. Jasmine is a mental euphoric and uterine tonic to strengthen and relieve painful cramps. I know from experience the fragrance of the blend will uplift the mother and child and anyone else in the birthing room.

The blend will mitigate the side effects of a traumatic birth! If difficulties occur, a healing method for the baby (or the baby as an adult—it is never too late) is cranial sacral healing modality. This is an energetic massage that subtly shifts the cranial plates to let go of blocked energy occurring from coming down a small, tight birth canal or from the use of forceps. I know in the case of my granddaughter, Audrey, who had just such a birth from her tiny mother, the three cranial sacral treatments realigned her cranial plates and reduced the pain. She no longer had severe colic and grew up to be a happy child.

What is your earliest memory? Can you remember your birth?

Several times in my life, I have found Rose oil *(Rosa damascena)* very effective at dissipating negative emotions or helping to release the memory of trauma. An Italian clinical, in vivo study done in 1999 by T. Umezo with Rose oil used the Vogel conflict test, a standard procedure to evaluate anticonflict effects of drugs. The Rose oil had a significant anticonflict effect, similar to benzodiazepines without any side effects or dependency.[4] The oil eases mental tensions and emotional conflicts.

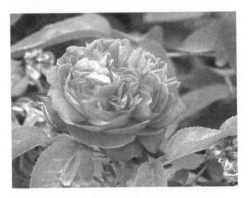

Rose

Central Nervous System

The new field of psychoneuroimmunology brings together at least three systems: the central nervous system, the endocrine system, and the immune system. Understanding how each of these systems function and correlate to each other gives a physiological basis to the mind-body connection. Essential oil therapy deals with the power of essential oils to strengthen the body via the immune system and evoke emotional stability through their work on the limbic brain, the central nervous system, and the endocrine system. This is an ideal modality for mind-body problems.

Let's examine briefly the central nervous system, the autonomic nervous system, the limbic brain, and the endocrine system. These are all extremely complex, yet I will attempt a short summary. The human body is such an awesome group of cells, organs, and systems unified into a magnificent whole. We need to honor this integrated balance!

The central nervous system is the master controlling and communication system. All human cells are linked to and provide information to the brain via the central and peripheral nerves. The millions of sensory receptors note changes both inside and outside the body, sending electrical impulses along nerves to the coordinating brain. There are forty-three major nerves that extend from the brain and spinal cord. Candace Pert's work makes us realize that other parts of the body, such as the immune system, also act as brains and coordinating agents.

The autonomic nervous system extends along the lower brain (such as the hypothalamus, pons, and cerebellum) and spinal cord, regulating involuntary activities. These are the activities that occur without conscious thought or control such as heart rate and digestion. The sympathetic nervous system releases two neurotransmitters, norepinephrine and adrenaline, which are stimulated by strong emotions of anger and fear. This system increases heart rate, blood pressure, and glucose levels for the fight or flight response. The parasympathetic nervous system releases acetylcholine neurotransmitters to act as the housekeeping system when the body is at rest. Working especially hard at night, these neurotransmitters help digestion and elimination, and slow down vascular activity.

An interesting study by Italian researchers in 2002 revealed that the inhalation of Lemon *(Citrus x limon)* reduced the effects of painful stimulation in rats as the oil increased the acetylcholine released in the hippocampus of the limbic brain. It was deducted that the connection between the olfactory system and the hypothalamus affected the essential-oil–induced changes in the acetylcholine release. This shows the connection between the autonomic nervous system, the limbic system, and the sense of smell (olfactory system).[5]

An ideal oil for both of the autonomic nervous systems is one of my favorites, Bay laurel *(Laurus nobilis)*. This detoxifying oil can stimulate the lymphatic system and tonify the liver and kidneys, which makes it very beneficial for the parasympathetic system. It warms up the central nervous system as a cerebral mind stimulant bringing mental courage. It opens us to new perceptions and creativity. This would help balance the primal headstrong sympathetic impulses.

The tissue of the brain includes nerves with billions of neurons that consist of a nucleus and hundreds of slender fibers called *dendrites* that receive electrical messages. These messages are sent to a single strand of the axon, which is on the opposite side of the neuron. It has axonal terminals at the end where chemical messengers called *neurotransmitters* are sent across the synaptic cleft to receptors on a receiving neuron. This is how communication in the nervous system is an electrochemical event! It is repeated endlessly from one neuron to the next. Since each neuron receives and sends signals to scores of other neurons, it carries on many chemical "conversations." Afferent neurons send signals to the brain and spinal cord, whereas efferent neurons send them out to the muscles and skin. A study in 1995 about linalool, which is a terpene alcohol and one of the largest chemical constituents in lavender and clary sage, showed how the action of linalool on glutamate, one of the most excitatory neurotransmitters, was sedative, anticonvulsant, and even hypnotic in the central nervous system.[6]

Some of the essential oils considered nervines are able to balance the central nervous system. This includes Lavender, Angelica *(Angelica archangelica)*, Vetiver *(Vetiveria zizanioides)*, and Roman chamomile *(Chamaemelum nobile)*. They soothe the nerves with esters and sesquiterpenes. A study by Leopold Jirovetz in 1990 at the University of Vienna, Austria, showed Lavender had a dramatic reduction of agitation on mice that had been injected with caffeine.[7]

A research scientist and biologist, Bruce Lipton, who spent much of his professional life studying the single cell, was amazed to realize that the cell's membrane functions like a computer chip. It operates as the cell's brain. This led him eventually to a community of billions of cells, the human brain and mind. He explored quantum physics. He began to look with awe at the power of the mind and its ability to heal our sick body. With a loving, positive orientation or a negative, destructive attitude, the mind overrides the body. He concluded that our beliefs, not our genes, control our lives. In *The Biology of Belief,* Lipton writes, "Young children carefully observe their environment and download the worldly wisdom offered by parents directly into their subconscious memory. As a result, their parents' behavior and beliefs become their own."[8] How marvelous our world would be if we had parents and teachers who would model how to use our conscious and unconscious minds to successfully copilot our lives. The information in the unconscious would be self-affirming and empowering. Thus the creative conscious mind could make decisions without being blocked and thwarted by the subconscious mind. Lipton continues, "For adoptive and non-adoptive parents alike, the message is clear: Your children's genes reflect only their potential, not their destiny. It is up to you to provide the environment that allows them to develop to their highest potential."[9]

Another significant study was done in India in 1976 on the oil of Lemongrass *(Cymbopogon citratus)*. Rats were injected with either 75 or 150 milligrams per milliliter of Lemongrass oil, which had a marked depressive effect on the nervous systems. Both concentrations of oil were analgesic and showed how similar the oil's activity was to tranquilizers like pentobarbitone.[10]

Neuron activity in the brain is divided into specialized functions. The gray matter of the cerebral cortex is one-eighth of an inch thick and has different areas designated for different tasks, for example, motor skills, olfactory, auditory, memory, higher intellectual, speech, and visual. We must remember that we humans, as a present-day species, use only 5 to 10 percent of these highly organized and proficient gray matter cells. What would we be like if we used even 20 percent more?

To keep our minds at top performance, we need to watch our blood sugar fluctuations. The brain needs a constant supply of blood glucose for energy. To avoid brain fatigue and mood swings, we need to keep our blood sugar up. The best diet includes whole foods that have few refined sugars and that are low in fats. The best brain food is low-glycemic carbohydrates such as green vegetables (spinach, zucchini, and chard), herbs (parsley, watercress, and nettles), fruits (apples, apricots, oranges, and pears) and whole grains, which are sugar stabilizing. Excellent examples of grains are millet, quinoa, brown rice, and oats. High-quality protein such as that found in beans, seeds, and nuts will also facilitate stable blood sugar.

Here are four oils that stimulate cephalic brain function:

Rosemary *(Rosmarinus officinalis)*, a brain tonic with its rich chemistry of monoterpenes and sesquiterpenes, 1,8-cineol, alcohols, esters, and ketones, all of which help to enliven brain cells and memory.

Basil *(Ocimum basilicum ct linalool)*, which relieves headaches, tones the nerves, and increases mental concentration.

Peppermint *(Mentha piperita)*, which brings mental concentration and relieves mental fatigue.

Thyme *(Thymus vulgaris)*, which stimulates the brain for a conscious intellectual mind, strengthens nerves, activates brain cells, and improves memory.

Perhaps we all need to make a brain-tonic blend for improving our brain functions.

A study was done in 1994 on the effects of Peppermint and Eucalyptus oil on headaches and the cerebral cortex. Peppermint oil was found to significantly reduce the pain of headaches, more than Eucalyptus. The combination of the two brought mental and muscle relaxation with increased cognitive performance.[11]

Endocrine System

The endocrine system has an incredible impact on the mind-body system. It governs our response to stress and seeks to regulate homeostasis in the body. Chemical messengers or hormones, secreted directly into the blood through ductless glands, are transported "leisurely" through the body. They deal with important processes on a long-term basis such as growth and development; electrolyte, water, and nutrient balance in the blood; and response to energy, sex, and pregnancy. A hormone can pick the right receptor site on one cell among millions. The body can release hundreds of different chemicals in minute quantity and amazingly orchestrate each one to create balance.

Essential oils function in a manner similar to hormones, traveling in the bloodstream to find the correct receptor site and "turn on" the biological activity associated with that oil in the cell. Like hormones, oils pass through the liver, where they are converted into inactive compounds that are excreted by the kidneys. René-Maurice Gattefossé called his book, *Aromatherapie: Les Huiles Essentielles, Hormones Végétales*. Vegetable or plant hormone is a great name for essential oils. He wrote (from the translated version, *Gattefossé's Aromatherapy*), "It is thus apparent that chemical phenomena which modify the composition of a plant's aromatic substances are closely linked to the plant's physiological functions. Experience has shown that factors, which intensify the chlorophyllous function, also promote the etherification of terpene in alcohols. This is, therefore, a biological process very similar to hormonal processes in animals [or people]. . . . Hormones are catalysts of vital functions, with a mechanism we still do not fully understand. . . . Essences are thus extremely powerful and their effects are manifold."[12]

The pituitary gland, called the master gland, is the size of a grape and hangs down from the hypothalamus in the limbic brain. The anterior pituitary produces six hormones that regulate other hormones, including ACTH (adrenocorticotropic hormone), which affects the cortex of the adrenal gland; TH (thyroid-stimulating hormone), which influences the thyroid gland; GH (growth hormone), which stimulates bones and muscles; PRL (prolactin), which stimulates milk production; and the two hormones that stimulate the ovaries, the luteinizing hormone (LH) and the follicle stimulating hormone (FSH). The posterior lobe of the pituitary gland secretes vasopressin, an antidiuretic hormone, and oxytocin, which stimulates contraction of the uterus during labor.

My choice for essential oils for the anterior pituitary would be Petitgrain *(Citrus x aurantium l. amara)*, which is relaxing and calming for the body's hormones and organs, and Geranium *(Pelargonium graveolens)*, the best endocrine harmonizer in general.

The pineal gland secretes the hormone melatonin, a mysterious one that affects the awareness of dark and light cycles and especially sleep cycles. For deeper sleep, I recommend Vetiver and Valerian *(Valeriana officinalis)*.

The thyroid gland produces a major hormone, thyroxin, affecting metabolism by the rate of glucose conversion to body heat, especially in the reproductive and nervous system. The oils of Myrrh *(Commiphora myrrha)* and Palmarosa *(Cymbopogan martini)* benefit the thyroid gland. The hormone calcitonin decreases blood calcium levels by causing calcium to be deposited in bones. The herbs of nettles *(Urtica dioica)* and comfrey *(Symphytum officinalis)* reinforce this action.

The thymus gland produces T cells for the immune system. The gland and immune system respond to Thyme *(Thymus vulgaris)*. Create an immune blend with Thyme, Lemon, and Niaouli *(Melaleuca quinquenervia viridiflora)* to rub on the chest and back. The white blood cells (T cells) created in the thymus will be stimulated into action.

The adrenals are two bean-shaped glands that drape on top of the kidneys. The cortex is glandular and the medulla (center) is neural tissue. The adrenal cortex produces corticosteroids including cortisone and cortisol to resist long-term stress by increasing blood glucose levels. The medulla produces adrenaline and noradrenaline. Spruce oil *(Picea mariana)*, Pine *(Pinus sylvestris)*, and the herb licorice *(Glycyrrhiza glabra)* balance the adrenal hormones to reduce tension and dis-ease or stress.

A famous mind-body loop is called the ACTH loop. Beginning (or ending) with depressed thinking, CRF (corticotrophin-releasing factor) is created in the hypothalamus. In people who commit suicide, ten times the normal amount of CRF is found in their brains. This hormone then activates ACTH in the pituitary, which goes on to stimulate the adrenal cortex that releases cortisol. Often adrenaline is released from the adrenal medulla to add to the stress hormone cocktail. The HPA (hypothalamic pituitary adrenal) axis initiates these hormones for extreme external threats. For example, these hormones affect the digestive system to redistribute blood from the digestive processes to the limbs for fight or flight emergencies. They also repress the immune system since it consumes so much energy when the body is under threat from internal enemies like viruses. All the focus is on fight or flight action.

The hormone cortisol is part of the ACTH loop. It has many effects over time, such as raising blood pressure, lowering immune function, creating insomnia, and weight gain. These physical actions trigger more depressed behavior, depressed mood, and depressed thinking, causing the hormone cycle to repeat itself. Each time it repeats, the physical effects are augmented, leading to serious heart disease, infections due to immune system dysfunction, and weight gain.

A study to illustrate some aspects of this loop was done in Japan in 1998. One group of mice was sensitized with sheep red blood cells and the other group had high pressure stress with immunosuppression, bringing down their PFC (plaque forming cell) count. The inhalation of Lemon, Oakmoss (*Evernia prunastri*), Labdanum (*Cistus ladanifer*), or Tuberose (*Polyanthes tuberosa*) brought their PFC count back to normal. The reduction of the PFC count was attributed to the activation of suppressor T lymphocytes in the immune system via the stimulation of the hypothalamus-pituitary-adrenal systems. This latter activation was blocked by the inhalation of essential oils, allowing the immune system to flourish again.[13]

This loop shows how depressed thinking can alter the autonomic and neuroendocrine output from the brain, modulating immunity. This loop is an incredible illustration of pyschoneuroimmunology. I have seen illustrations in some family members and students.

Using essential oils such as Ylang-ylang (*Cananga odorata*), Frankincense, Spruce (*Picea mariana*), Rose, and Bergamot (*Citrus x bergamia*) in a blend at any point in the cycle can lift the mood, break the flow of hormones, and diminish the physiological symptoms. A 1995 in vivo study on how Bergamot influenced the central nervous system exhibited important sedative and anticonvulsive effects.[14]

I created a deep, colorful-smelling blend of woods and roots called "Break the Cycle" to address the effects of this hormonal ACTH loop. It has Frankincense to regulate the hypothalamus and help us let go of past obsessions, Angelica to detoxify the body of poisons and open the mind and psyche to higher clairvoyance, and Galbanum (*Ferula gummosa*) to benefit the body's chronic conditions and to relieve emotional nervous tension and stress. This mysterious blend of five oils (three mentioned) helps to break the spell of the negative mind-body hormones.

The pancreas is another important source of two hormones—insulin and glucagon—that affect the amount of glucose in the bloodstream. Insulin decreases blood glucose levels and glucagon targets the liver to release glucose. There has been a huge increase in diabetes in the United States in the last twenty years, which is attributed to an increase in the consumption of sugar and high-density glycemic foods such as white flour products. The pancreas does not produce the insulin hormone in type 1 diabetes, so very little glucose gets into the cell, building up instead in the blood. In type 2 diabetes, which is the most common (thirty million in the United States today), the body's cells become less responsive to insulin. The signal insulin usually sends to glucose transporters to take glucose into the cells becomes blocked. This often leads to a stroke or heart disease.

Essential oils are effective agents to prevent and balance diabetic situations in the body. Rosemary was shown to suppress the insulin response (type 2 diabetes) in rabbits whose plasma glucose levels remained at 55 percent for two hours. In his clinical trial, Al-Hadder concluded, "Rosemary created hyperglycemia and inhibited insulin release in rabbits with artificially induced diabetes."[15]

Jane Buckle, an English nurse and aromatherapist, writes about oils for a hypoglycemic effect (like insulin). She describes a 1958 study on rabbits by N. Revoredo in which Lemon Eucalyptus *(Eucalyptus citriodora)* is used for this effect. Ylang-ylang is stated as helpful for diabetes by Pierre Franchomme and Daniel Pénoël in 1991 and Shirley Price in 1995. Jean Valnet writes in 1993 that Geranium benefits the high glucose condition of diabetes.[16]

In women the ovaries produce female eggs and two hormones: estrogen and progesterone. Both FSH (follicle-stimulating hormone) and LH (luteinizing hormone) trigger the secretion of estrogen in the ovaries. Estrogen stimulates the secondary sex characteristics such as maturation of breasts and reproductive organs and prepares the uterus to receive the fertilized egg.

Today we live in an estrogen soup. Many foods such as sugars and starches and plastics emit estrogenic substances into our bodies. John Lee, a doctor in Marin County, California, described women with elevated estrogen and low progesterone as more susceptible to cancer, blood clots, and weight gain. Miscarriages are often due to insufficient progesterone. Synthetic estrogen (as found in HRT, hormone replacement therapy) leads to uterine and breast cancer, as several studies have shown. One HRT is made from the urine of a mare (a female horse).[17]

Many essential oils can help with premenstrual syndrome and menopause. Both of these are caused by fluctuations in estrogen (estradiol, estrone, and estriol) and progesterone. Women need to have a balance of the two hormones for stable menstruation and easy menopause. The uterus makes prostaglandin (pain-producing compounds) to help with labor and the same ones can cause havoc as menstrual cramps. Jane Buckle writes, "Anything that interferes with cellular activity within the cell can indirectly affect the hormonal and endocrine system. Calcium regulates cellular activity (Alexander 2001). Components within essential oils can interfere with the release of calcium at a cellular level."[18] Thymol, menthol, anethole, and eugenol, which are in oils such as Thyme, Peppermint, Fennel, Bay laurel, and Clove *(Syzgium aromaticum),* show this ability to interfere with the release of calcium.[19]

A study done in 1996 showed that Peppermint affects the absorption and secretory mechanisms of the epithelial cells in the small intestine by inhibiting the availability of calcium.[20] Fennel has 75 percent anethole, which is often considered a precursor to phytoestrogen. A study of Fennel

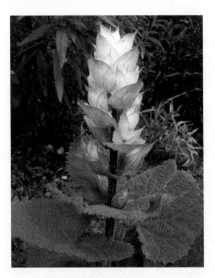

Clary sage

in 2001 showed a reduction of uterine contractions by Fennel, which significantly inhibited the intensity of oxytocin and prostaglandin-induced uterine muscle contractions.[21] This would mean less pain in the PMS cycle. Anethole, the main chemical constituent in fennel and anise *(Pimpinella anisum)*, has estrogenic qualities with minimal hepatotoxicity.[22]

Clary sage *(Salvia sclarea)* has a diterpenol called *sclareol.* A large molecule in sclareol acts as a steroid in the body and reduces the effect of the prostaglandin or cramping pain in PMS. *Salvia sclaria* and Sage *(Salvia officinalis)* are also considered to have estrogen-like properties. Paul Belaiche, a French physician and student of Valnet, suggests the use of Geranium in his book devoted to female problems for mood swings and nervous tension.[23]

Essential oils for mood swings and depression

4 drops Jasmine *(Jasminum grandiflorum)*

5 drops Rose *(Rosa damascena)*

3 drops Geranium *(Pelargonium graveolens)*

10 drops Bergamot *(Citrus x bergamia)*

3 drops Ylang-ylang *(Cananga odorata)*

1 ounce apricot kernel oil *(Prunus armeniaca)*

1 ounce evening primrose oil *(Oenothera biennis)*

The oil for progesterone is one used as an herb throughout the ages, Vitex *(Vitex agnus-castus)*. Both herb and oil will bring results. Progesterone acts with estrogen to bring about the menstrual cycle. It quiets the muscles of the uterus so the embryo will not be aborted. It helps prepare breast tissue for lactation, reduces depression, boosts immunity, and increases memory. From research, Vitex has been observed to interact directly with the pituitary gland.

This herbal formula will stimulate more progesterone production in menopause.

Menopause herbal remedy

wild yam *(Dioscorea villosa)* in a cream

1 drop Vitex *(Vitex agnus-castus)* tincture or essential oil

4 drops red raspberry leaf *(Rubus idaeus)*

3 drops blessed thistle *(Carbenia benedicta)*

Mix tinctures and essential oil together. Once a day, rub wild yam on stomach and then orally take the tincture mixture.

Essential oils for hot flashes during menopause

> 10 drops Clary sage *(Salvia sclarea)*
> 6 drops Geranium *(Pelargonium graveolens)*
> 3 drops Sage *(Salvia officinalis)*
> 8 drops Lemon *(Citrus x limon)*
> 4 drops Cypress *(Cupressus sempervirens)*
> 2 ounces distilled water in a spray bottle

Blend, shake, and spray on face, neck, and lower abdomen.

We need more study on the "psycho" part of psychoneuroimmunology, including how essential oils interact with the delicate yet powerful hormonal processes in the human body. As of this moment, we know that the oils bring a steady balance to the ongoing flow of hormones in the river of the bloodstream and the cells with which they connect.

Mind-Body Pain

Another shining piece in the glittering mosaic of the mind-body enigma is the work of John Sarno, a physician in the northeastern United States who has had years of experience working with people in pain. He has come to some rather startling conclusions. In *Healing Back Pain: The Mind-Body Connection* and *The Mindbody Prescription: Healing the Body, Healing the Pain*, Sarno states the theory that strong, painful, threatening emotions like rage, grief, and shame are repressed in the unconscious. He believes most people need a strategy of avoidance that allows them to keep the feelings hidden by using physical pain and disease to replace emotions of rage and fear.

We all have been conditioned not to express emotions, especially fierce, negative ones. Pain becomes a distraction for the conscious mind to control anger, fear, and grief by pushing them into the subconscious. Often this causes physical ailments later in life. This is especially true of chronic pain such as backaches, arthritis, fibromyalgia, and knee problems. Many doctors do not understand how the mind affects the body so they do not want to be involved; they prefer drugs or surgery as an expedient method to solve pain. Yet more and more evidence is being found to support this mind-body causation of the common ailments that involve pain.

John Sarno has successfully treated over ten thousand people who have TMS (tension myositis syndrome), which is a painful but harmless change of state in muscles. He treats them by explaining that their pain is caused by tension, mental stress, and nerves originating in the central nervous system. He relates how a person's thought patterns start the process of wanting to avoid feelings. The autonomic nervous system centers are activated and within milliseconds, the circulation to the neck or back is reduced, depriving the tissues of oxygen, the result of which is back or neck pain. He claims the pain is a defense mechanism to divert a person's attention to the body, so the awareness of certain repressed negative feelings can be avoided. This process can play a part in arthritis, cancer, and heart disease. Sarno's 1987 study showed that even patients with disc herniation who attended his class were 88 percent pain-free one to three years later. It's hard to argue with such success.[24]

We need to remember that pain is a reminder to look at hidden emotions. Acknowledging our feelings, no matter how terrifying, offers a release of tension in this mind-body loop. Candace Pert concluded from her work that feeling all of our emotions is important to keep the peptides flowing in the mind-body; otherwise the emotion is repressed and blocks the flow literally with painful results. This is similar to the Chinese belief that energy blocks in the meridians create too much heat or cold with the consequence of impending disease.

I think some helpful tools as part of any treatment are to write in a journal and talk about your feelings to a counselor or friend when hidden emotions bubble up to the conscious mind. Some mind-body doctors also recommend breaking free of the chronic pain cycle by positive messaging to yourself, through repetition and attention. All of these methods are greatly enhanced by meditation and essential oils.

Here is a meditation to begin each day when experiencing a painful back or neck.

Find a quiet place to sit and feel comfortable. Begin with eyes closed, breathing deeply and paying attention to the breath. As you focus on the incoming and outgoing of the breath, your mind comes into the present moment. Here the greatest awareness and healing can take place. Let your relaxed mind zero in on the pain and see the emotions behind it. Bring those emotions forward to objectively see them. Experience the connection between the emotion and the physical sensation of pain. Smell a favorite oil like Rosewood *(Aniba rosaeodora)* or Juniper *(Juniperus communis)*. See yourself dissolve the emotion in the fragrance. See the pain released from your body. Repeat any part of the meditation until it feels complete. See yourself as being lighter with no dark emotions holding you down. Rub Frankincense between your hands and massage it energetically over the area of the emotional pain with the intention of releasing your pain to higher forces. See yourself in your mind's eye as healed.

This is a powerful mind-body meditation technique.

One of my favorite aspects of essential oils is their holistic effect. Since most of our problems have holistic origins—mental, emotional, and physical—the oils are ideal for treating someone with TMS. The oils would help the patient's mind relax and be open to the suggestion that the mind chooses to mask emotional turmoil with physical pain.

A study by N. Hadfield described in the *International Journal of Palliative Nursing* (2001) focused on the role of aromatherapy massage in reducing anxiety in patients with malignant brain tumors. Patients were offered a foot, hand, or neck and shoulder massage with Lavender or Roman chamomile. The results of the test demonstrated a reduction of blood pressure, pulse, and respiratory rate. It concluded that essential oils and massage affected the autonomic nervous system and induced relaxation.[25] These two oils would be beneficial for John Sarno's patients, physically and emotionally.

An example of a case study is one of my lovely students, a woman in her fifties who experienced the death of her mother and all the emotional fallout in her family and herself due to this loss. Soon after the mother's death, she began getting respiratory infections, swollen jaw and face, and pains in her back. Some doctors thought she needed surgery and put her on many antibiotic and painkilling drugs. She had trouble sleeping and felt emotionally overwhelmed and depressed. She could barely get to classes. She did begin using essential oils in steams such as Thyme, Lemon, and Tea tree. All three of these oils are strong bactericides and strengthen the immune system. The Thyme oil is also an antidepressant while fortifying the nerves and activating brain cells.

A study done in 1992 by Feher et al. examined the effects of Thyme on nerve elements. "It was concluded that the neuropeptides containing nerve fibers may influence blood flow and mobility. The thyme oil had a beneficial effect on the quantity of these neuronal elements."[26]

Partly due to her new use of essential oils, my student began to recover from all the infections and nerve dysfunctions. She began to acknowledge the feelings she had due to her mother's absence and her siblings' greed and fear. Slowly the jaw and back pain disappeared and she began to feel normal again. She still does steams, especially with Frankincense, Lavender, and Orange. She feels these oils are bringing her into balance. Looking at these oils holistically:

- Frankincense *(Boswellia carteri)* is revitalizing, regulating the body's secretions such as in the lungs. It elevates the mind to relieve anxious and obsessive states linked to the past. It helps to awaken the spiritual purpose for an individual.
- Orange *(Citrus sinensis)* calms digestion, activates the lymph system, and stabilizes nervous states. It helps with insomnia and spreads sunshine on gloomy thoughts.
- Lavender *(Lavandula angustifolia)* balances the central nervous system, relieves pain, and reduces anger, exhaustion, and stress.

Depression

Most doctors prescribe antidepressant drugs or serotonin-enhancing pharmaceuticals like Prozac or Zoloft for their depressed patients. Depression has been steadily increasing in North America since the beginning of the twentieth century and the industrial age. As we saw with the ACTH loop, depression affects general health by suppressing the immune system and altering brain chemistry. It creates low energy, foul moods, poor relationships with family, and often insomnia.

Some more natural alternatives to drugs are these recently researched supplements.

- Saint John's wort *(Hypericum perforatum),* an herb that is well known to benefit mild to moderate depression. It can take three weeks to show benefits. It can cause interference with some prescription and over-the-counter drugs. Take by itself or with essential oils.

- B vitamins, all of which can boost moods by facilitating neuro-transmitter functions. A
- B-complex that includes B6 and B12 is often the best. There are no risks.
- Essential fatty acids, found in salmon and other deep-water fish. They are part of every human cell membrane and are vital for brain cells. The omega-3 and omega-6 fatty acids in fish oil give a boost to many aspects of the mind-body functioning. They are very safe if purified of heavy metals.
- The herb golden root *(Rhodiola rosea)*, an adaptogen used in Russia and Scandinavia, can help the ability to withstand a variety of stressors, similar to American ginseng *(Panax ginseng)*. It may be supportive of mild to moderately depressed people. Take small doses.

Medical doctors may eventually accept essential oil therapy and herbal therapy as effective alternatives for depression. According to the research by Steve Van Toller at the Warwick Olfaction Research Group in England, the effect of fragrance on the brain is similar to that of some of the anti-depressant drugs. Certain scents, such as an ancient Biblical one, Galbanum *(Ferula gummosa)*, alter the brain chemistry that causes chronic depression, anxiety, or other mood changes.[27]

Returning to the important study of Japanese scientists (Komori et al.) discussed in Chapter 17, "Immune Stimulating Effect of Essential Oils," is appropriate here. It shows the antidepressant benefits of the citrus oils (Orange, Bergamot, and Lemon) plus their boost to the emotional immune system. The results support the concept that human depression is based on homeostatic dysregulation and citrus oils improve the homeostatic balance more than antidepressant drugs. It was concluded that citrus oils were of psychoneuroimmunological benefit for the treatment of emotions and the immune system.[28]

Essential oil therapy deals with the power of essential oils to strengthen the body via the immune system and invoke emotional stability through their work on the limbic brain, central nervous system, and endocrine systems. Previously we thought the nervous system and immune system worked independently, but now we know that they communicate via chemical messengers (peptides) and nerve tissue. We are discovering how our emotions can suppress the immune system by triggering certain hormonal messengers that switch off the white blood cell activity. Although she lacked this scientific knowledge, Theodora of Constantinople in the sixth century used the essential oils in her bath to calm her emotions and to revitalize her body and senses, which helped her take action in a crisis.

Death

I was honored to be a hospice caregiver in Petaluma, California, in the early 1980s. I worked with several families attending to the physical and psychological needs of the dying patient. For some families, death was a frightening ordeal. One family accepted their father's passing with grace and integrity. Working with the dying was a powerful experience because the physical body alone was no longer the emphasis of life. Rather, the emotions, the mind, and the soul emerged as the focus. Hospice is truly a mind-body catharsis service. How to support someone in making this monumental transition required paring down to the essentials. What really mattered was how much forgiveness and love could be expressed. This was important in the patient's relationship with herself and with family members. Making the journey to life after death a peaceful, soul-enriching one was paramount. Entering the cocoon of death in a gentle, caring way and letting go of all the fear, anger, jealousy, and angst of mortal life is the goal. Some essential oil to enhance this process would be Marjoram (*Origanum majorana*), Frankincense, Grapefruit (*Citrus x paradisi*), and Spikenard (*Nardostachys grandiflora*) in a 4 percent solution. Mix in a spray bottle with water to spritz the face, hands, and chest several times a day.

I sought to create a space for the dying person to be self-appreciative and finish the unfinished business in significant relationships. Most of all, I tried to bring about circumstances allowing the inner spirit to carry the soul to the new destiny. The caterpillar-cocoon-butterfly image is a key visualization to have here. Oils of Rose, Geranium, Bergamot, and Neroli (*Citrus x aurantium l. amara*) in a body lotion applied to the neck and heart area would be most beneficial for both client and caregiver.

During this period of my life (three and a half years), I read some of Elizabeth Kübler-Ross's work. A favorite quote is "People are like stained glass windows: they sparkle and shine when the sun's out, but when the darkness sets in, their true beauty is revealed only if there is . . . contact with the light within."[29] After reading her books and hearing her speak, I realized Kübler-Ross is a true guide into contact with the spirit. She holds a light out for those of us stumbling through the wilderness of the death and mourning process with loved ones. Her classic five steps of the grief cycle (denial, anger, bargaining, depression, and acceptance) can be applied to many transitions in life. One of the key messages I received from her is to be gentle and forgiving with ourselves, as many intense emotions appear. Accepting the stages of anger and denial is not easy. Tuning in to the wisdom of our inner spirit is vital in times of losing loved ones.

Power of Self-Healing

As health care workers, we need to keep our own light burning. Here is a favorite quote from another woman involved in this field, Joan Borysenko, who set up the Mind/Body Clinic at Harvard Medical School. "The work of healing is in peeling away the barriers of fear and past conditioning that keep us unaware of our true nature of wholeness and love."[30] Both Joan and I believe in healing the mind by meditating every day.

One of the best tools, the practice of meditation, is heightened by the addition of aromatics. I use essential oils to deepen my meditation practice so it becomes more relaxing and effective. Meditation is a spiritual practice because it allows your mind and body to relax while you bring your consciousness into the present moment. In that place the past is forgotten and the future is not a concern. I find fragrance helps with this practice by intensifying an awareness of the present. Certain oils lift your mind to higher thoughts. Sandalwood *(Santalum album* or *Santalum spicatum-Australia)*, which has traditionally been used for spiritual practices; Neroli, which is soothing to the nervous system to relieve any anxiety and entice you to feel uplifted with its sweet, spiritizing scent; and Elemi *(Canarium luzonicum)*, which brings feelings of deep peace, are all beautiful instruments. Try infusing these oils into the air with a debulizing diffuser near the place of meditation. A favorite method of mine is putting a few drops of the above oils on a piece of tissue and inhaling frequently as I meditate. An easy method is to put a few drops in the palm of each hand and rub together, creating an aromatic friction to be inhaled.

It seems to me that working with the mind for human evolution and personal progress is vital. Our thoughts have magnetic qualities, attracting the same energy we are sending out into the universe. Energy follows thought. If we think about what our true purpose is while living here on this earth, we will begin to resonate and make decisions that manifest this true purpose. Keeping our minds focused on what we are meant to express in life, what we are meant to be, and what we are to act out brings radiance. We start to feel happier and more peaceful, following our unique soul's purpose. This requires taking responsibility for our thoughts, feelings, and actions. It means being present, not letting the mind drift into regretting the past or fearing the future. It means beginning a relationship between your personality and your inner spirit.

A very special book, *The Urantia Book,* relates: "Mind is a temporary intellect system loaned to human beings for use during a material lifetime. Human consciousness rests gently upon the electro-chemical mechanism of the brain below and delicately touches the spirit energy system above."[31]

Larry Dossey has written many books on the expansive power of the mind for more healing in prayer. In *Healing Words: The Power of Prayer and the Practice of Medicine,* he discusses the validity of joining scientific research of the Western medical world with the religious practice of prayer. He writes, "... investigating prayer does not imply 'bringing God into the laboratory' but 'bringing the laboratory to God,' requesting and inviting the Universe to reveal its workings."[32]

Seeking the inspiration of the universe can lead to some omnipotent experiences. For example, Dr. Dossey relates some studies showing how in prayer the mind—when thoughts are divinely attuned—is able to bring about healing on the other side of the planet. Mind can be used for good or evil. Using the mind to build a life based on unconditional love for self and humanity as the underlying principal brings courage and honesty. It means forgiving the mistakes, looking into the darkest regions of the soul, and freeing the mind from fear.

Once this mind-spirit relationship is developed, understanding the greater design of life begins to take over. Working with the universe becomes an everyday occurrence. Then the mind can manifest abundance instead of lack, wonder and curiosity replace worry, and inner joy supplants loneliness and depression. The combination of thinking spiritual thoughts and expressing emotions (especially positive ones), eating well, exercising, using essential oils, and practicing meditation help us let go of emotional and physical blocks to becoming the radiant, balanced beings we really are.

Elizabeth Kübler-Ross used the imagery of the children who were killed in the Nazi pogroms to describe the experience of life after death. These children drew butterflies on the walls of their prison cells. They intuitively knew they were leaving the cocoon of life on this planet and their souls would be free. During our present-day life, we can experience the mind as a butterfly, going from flower to flower and person to person, drinking in fragrant nectar from a divine source and offering the other humans we encounter the joy of our unique, nourishing, body-mind-spirit journey.

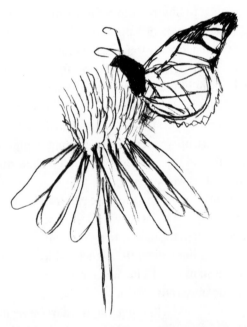

Butterfly on Echinacea flower by Audrey Rood

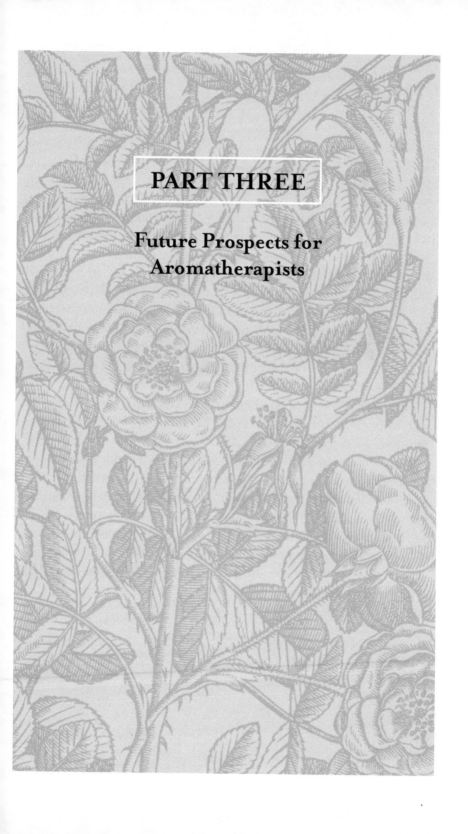

PART THREE

Future Prospects for Aromatherapists

THE FUTURE OF ESSENTIAL OIL THERAPY LOOKS BRIGHT. The flowering of the therapy will include more research and support in the health care field. In the general population globally, it can grow slowly with the birth of more essential oil colleges. Many more practitioners will arise who will utilize their intuition and their internal pendulum. They will be grounded in a rigorous, far-reaching education. The practitioner will know the botanical origins and the chemical constituents of the oils, the history of aromatics, and the human body and mind with all their interactions to reveal the therapeutic value of plant medicine and to impact the efficacy of an aromatherapy practice.

The time will come when people experiencing depression will be given a prescription of uplifting essential oils. The oils will be part of any immune-boosting regimen for fighting viral infections. The oils will be considered indispensable in supporting many mental illnesses. The oils and herbs will give comfort and healing to people with pain and increase vitality for any circulation problems. They will offer a sparkling elixir of citrus, wood, and herbal liquid scents for those who are healthy, needing more energy.

Practitioners will be artists, doctors, researchers, and alchemists, providing transforming fragrant blends and herbal cocktails for all clients. The practitioners will create the resurgence of phytoaromatherapy with their medicines of the earth which promote life and restore the equilibrium of an organism.

CHAPTER TWENTY

Energetic Medicine

One sees clearly only with the heart. Anything essential is invisible to the eyes.

—Antoine de Saint-Exupéry, *The Little Prince*

WHAT AN EXCITING TIME for the development of our awareness about energy beyond the physical realm and how to heal on that level! It all started with Albert Einstein's theory of relativity, which broke the mold of Newtonian linear thinking. Einstein's amazing work led to the field of quantum physics. Of course the whole exploration really began with the ancient schools of healing, like the Chinese, who developed acupuncture and the energy meridians; the Egyptian temples with their spiritually uplifting aromas; and the Greek schools of Asclepius with their psychic channeling.

Einstein blew apart the Newtonian model of seeing ourselves only as solid objects under the influence of gravity. Einstein saw mass as energy slowed down and time as relative not linear. The human body like all matter is really energy at its core or $E = mc^2$.[1] All cells are composed of atoms, which have dancing electrons whirling around the nucleus of protons and neutrons. The body's cells have different patterns or vibrations—the brain's nerve cells waltz and the cardiovascular cells tango. Have you noticed how time changes according to our mood or external circumstances, like becoming unconscious of time while driving a car? This opened the physicists to the nature of the subatomic world, that is, light is a particle but also a wave. Particles transmute to energy and vice versa. Matter, they found, is completely mutable.

On a personal level, people are no longer good or evil, but shades in between. We still cling to the old dualistic idea of good and evil as we see manifested over and over again in movies, videos, comics, and even politicians. In this new reality, our minds, emotions, and characters are mutable too, changing with the thoughts we choose. We create more honorable personal characters by the decisions we make and how connected we are to our inner spirit.

Our own energy field, which we call the *aura*, is inside and outside of linear time and 3-D space. Auras are dynamic webs of energy. Our higher energy fields are composed of vibrational energy with different frequencies, making up the seven levels of our human aura. An important principle in physics is that energy of different frequencies can coexist within the same space without destroying or interfering with the other frequencies. As a result, the seven aura layers can synchronize as one united energy field for each person. Meditation transcends limits of the linear mind and allows us to integrate our auric levels and feel connected to all things.

Human Aura

Here is a brief summary of the first three levels of the human aura (the etheric body, the astral body, and the mental body), according to clairvoyants who see and experience them, and some of the alternative medicines that treat them.

The etheric body, the first layer of the aura, carries information to guide the cellular growth of the physical body. It works closely with the body's functioning. Barbara Ann Brennan[2] and John Perrakos,[3] two perceptive clairvoyants, observed how a plant projects an energy field matrix in the shape of a leaf prior to the growth of a leaf. This would be the etheric body of the plant.

In acupuncture there is a connection between energy meridians and the organs of the body, which are activated by the needles inserted almost painlessly into the skin. The needles stimulate the *qi (chi)* or life force energy to create a flow when the organs along a meridian are blocked or becoming diseased. This ancient Chinese practice, first developed in 2600 BC by Huang Ti, who wrote *The Yellow Emperor's Classic of Internal Medicine*, is becoming very popular due to its success at restoring health. Along with the Chinese herbs that are recommended for tea, acupuncture is a physical body and etheric body interface.[4]

The astral body, the second aural level, is concerned with the emotions and has a fluid structure of many changing colors. Different emotions create certain colors; for example, love forms a rosy pink or green color while confused, negative feelings turn the colors muddy. This level is a link between the mind, the emotions, and the physical body in mind-body illnesses (or health).

Edward Bach in England first developed "flower remedies" about 1910.[5] Since then many other parts of the globe (such as northern California, Alaska, and Australia) have created their own local remedies to alleviate emotional stress and disease. In his work as a physician, Dr. Bach became aware of how many of his patients had emotional components to their physical problems. Subsequently he was led to wander the English meadows, finding healing dew on flowers. He then began experimenting, putting plant material such as flowers on top of spring water in a crystal bowl for six hours in sunlight. The water became infused with the vibrational imprint of the flowers. He bottled it with a dropper so the liquid could be taken under the tongue. He experienced all the symptoms and cures of many human illnesses. Up to six remedies could be blended for the emotional healing of the patient. Here are some of his remedies: larch for people with low self-esteem, mimulus for those with known fears, gorse for those who suffer feelings of despair, heather for those who are self-obsessed, mustard for those who suffer depression without cause. Bach flower remedies are an important emotional energetic medicine that affects the astral level of the aura.

The third layer of the aura is the mental body, which has a yellow glow that cascades down to the physical level. If the mental body functions well with the endocrine and nervous centers, a person is able to think clearly and to focus mentally with force, vigor, and clarity. Healing at this level produces stronger, longer-lasting effects.

Homeopathy affects the mind's perception of pain and even the mental condition of schizophrenia as well as physical ailments such as infection and malaria. It works on the higher auric levels' vital force with natural substances to restore the balance of the mind and the body. "Like cures like" was Samuel Hahnemann's belief when he developed this medicine in 1785.[6] A physician, Hahnemann had a lack of faith in his profession, especially in the heroic medicine of his day. He believed that a medicine that produced the same symptoms of the disease would increase the body's vital energy to vanquish the disease, similar to a vaccine. He believed the smaller the dose of plant, mineral, or animal medicine, the more effective it was. Homeopathy substances are still diluted down to parts per million so the medicine contains only the vibration of the original substances. The remedy is added to a sugar pill that is placed under the tongue for absorption into the physical body and the first three auric levels. These homeopathic remedies are still used around the world today due to their effectiveness without any side effects.

Essential oils fit into this new era of energy fields with their ability to transform and balance our energy in the same way they heal and balance our cellular matter. On the energetic level, we can use less quantity of oil for great impact. The oils also work harmoniously with acupuncture, Bach flower remedies, and homeopathy. Essential oils with flower remedies and acupuncture are natural companions. Using the correct oils on the needles to treat certain conditions will only enhance the effectiveness of the acupuncture treatment. Applying Tea tree *(Melaleuca alternifolia)* to needles before insertion, instead of alcohol as is practiced today, would prevent infection and offer immune-strengthening results. When stimulating certain organs like the stomach and the spleen, using Ginger *(Zingiber officinale)* on the needles would augment the healing treatment.

Combining essential oils with flower remedies can "potentize" the healing properties of both in their liquid menstrum. For example, adding Jasmine *(Jasminum grandiflorum)* and Bergamot *(Citrus x bergamia)* to a tincture of mustard and gentian Bach flower for treating doubt and depression would increase the results with more light and hope for the client.

Some homeopaths believe that camphor-bearing oils such as Rosemary *(Rosmarinus officinalis)* and Lavandin *(Lavandula x intermedia)* are detrimental to homeopathic remedies. More research needs to be done. However, homeopathy and essential oil therapy—two mostly plant-based alternative medical approaches—are extremely compatible. For example, using strengthening oils like Eucalyptus *(Eucalyptus globulus)* and Thyme *(Thymus vulgaris)* with the homeopathic remedy silicea could help someone struggling to overcome fatigue and infection. We are just at the beginning of our ability to understand how and why all of these four energetic medicines work. Much more research and many more experiences need to be documented and shared.

The outer levels of the aura are more difficult to perceive, even by talented clairvoyants. The outermost layer absorbs life-giving energy (*ka* to the Egyptians, *qi* to the Chinese, and *prana* to the Hindus), sending it down through the inner layers to the human body. Conversely the physical body and mental thoughts send vibrations up through the auric layers. The memory of an emotionally charged trauma or accident stays in the aura for some time, unless it is cleared by meditation and essential oils. Psychics are able to observe negative thought forms and disease in the outer layers of the aura before manifesting as illness in the human body.

Using essential oils and crystals to clean and energize the aura will help release the patterns of illness. Here is an exercise that my students do in our energetic healing class:

Ask the client to lie down (ideally on a massage table), breathe deeply, and visualize his body surrounded by his favorite color. As the client relaxes, choose an essential oil that fits his condition, perhaps Neroli *(Citrus x aurantium l. amara)* for nervous anxiety and to purify the higher levels of the aura, Elemi *(Canarium luzonicum)* to regulate secretions and unify all levels of the aura and chakras (balance one's spiritual practices with every-day responsibilities), or Sandalwood *(Santalum album* or *Santalum spica-tum)* to stimulate the immune system and open the higher auric levels and the crown chakra. Rub the oil between your hands and ask for the high-est good for your client. Then sweep your hands from the toes to the head and back again several times, never touching the body. Ask the client to turn over while applying more oil to your hands and repeat the above exer-cise. Visualize the aura being cleansed of all negative thought patterns as you do this exercise. The oil with your intention has powerful healing effects.

Patricia Davis writes, "The saying 'Thought precedes form' is a pro-foundly true statement and we influence our health, both physical and subtle, by our thoughts."[7] Affirmations of confident thinking, meditation, and prayer can help clear the aura of all tendencies toward disease and heal the energetic etheric-physical body complex with harmonious divine energy. Practicing the mind-body meditation for releasing pain (see Chapter 19, "Essential Oils and the Mind-Body Connection") can work for other maladies. It is most important to acknowledge the emotional pain and bring the mind into the present.

Just to remind the reader, essential oils are complex compounds of chemical constituents making the signature aroma and properties of the parent plant. These aromatic molecules have their own individual rates of vibration that relate the life-energy of the plant for this higher healing on the oscillation energy of humans.

A simple example of working on this elevated level would be applying 3 drops (0.5 percent dilution) of Lavender *(Lavandula angustifolia)* in apricot carrier oil *(Prunus armeniaca)* to the spinal cord from the neck to the base of the spine to activate all seven auric levels and chakras.

The aromas, colors, and viscosity of oils reveal their subtle properties. When we dilute the oils past the place they have a physical outcome we can experience their higher vibrations. In the subtle energy work, it is important to dilute them to 0.5 to 1 percent, 2 to 3 drops in 8 milliliters (0.27 ounces) of carrier oil. (See chart in Chapter 13.) Use this formula for all the blend examples that follow in this chapter.

Chakras

Another vital part of our energy field is the chakras. There are seven major energy circles from the top of the head to the bottom of the spine that move clockwise or counter clockwise. Hindu yogis in India first discovered them. They are connections between the gross physical body and the subtle aura levels. Chakras make the aura brighter or dimmer with their capacity for transmission as well as reception. Each chakra goes out to the seven fields of energy in the aura. Energy from the higher vibrational levels is stepped down the chakras to the special nervous and glandular centers in the physical body.

The health of each organ system depends on proper functioning of the associated chakra. For example, the throat chakra brings in subtle energy for a stable thyroid, and the solar plexus creates a balanced digestive system. Each layer of the aura is paired with a chakra, for example, the etheric layer with the base chakra. Each of the seven chakras has a front-of-the-body part that is related to the person's feelings and a back part that is related to the person's will. Energy flows into all chakras from the universal energy source. They are like whirlpools of dazzling energy unless our emotions and thoughts have shut them down. When we block our personal experience and feelings, we disfigure our chakras. This leads to disease and distorted consciousness. We still have much to learn about these centers.

An exercise to test the openness and movement of the chakras is another one we do during class on each other. We ask our partner to lie down on the floor or on a massage table. We have a pendulum—a crystal (ideally a quartz crystal) on a string. We say a prayer for the client and ask that his or her highest good be served. Then we hold the crystal over each of the seven chakra centers, one inch from the body, and note the swing or lack thereof. It is best to draw the outline of a human body and draw the action of each chakra on a piece of paper for reference. With a healthy, open chakra, the pendulum will spin in an active, clockwise direction over the chakra. For those whose chakras are closed or partially closed, the crystal will spin counterclockwise. Using essential oils on the crystal, we can magically realign the crystal spin to move clockwise and greatly activate it. This action can open and realign the chakra, which is a clear demonstration of the power of essential oils on the energetic level with only one drop of oil.

Here is a brief description of the chakras and the oils that resonate with each one.

FIRST CHAKRA, BASE OR ROOT

The first chakra, related to survival needs, reflects how grounded we are and how bonded to mother earth.

Color is red.
Endocrine glands are adrenals.
Element is earth.
Organs are kidneys, urinary system.
Oils are Myrrh (*Commiphora myrrha*), Patchouli (*Pogostemon cablin*), and Cedarwood (both *Juniperus virginiana* and *Cedrus atlantica*).

SECOND CHAKRA, SACRAL

The second chakra relates to the quality of a person's sexual energy and the expression of emotion.

Color is orange.
Endocrine glands are gonads in male and female.
Element is water.
Organs are reproductive system.
Oils are Jasmine (*Jasminum grandiflorum*) and Ylang-ylang (*Cananga odorata*).

THIRD CHAKRA, SOLAR PLEXUS

The third chakra supplies energy for our will and personal power, and our expression in the world.

Color is yellow.
Endocrine gland is pancreas.
Element is fire.
Organs are stomach, liver, gall bladder, and digestive system.
Oils are Ginger *(Zingiber officinale)*, Rosemary *(Rosmarinus officinalis)*, and Lemon *(Citrus x limon)*.

FOURTH CHAKRA, HEART

The fourth chakra relates to the expression of love and compassion for self and others.

Colors are green and rosy pink.
Endocrine gland is thymus.
Element is air.
Organs are heart, circulatory system.
Oils are Rose *(Rosa damascena)*, Bergamot *(Citrus x bergamia)*, and Thyme *(Thymus vulgaris)*.

FIFTH CHAKRA, THROAT

The fifth chakra relates to the expression of one's truth and taking responsibility for one's life.

Color is blue.
Endocrine gland is thyroid.
Element is ether.
Organs are lungs and respiratory system.
Oils are Chamomile *(Chamaemelum nobile)* and Palmarosa *(Cymbopogan martini)*.

SIXTH CHAKRA, THIRD EYE

The sixth chakra relates to the rational mind and psychic ability.

Color is magenta.
Endocrine gland is pituitary.
Organs are eyes, ears, and nose.
Oils are Clary sage *(Salvia sclaria)*, Bay laurel *(Laurus nobilis)*, and
Helichrysum *(Helichrysum italicum)*.

SEVENTH CHAKRA, BRAIN

The seventh chakra is our highest wisdom and our spiritual connection
to God.

Color is violet.
Endocrine gland is the pineal gland.
Element is spirit.
Organs are the frontal lobes of the neocortex.
Oils are Frankincense *(Boswellia carteri)* and Sandalwood *(Santalum
album* and *Santalum spicatum)*.

Growth in the Energetic Healing Field

To see an event in the future, one goes beyond linear time. We will dedi-
cate this part of the book to our newly discovered energetic abilities. Our
higher auric frequencies are more connected to others' higher bodies and
we can raise each other's consciousness by sending loving, positive thoughts.
Energy flows through us as moods, thoughts, and attitudes. As Barbara
Ann Brennan implies, we are all valuable parts of the whole (universe).
We are holograms, capable of being parts that are exact representatives of
the whole (universe). We can tap into the creative powers of the universe
to instantaneously heal anyone anywhere with our thoughts and intentions. The essential oil therapist's intentions are important in this subtle
work.

Awareness of all of the above exciting energetic information opens up
incredible new vistas for the modern day healer. Some pioneers using
essential oils as vibrational medicine to expand awareness are Patricia
Davis and Valerie Worwood; both began the exploration with studies of
how the oils work on the human aura and the energy centers, and have
written books about their studies (*Subtle Aromatherapy* by Patricia Davis

Fragrant Heavens: The Spiritual Dimensions of Fragrance and Aromatherapy by Valerie Worwood). Patricia now dedicates her time as an artist and aromatherapist to the pursuit of wisdom and experience on the higher energetic levels.

Other "energetic" medicines besides homeopathy, acupuncture, and flower remedies are color therapy, Reiki, qigong, acupressure, sound healing, zero balancing, and cranial sacral.[8] These will play an increasingly important role in health care. One of my graduates relayed a story of how he attended a sound conference. Instruments sensitive enough to pick up his voice vibrations tested his voice sound and interpreted them by conveying his strengths and weaknesses. He was astounded by how a voice energetic imprint can so accurately reveal all of one's essence. They then used sound to heal his vibrational personality. He experienced a profound change.

The fantastic value of essential oil therapy is that it is effective on a physical, cellular level; on an emotional, glandular level; on a mind, neurotransmitter level; and on a spiritual, auric level. We are just beginning to discover the broad range of the effects of essential oils—on their own and in combination with all of the other alternative medicines. The amazing story will unfold as we continue to evolve and open to our spiritual potential as human beings.

We are coming into a time when the intuitive abilities will be acknowledged as important as the rational and scientific. Here again, the fragrant oils' affect on the limbic brain, where mood and memory and creativity are stimulated by odor molecules, will give credence to the insightful shamans of the future. The answer is for both sexes to find an inner symmetry between these male and female characteristics.

A wonderful model for these two approaches is Hildegard of Bingen, who holistically approached life and healing. Here is an example of her prescription: "Take equal parts sage, mint, and fennel, soak it overnight in good wine. When the stomach is so weakened through food, almost filled with pus, drink from the mixture after having eaten and before the night. The stomach will be healed and cleansed and the appetite for food returned."[9] Hildegard had no fear of doing research and speaking out in a man's world, yet she also cultivated her intuitive inner life that expressed itself in art, gardens, music, and visions.

Case Study: A Holistic Approach

A.J., a student of mine, is a massage therapist who works holistically, that is, she includes treatment of the energy level with her clients. Her client, G.R., is an older woman, age seventy-five. She was very fatigued and in pain from a sprained ankle and a recent car collision. She was emotionally depressed because in the past month she lost her beloved dog of fourteen years to whom she was entirely devoted.

A.J. began the session with a footbath in her whirlpool tub to which he had added 2 drops of Peppermint *(Mentha piperita)* and 1 drop of Cardamom *(Elettaria cardamomum).* G.R. was given a cup of peppermint tea to drink during the aromatherapy interview.

A.J. chose the following blend of oils to relieve aches and pain, to assist circulation, and to uplift G.R.'s spirit:

> 3 drops Lemongrass *(Cymbopogon citratus)*
> 5 drops Eucalyptus *(Eucalyptus globulus)*
> 4 drops Juniper *(Juniperus communis)*
> 5 drops Rosemary *(Rosmarinus officinalis)*
> 5 drops Mandarin *(Citrus reticulata)*
> 4 drops Cypress *(Cupressus sempervirens)*
> 2 ounces macadamia or safflower oil

By the time G.R. lay on the massage table, A.J. had prepared the blend, mixing it with 2 ounces of carrier oil. A.J. placed four quartz crystals in the four corners of the massage table, with each one pointing inward. Under the table she placed a rose quartz crystal to release fatigue and depression. A.J. started the treatment by opening up to the spiritual energy with Reiki, a healing art that uses a laying on of hands. "The moment we started, I knew all was in order. My intent was so incredibly strong and sincere, and her trust and faith in me was equally deep." A.J. then proceeded with a nurturing facial massage using the essential oil blend. She worked on her client's hands and up her arms to the throat chakra. The oil blend seemed perfect. She then massaged the oil into G.R.'s feet, using traditional reflexology strokes while focusing on the hurt ankle. She balanced her with a few polarity positions. G.R. was very peaceful and relaxed so A.J. took her on a guided meditation that allowed her to heal herself and her pain with each cleansing breath.

After her treatment, G.R. said the pain was completely gone. A.J. thought this was predictable since she was so relaxed. The best indication of the results of this session came forty-eight hours later when G.R. called A.J. with such joy and appreciation to say the pains were still diminished. They scheduled another session in two weeks, using the same blend with the same results. G.R. also felt emotionally revived and mentally more alert than she had been for a long time. This is a wonderful example of an energetic treatment with holistic results!

Today's Integrative Approach

The approach of Western medicine has brought much knowledge about different physiological systems, but it has led to an overspecialization of medicine. Not only do we have the demise of the general practitioner that existed for Elizabeth I, but also the ability to see and heal the whole person has been lost in the last century. Many of us are finding this is the time to ignite such feminine values as service, caring, natural medicine, and honoring the earth. It is time for male and female approaches to many aspects of life to enrich and to begin truly listening to each other. We can benefit from the differences and co-exist in expanded awareness. As described in Chapter 4, "Women in the Life of Jesus," Jesus of Nazareth was a beautiful model of the integration of both genders and had an astonishing ability to see and hear each individual he encountered with compassion and love.

The health field is one area where this broad acceptance of people, male or female, with special abilities is especially appropriate. Allopathic medicine, plant therapies, and energetic healing can work in concert together. Allopathic medicine is important for emergencies and disease-crisis intervention. The preventive, restoring, holistic approach of essential oils, acupuncture, yoga, and Reiki in maintaining health is also vital to clinics and hospitals and people's homes today. Energetic medicine of homeopathy, flower essences, and sound healing offers deep, sensitive, effective healing on a higher vibrational level. All of these approaches can be complementary, instead of exclusive and antagonistic, creating true integrative medicine.

Another important cooperative, energetic modality of essential oil therapy is reflexology, a healing system of touching and massaging the feet.

Eunice Ingham, another important woman who is relatively unknown today, was a physiotherapist and a student of William Fitzgerald's zone theory in the 1930s. Eunice discovered feet were the most responsive to healing touch and mapped out the entire body on the feet. The art and science of reflexology was born—in the tradition of the Egyptians (Imhotep is considered the grandfather of both aromatherapy and reflexology, 3000 BC), the Native Americans, the Russians, and the Chinese, who all worked on the feet to promote good health.

Both reflexology and essential oil therapy can be considered preventive or restorative healing arts. The goal of both is to return the body and mind to a state of homeostasis when the modern disease of stress has created imbalances. Reflexology is the application of pressure by the hand to reflex points located in the feet, resulting in an even flow of energy or *qi* (as it is called by the Chinese) throughout the body. Eva-Marie Lind, an aromatherapist, said, "Too little Qi shows itself in the form of fatigue and toxemia. Too much Qi can produce pain and inflammation and can lead to more chronic degenerative diseases."[10] The seven thousand nerves located in the feet are receptive to receiving the essential oils to affect different parts of the body. When the correct essential oil, such as Cardamom, is applied and massaged into the correct zone on the foot for stomach or intestinal area, then relief from digestive problems can be realized. Rubbing Lavender or a blend of Lavender and Neroli, which are nervines, on the inside arch of the foot can help relax the central nervous system. Using Celery seed *(Apium graveolens)* to rub on the bladder and kidney points can help with urine retention. Applying 2 drops of Eucalyptus on the lung areas can act as a decongestant and reduce infection in the pulmonary tract.

The organs are laid out on the foot as they are in the body. The inside of the foot is like the curve of the spine, the toes are like little heads, and the ridge under the toes is a natural shoulder, neckline. Reflexology improves circulation, helping to release the toxins that gravity stores in our feet. It reduces stress and induces deep relaxation of the central nervous system.[11] Essential oils, carefully chosen, can enhance the nurturing power of touch and the freeing of energy flow in the body and mind. This is an example of how essential oil therapy creates a powerful team effect between two synergistic healing modalities!

In Closing

The field of energetic medicine is ready for dynamic expansion in the next twenty-five years. It promises a new approach to medicine that presents immediate spiritual as well as physical insight into an individual's health. The forms of healing offered to patients will be less technological, less aggressive, more humane, and more instantly effective. Essential oils as the energetic gifts of nature will vivify many energy modalities as this exciting field unfolds.

CHAPTER TWENTY-ONE

Integrative Medicine

The doctor of the future will give no medicine, but will interest his patients in the care of the human frame, in diet, and in the cause and prevention of disease.

THOMAS EDISON, 1902

THE FUTURE OF THE AMERICAN MEDICAL world calls for a new, startling approach and philosophy. We are ready to change American health care from just sick care to include well care. Most Americans are weary of "finding a bug, using a drug" kind of medicine. Western medicine has developed miraculous abilities to surgically save heart patients, to scan the body with X-rays and MRIs (magnetic resonance imaging), to provide implants of many organs, to arrest some bacterial infections with penicillin and other antibiotics, and to offer emergency interventions for appendicitis and broken bones. Yet this focus on emergency care supplants the American desire to build a long-term health care philosophy based on natural principles for each person. Most of the time concentrating on symptoms of disease with pharmaceutical drugs and all their side effects is less effective than fortifying a strong immune and cardiovascular system with natural supplements, herbs, and oils. To foster lifestyles that are preventive is the banner of the future.

Today Americans have very high rates of diabetes, heart disease, strokes, lung disease, and cancer considering the modern technologically advanced medical system. The prevalence of disease is due to a variety of factors: poor nutrition (fast foods and overly processed foods), lack of exercise, alcohol consumption, polluted air and water, tobacco, and high stress levels. Stays in hospitals consist mostly of surgery and a new regimen of pharmaceutical drugs. Due to so many emergency interventions, this invasive approach seems necessary. Often a patient succumbs to staph infections or even MRSA (methicillin-resistant *Staphylococcus aureus*) from a hospital visit. There is little thought or action spent on preventive health in the allopathic medical world. The cost of medical care in the United States is higher than most countries. Here a person spends an average of $7,200 annually for medical care, yet Americans trail the English in life expectancy, where health insurance is provided for all. Forty-eight million people are unable to afford health insurance and others have high deductibles. This boosts unpaid patient bills and makes hospitals unprofitable. Due to the costs and lack of satisfying care, many are forced into layoffs of personnel and closing their services. The American medical world is in crisis.

Offering universal medical insurance to every American is vitally important, yet also imperative is improving the quality of health care: deepening and expanding it. Due to the costs and lack of satisfying care, many people today are seeking natural modalities to keep their families healthy in a holistic (physical, emotional, mental, and spiritual) sense. The once-personal bond between patient and doctor has been replaced by a multi-billion-dollar-per-year medical industry that offers little compassion in its care and that results in 783,936 iatrogenic deaths annually (2001). These deaths, induced by a physician or medical procedures, include 106,000 from the adverse effects of medication.[1]

"Traditionally, hospitals have been organized for doctors, for auxiliaries, for insurance companies—everybody but the patient.... The total institution is like a concentration camp ... that is overwhelmed with volume and stress and strain and people not dealing with their own feelings.... We're the only country where the more we spend, the less people are satisfied with health care.... patients tell us they want a more personal relationship with their doctors." Ron Anderson, chief executive officer of Parkland Hospital in Dallas, Texas, spoke these words to Bill Moyers during an interview.[2]

Even the spa market is going through a fundamental shift. People want products and services that have a positive effect on their health and environment. Clients no longer want to be in a luxurious pampering palace full of synthetic products and buildings. Instead, they want a stress-free zone that provides eco-friendly products and a sanctuary based on sustainable resources. A spa now sees its job is to provide a caring staff with healthy food, reasonable exercise, and a therapeutic touch in a beautiful, nurturing environment.

Integrative medicine offers the most hope for treating specific diseases and, best of all, for helping clients sustain the healthy habits that greatly reduce costs and improve the joy of living. Andrew Weil shaped the term *integrative medicine*. Part of his vision is the collaboration of a physician trained in Western medicine working with an acupuncturist, a nutritionist, an osteopath, an essential oil therapist, a Western herbalist, and many more possible combinations. He suggests merging the best of treatments in one clinic with the benefits of diagnostic techniques that Western medicine offers plus essential oils in the air and in blends to apply to the skin for eliminating infection and promoting relaxation, specific food and supplements from a nutritionist, and the analysis of the emotional state by a psychologist.[3] This is a winning approach to health care. A client with a minor illness or even a major disease would find all the advice and treatment needed to decrease pressing symptoms and moderate future lifestyle choices for continued holistic harmony.

Here is an exciting idea to contemplate! We can fashion hospitals into therapeutic sanctuaries, places of healing with some direction from the Aesclepion model of ancient Greek hospitals (800–200 BC). The ailing Greek citizen was offered a space for rejuvenation and holistic cures with plant medicine, nutritional guidelines, emotional mind offerings, and relaxation techniques. These modalities alongside the "emergency" techniques will provide more balance and deeper healing. A hospital spa could combine the sound medical practice of trained physicians with the power of complementary therapies and equally trained practitioners. There would be a green nuance by using high-quality, natural, organic products and sustainable energy resources for water and heat. Solar panels could provide much of the electrical needs at low cost. The buildings could be constructed with nontoxic, sustainable materials.

The concept of a medical spa would allow a hospital to enhance its revenue without financially bleeding the customers, appealing to health-conscious clientele as well as to those with emergency illnesses. Memorial Hermann Wellness Center in Houston, Texas, offers aromatherapy, body polishing, dry brushing, body wraps, reflexology, pre- and post-natal massage, and some mind-body treatments along with traditional medical offerings. Essential oils are part of many of these services because of their delightful smells, but also their desirable qualities of being antimicrobial, pain relieving, anti-inflammatory, emotionally uplifting, and so much more.

Scott Morcott, a doctor at the Condell Medical Institute in Libertyville, Illinois, said, "Healthy habits such as good nutrition, regular exercise, and relaxation techniques like yoga, massage, and aromatherapy ... ward off illness."[4] Some hospitals are building new treatment rooms with a view of a healing garden. Some spas provide ayurvedic treatments, hydrotherapy skin care, and massage. Many European hospitals that treat cancer use complementary approaches alongside traditional methods such as chemotherapy and radiation. Acupuncture is effective in controlling chemotherapy-related nausea, vomiting, fatigue, and postoperative pain. This ancient Chinese modality puts forward the use of Chinese herbs. Essential oils of Ginger *(Zingiber officinale)* and Peppermint *(Mentha piperita)* mitigate nausea. Milk thistle *(Silybum marianum)* supports the liver, Hawthorne berry *(Crataegus monogyna)* strengthens the heart, and Licorice root *(Glycyrrhiza glabra)* is a demulcent for the digestive system. A holistic style with herbs and oils proffers the patient accordingly much more custom care in cancer treatment. Patients are entitled to know options and make choices. Both practitioners and patients are empowered by integrative medicine.

Here is a possible scenario in an integrative medical clinic. A woman makes an appointment for a medical overview. She arrives at the clinic where fragrant plants like rhododendrons and roses are growing by the front door. The air in the reception room has a soft aroma of Lavender, Lemon, and Cedarwood. She is warmly greeted on arrival and ushered into a room with six practitioners waiting to meet her. She is introduced to each one and begins to share her physical and emotional conditions. She reveals she is suffering from headaches, joint pain, depression, insomnia, and constipation. She has much stress at work and at home with an unhappy marriage. Each of the practitioners—an acupuncturist, a medical doctor, a psychotherapist, a nutritionist, a massage-Reiki therapist, and an aromatherapist-herbalist—ask her questions and fill out their own specific forms. They spend forty-five minutes giving her complete attention and care. Then they ask her to enter another room where she submerges into an aromatherapy bath and drinks a cup of tea. The practitioners utilize the next thirty minutes consulting with each other, devising a strategy of healing for this new client. Each practitioner will work with her, offering their specialty. When she emerges from the bath, feeling refreshed, she is given a paper with suggestions on how to proceed and possible appointments to make.

At the reception desk she receives a bill for this initial group consultation; the fee will be partially paid by the universal health insurance plan. She decides to make an appointment with the lab for blood tests, with the psychiatrist for her marriage problems, and with the acupuncturist for pain issues. Later she will consult with the aromatherapist for insomnia and stress, and then use the suggested oils in a massage with the Reiki practitioner. A large percentage of the cost will be covered by her health insurance.

Overall, the client experiences an immediate uplift from the supportive, sweet-smelling environment and the people at this clinic. She is filled with the hope that some of her troubles can be resolved. The practitioners like the direct contact with her and the creative problem-solving atmosphere of the clinic. They like asking her to be part of the health care team and finding solutions that are on-going and self-empowering.

Unease with the present-day medical system of seven-minute doctor visits and expensive insurance that only partially covers diagnostic tests creates a populace interested in exploring alternative medicine. People want to be seen and heard by their doctors. A team of integrative health workers can provide perspectives from many diverse healing modalities. They can truly examine an entire person: the physical, emotional, mental, and spiritual levels. They can find the imbalances and realign the person's physical chemistry with Rolfing massage, shiatsu, and reflexology. For the person's emotional disturbances, sound therapy, Bach flower essences, hypnosis, and guided imagery can harmonize. Meditation, prayer, and Reiki massage are possibilities for the spiritual level. Two modalities that balance all the PEMS levels (physical, emotional, mental, and spiritual) are nutrition, healthful eating for optimal well-being, and essential oil therapy, the gift from the plant world to soothe, detoxify, revitalize, and uplift.

How can clinics, hospitals, and private practices best draw on the healing properties of essential oils? The first, most apparent use is to provide calming, pleasing fragrances in the air. A hospice clinic or a hospital can provide a diffuser that is easy to clean and refill in every patient room. The patient will benefit in mood and health with an antibacterial and emotionally uplifting blend of oils.

Some studies have looked at the mental and emotional effects of oils in the air. A Japanese experiment by Miyazaki et al. in 1992 showed the speed of performing a mental task was increased while the rate of mistakes was decreased when inhaling essential oils, including Orange *(Citrus sinensis)*.[5] In 1993 C. H. Manley used an electroencephalographic method to measure brain-wave responses to odorants at the frontal location on the scalp. Essential oils were inhaled, causing changes in the magnitude of CNV (contingent negative variation) from baseline of participants' EEG (electroencephalogram). Stimulating oils that increased CNV were Basil *(Ocimum basilicum)*, Clove *(Syzgium aromaticum)*, Peppermint *(Mentha piperita)*, and Lemongrass *(Cymbopogon citratus)*. Oils that decreased CNV were Bergamot *(Citrus x bergamia)*, Roman chamomile *(Chamaemelum nobile)*, Lemon *(Citrus x limon)*, Sandalwood *(Santalum album* and *Santalum spicatum)*, and Marjoram *(Origanum majorana)*.[6]

With the use of specific oils, staph infections can be diminished. Presently this is a crucial problem in many U.S. hospitals. Offering staff liquid soaps and lotions with antibacterial essential oils, not synthetic antibiotics that create resistance, with mandatory hand washing before and after procedures, would greatly reduce the spread of this dangerous contamination. Such oils as Marjoram, Thyme *(Thymus vulgaris)*, Lemon, and, of course, Tea tree can be blended for safety in hand-cleaning products.

A 2004 study described by Rachael McGraw in *Medical News Today* found that essential oils can kill the deadly MRSA bacteria. The study took place at the University of Manchester in the United Kingdom. Jacqui Stringer, Clinical Lead of Complementary Therapies at Christie Hospital, summarized the findings: "The reason essential oils are so effective is because they are made up of a complex mixture of chemical compounds which the MRSA and other superbug bacteria find difficult to resist." She went on to remark that antibiotics are single components that MRSA quicky resist.[7]

Other studies show that essential oils greatly reduce airborne bacterial count. A 1995 study by C. F. Carson found Tea tree and *Eucalyptus globulus* very effective for eliminating MRSA infections in the air or on the skin.[8]

Direct application of oils on patients could begin with hand and foot massages. Using an aloe vera lotion for its skin-healing properties as a base would be best. Depending on the needs of the patient, adding 5 drops of Helichrysum *(Helichrysum italicum)*, 3 drops of Roman chamomile, 2 drops of Carrot seed *(Daucus carota)*, and 2 drops of Rose *(Rosa damascena)* to the unscented lotion or massage oil is healing for a burn victim or a patient with skin abrasions, skin allergies, or skin irritation from radiation or chemotherapy.

For a patient with lung problems, applying oils to the area of the foot for lungs would add a second dimension to the reflexology massage on the feet. If a person suffers from pneumonia, Eucalyptus *(Eucalyptus globulus* or *Eucalyptus radiata)*, Myrtle *(Myrtus communis)*, Ravintsara *(Camphora communis)*, and Cypress *(Cupressus sempervirens)* would relieve infection and excessive congestion.

Essential oils also excel in the unpleasant reality known as pain. Pain can be self-inflicted, as discussed in the mind-body chapter, or as a symptom of a serious disease. There are many diverse kinds of pain. In general, pain receptors (prostaglandins) are activated in the dermis of the skin or in deeper, muscular-skeletal tissues. Deep somatic pain often feels like aching, yet localized pain. Surface pain usually has a sharp, burning quality.

Instead of ingesting over-the-counter drugs that dull pain yet have side effects, remedies based on herbs and essential oils are natural, effective analgesics. They can be used in hospital spa settings and in daily routines to maintain a healthy body. Essential oils and herbs can be used synergistically in baths, massage oils, and compresses after exercise or during the stress of living.

In a 2006 article, "How to Integrate Clinical Aromatherapy in a Hospital Setting," Jane Buckle describes a three-week study of elderly patients with arthritis and chronic pain. She suggests the use of a massage oil with 10 drops of Frankincense *(Boswellia carteri)* and 4 drops of Lavender *(Lavandula angustifolia)* in a 2-ounce base of calendula-infused almond oil. When this blend was used as a hand massage on thirty elderly patients, their pain was reduced and their sleep increased. Buckle also describes two controlled three-week studies on arthritic patients using either 4 percent Marjoram or 4 percent Black Pepper *(Piper nigrum)* in an apricot carrier oil. Both oils substantially reduced the symptoms of pain, but Marjoram was found to be slightly more effective. Patients in the Marjoram study showed 27 percent more dexterity, 29 percent increased strength, 32 percent reduction in stiffness, and 32 percent reduction in pain. The Black Pepper study showed the results to be 2 to 4 percent less effective than the Marjoram.[9]

For other sufferers, an aromatic remedy for headaches is to blend 3 drops of Peppermint *(Mentha piperita)* and 6 drops of Rosemary *(Rosmarinus officinalis)* in a warm water basin. Dip a compress of cotton in the fragrant water and apply on the forehead and back of neck.

Important Educational Standards

To successfully accomplish these empathetic treatments, educational training in essential oils and reflexology would bring maximum effectiveness. Just as aromatherapy is part of nursing training in the United Kingdom, all American registered nurses should receive 400 hours of instruction in essential oils and reflexology. The following is part of the COBHA (College of the Botanical Healing Arts) curriculum and the AIA (Alliance of International Aromatherapists) suggested outline for clinical level education. I was a member of the AIA Education Committee, 2006–2008.

- Anatomy and physiology covers the twelve systems of the body and the olfactory and immune systems. It contains pathologies of all these systems plus essential oils, herbs, and nutrition that support the healing of these imbalances and illnesses.
- World history of aromatics includes ancient cultures and modern developments in Europe, America, Australia, Japan, and the Middle East.
- Integrative therapies explores psychoneuroimmunology with essential oils for therapeutic rebalancing of the nervous, endocrine, and immune systems. The mind-body interaction is studied on a chemical, molecular, and emotional level for its crucial understanding of certain diseases.
- Botany includes binomial taxonomy, botanical families containing essential oils, germination, photosynthesis, and Mendelian genetics.
- Organic chemistry focuses on the main pharmacological effects of the primary chemical constituents in essential oils. It includes understanding the GC-MS (gas chromatography–mass spectrometry) analysis of each essential oil studied (seventy oils).
- Clinical science offers classes in pathology; treatment of bacterial, viral, and fungal infections; parasitical testing; aromatograms; and

nutrition, including diet as a means of overcoming disease, using enzymes, and cleansing the body.

- Energetic medicine delves into how essential oils act on the human energy field.
- Business skills is taught so a graduate can establish an aromatherapy practice: the value of networking, marketing, basic accounting skills, trade-name registration, communication of the benefits of essential oils to the public and health care providers, and creation of business cards and brochures.
- The whole course provides profiles on at least seventy essential oils and thirty herbs with safety information and a list of cautionary oils. An important aspect focuses on consultation skills, compassionate listening, formulating an aromatic and herbal intervention, record keeping, interdisciplinary cooperation with other practitioners, and follow-up care for the client. A code of ethics for a professional business practice is included.
- A live clinical practice of at least forty-five hours is mandatory at the end of the study. It involves treating local residents for one-hour and half-hour sessions. A class is offered in conjunction with the clinic to discuss how each treatment session is received. Support from fellow students is part of the process of learning and growing from the experiences.

Clinical aromatherapy education on a professional level is critical. This will open the door to career opportunities in family health and community clinics. Receiving 400 hours minimum of live classes seems imperative for the ability to offer clients a clinical approach to their physical and emotional problems. A minimum two-year study of at least seventy essential oils, thirty herbs, and an in-depth focus on nutritional solutions seems important if graduates are to offer clients preventive medicine. It would be valuable for every state to have such an educational school and program. Job opportunities in private practices, health clinics, hospitals with alternative medicine, physical therapy clinics, pediatric offices, and burn clinics will become available when education provides clinical competency. This two-year study can be available to nurses and doctors in the United States to augment their tools for healing. Jane Buckle states in *Clinical Aromatherapy*, "The Royal College of Nursing (RCN) in England issued guidelines for nurses wanting to use aromatherapy. These state that a nurse 'should know his/her subject and have received training.'"[10]

According to Aurora Ocampo, RN, at Beth Israel Medical Center, "Traditionally, nursing is committed to caring for the whole person—body, mind and spirit. Aromatherapy is believed to work at psychological and physiological levels. I have found that by incorporating this healing therapy into my nursing practice, patients were not only able to reduce their levels of stress, but also to significantly improve their quality of life."[11]

Soon we need to set up licensing of aromatherapists in many countries, including the U.S. The number of hospitals that are incorporating essential oils into their treatment program is increasing. The demand for educated therapists and quality essential oils will be increasing.

The future of health care is a vision of hope and whole body medicine. We will look back at the present moment as a time when medicine was dominated by pharmaceutical drug companies and the insurance industry. The drug companies offer expensive, sometimes dangerous medicine with iatrogenic, chemical side effects that often leading to death. In 2009 close to fifty million Americans are without health insurance and an additional twenty-five million are "underinsured." Medical bills cause more than half of personal bankruptcies in the U.S. The hospitals employ doctors who have little training in nutrition and who deny the validity of mind-body ailments. Only 2 percent of medical students become primary-care physicians because pay is less than for specialists. As it is, young doctors need twenty years to pay back medical school debt. Primary care physicians and staff spend much time with insurance paperwork. They use high-tech methodologies at the exclusion of humane one-on-one care. However, nurses and doctors of this time receive high marks for diligence in a difficult situation.

Sanoviv Medical Institute in Baja California, Mexico, is an exception. It combines conventional therapies with complementary ones and treatment with lifestyle prevention. The focus here is on healing, not drugs, with a belief in the body's innate power to heal itself. They begin with a detoxification program and each guest undergoes a series of diagnostic tests. Their doctors, dentist, and psychologist work with experts in many alternative-heath fields to create a comprehensive program tailored to each individual's needs. This includes a custom nutrition, detoxification, and exercise program. To treat the root cause of disease rather than suppress it with drugs is a blessing.

Another integrative medicine center, Tree of Life Rejuvenation Center in Patagonia, Arizona, is run by my friends, Gabriel and Shanti Cousens. They offer spiritual fasting with fresh, low-glycemic, high mineral content organic juices. Activities include daily meditations, yoga classes, aromatherapy treatments, live foods prepared with love, walking a labyrinth, native sweat lodge, qigong movements, and medical consultations for those with chronic illness. Gabriel has written seven books on heath and diet. One guest said, "Gabriel Cousens, MD, is in the gem business: you arrive rough and leave beautifully crafted, ready to take your light and joy out into the world."[12]

Integrative medicine works well for stress and aging, as well as for critical diseases. Doctors, scientists, and aromatherapists know that hormones like cortisol and adrenaline from the adrenal glands play a crucial role in chronic stress. Our perception of stress regulates how destructive and aging it can be to our bodies and minds. If we regret past actions or fear future events, we set into action the ACTH loop of constant secretion of cortisol; over time, this can be harmful to blood pressure, immune functioning, and free radical production, which in turn can lead to more aging, weight gain, and other health problems. This was discussed in Chapter 19, "Essential Oils and the Mind-Body Connection." Integrative medicine can break the cycle.

Dr. Andrew Weil wrote, "One of the cornerstones of integrative medicine is the idea that physicians and patients can work on all levels of lifestyle ... treating the whole person, the physical as well as the mental, emotional and spiritual dimensions ... to uncover the root causes of illness or discover powerful ways to optimize health."[13]

Aromatic Gardens

*When I pick and crush in my hand a twig of Bay, or brush
against a bush of Rosemary, or tread upon a tuft of Thyme, or
pass through incense-laden branches of Cistus, I feel that here is
all that is best and purest and most refined, and nearest to
poetry, in the range of faculty of the sense of smell.*

—Gertrude Jekyll

Walking on a flagstone path through fragrant glades of wisteria and jasmine can make springtime an olfactory feast. Continue on the path past roses, luscious in the warm sun, and lavender flower tips gently blowing in the breeze, together creating a rose-lavender plant blend. Take another path past spicy rosemary, sage, and licorice-infused fennel. Rub them between your hands and inhale the savory mixture. Low-growing thyme, the purple flowers of hyssop, and pungent peppermint all welcome the nose to enjoy a multitude of delightful aromas. Fragrances can beguile and intrigue us with their immediate, mysterious presence. A few citrus trees like orange and lemon with their delicious-smelling flowers bring olfactory delight. Other trees enveloped by the wind—bay laurel, spruce, and cedarwood—wave above the fragrant chorus in the garden below. All of these living plants are begging to be distilled into essential oils and hydrosols.

A living plant is a vibrant organism involved in a continuous cycle of transformation through absorption, assimilation, and exhalation. The process of photosynthesis requires an intake of sunlight, CO_2, and H_2O when the chloroplasts boost the chlorophyll's electrons to a high-energy potential to create ATP (adenosine triphosphate) and triose sugar, which is produced for the plant to use as energy and food, and then oxygen is

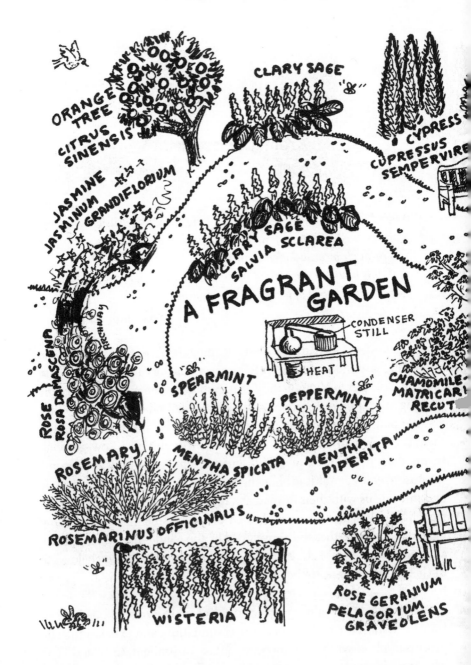

Fragrant garden

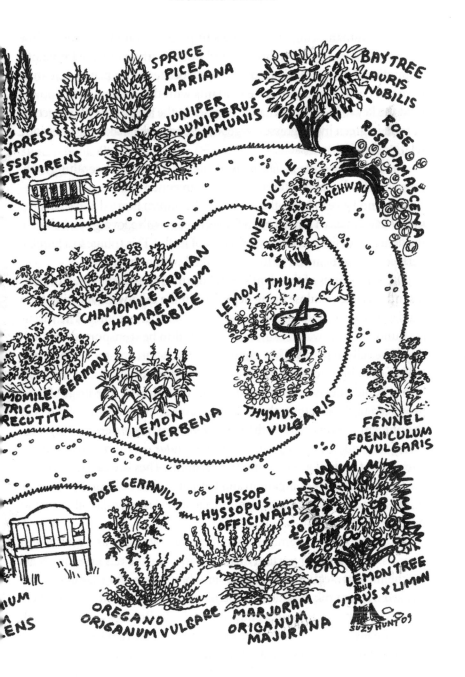

I's reign, became so popular that even the smallest country houses had their still-rooms. Old garden still-house books were full of fragrant recipes for rosewater, honey of violets, lily of the valley spirit, conserve of the flowers of lavender, and lavender water, syrup of clove, carnations, jasmine water, sugar of damask roses, musk rose water, spirit of rosemary, Madonna lily water, balm water, cowslip syrup, and elder flower water.... In her still-room, the lady of the house made perfumed powders, waters, wash-balls, spirits, pomanders, scented ointments and sweet bags ... filled with rose petals, mint powder, and powder of cloves."[4]

A distillation of rosemary in a copper still, which we do every year in January at the College of Botanical Healing Arts, manifests invigorating bottles of Rosemary hydrosol. It can be used in a bath, as a mist on the face and hair, as a poultice for a headache on the forehead, to rub over the liver area for detoxification, or to help regenerate paralyzed limbs.

All the aromatic plants, shrubs, and trees can be planted in a clinic or hospital garden. Putting benches along curving paths where people can sit and take pleasure in the smells of the familiar and exotic plants is important. Letting people sit next to different species of lavender would reduce stress and create balance in their mind-body system. Putting in metal arches for plants like roses and jasmine to climb offers vertical, curved movement in the garden and the chance to smell them while walking the path. Sealing the garden off from car traffic with stone walls, hedges of lemon verbena or small junipers, bamboo, or wooden fences will give the garden a sense of serene privacy. Make paths with gravel or fired clay stepping stones that curve through the scrumptious trees and vines. Create a small garden within the larger one by standing a small statue or sundial in the center of a circle and planting low-growing herbs in wedges around it. Different thymes like lemon and *Thymus vulgaris*, parsley, spearmint, marjoram, lemongrass, garlic, coriander, basil, chamomile, tarragon, and yarrow are all possibilities.

I must mention my father here as an important influence in my life by his love of gardens. He spent his early years in upstate New York along the Saint Lawrence River with many secret "offices" and "meditation rooms" in the woods near his home. As an adult he became a historian, teacher, and lover of the arts. He carried the attraction for the wilderness into his older years by planting rock gardens wherever we lived. He would explore areas with unusual rocks, load up the car (sometimes to my mother's chagrin), and bring them home to create a rugged but handsome garden with flowering plants and ferns in between the stones and boulders.

Inspiration can come from some famous scented gardens of the past like the Hanging Gardens of Babylon (2500 BC) that Nebuchadnezzar built for his homesick wife. As described in Chapters 1 and 3 on Hatshepsut and Cleopatra, the Egyptians were experts with aromatic plants. In the temple of Amun-Re at Karnak, a room called "Botanical Garden" contains 256 different types of plants. The earliest medicinal gardens were formed by Egyptian priests in their walled garden retreats. The Ebers Papyrus reports on hundreds of healing plants in 1550 BC. The Greeks were inspired by trips to Egypt that led to the use of aromatic plants in the medical repertoire of Hippocrates and Herodotus. Aesclepion temples were the places of healing where the early Greeks (800–200 BC) went for physical, emotional, and spiritual renewal. The gardens at these temples were rich in aromatic plants, trees, and peacocks. The Romans received inspiration from the Greeks. As the ruins at Pompeii reveal, gardens grown with a large variety of flowers and herbs for medicinal and culinary purposes surrounded most of the buildings. The Romans also used these plants to create perfumes such as rhodinum, a lovely fragrance of Myrrh, Fennel, and Rose. As described in Chapter 7, Trota worked closely with her garden's treasure for healing remedies in her teaching and medical practice. The formal rose garden and the medicinal herb garden for distillation were prominent under Elizabeth I.

In more recent times, advances in technology and new drugs have been the focus of medical institutions. However, some in the medical community are rediscovering the healing power of gardens. Healing gardens can be found in a variety of organizations including substance abuse treatment centers, long-term care facilities, outpatient clinics, retirement homes, and hospices. In Santa Cruz today, the Homeless Garden Project benefits many emotionally dejected people with the healthy joy of gardening and the financial assistance from selling its produce and flowers. The Center for Victims of Torture in Minneapolis developed a garden to aid in the healing process of people who have suffered psychological and physical abuse. Oregon's Portland Memory Garden provides a safe and enjoyable setting that addresses the restorative power of gardens for Alzheimer's patients.

In 1879 at Philadelphia's Friends Hospital, a physician noticed that psychiatric patients working in the fields and flower gardens were calmer and emotionally uplifted. More recently doctors at the Jupiter Medical Center in Jupiter, Florida, found that cardiology patients in rehab who had a view of the healing garden from their room took less pain medication and had shorter hospital stays than those who could not see the garden. Hope in Bloom is a nonprofit organization in Massachusetts that installs gardens without cost at the homes of women with breast cancer. The gardens are designed to give these women a tranquil place to escape from the world of doctors, hospitals, and sickness.

Wendy Johnson wrote, "Every paradise garden I know is rooted in real work and real bounty. The two beget each other. Every garden worth its salt becomes paradise by being both a safe refuge from the madness of the world and a field of action within the cacophony of this very world."[5]

Research reveals that working in the garden can benefit everyone. The physical efforts of gardening—digging, planting, bending, and walking—are great ways to keep the body healthy. Weeding burns calories and prevents osteoporosis. Studies show that gardening can lower blood pressure and cholesterol, which reduces heart disease, the number one cause of death in the U.S. Hospitals have TVs, cafeterias, and sometimes a fish tank. When a hospital adds a healing garden, the resulting sensual interaction with nature can bring satisfying results for patients, nurses, and doctors. The rich aroma of fresh earth and the delightful scent of sweet-smelling herbs fill the air we breathe while the fruit of an orange tree tantalizes our taste buds. We can touch the velvety smoothness of a rose petal or the leaf of a lamb's ear plant. Breathing in the oxygen that plants produce, and watching and nurturing plant growth all enhance our well-being.

European monasteries created complex gardens to offer their communities medicine and replenish the spiritual needs of the sick. This was true of Hildegard. "The idea that gardens are beneficial to patients in health care settings dates as far back as the Middle Ages, when European monasteries created elaborate gardens to provide medicine as well as fulfill the spiritual needs of the ill. Today, we know that being surrounded by nature plays a significant role in patient outcome," said Evangeline Lausier, staff physician at Duke Integrative Medicine in Durham, North Carolina.[6] Adding the dimension of a medicinal garden where herbs can be harvested as medicine and plants distilled for hydrosols and essential oils gives a health care facility extra benefits. Using the garden for beauty, restoration, and practical medicine is the subject for another book.

CHAPTER TWENTY-THREE

Molecules of Light

We come to drive away darkness,
in our hands are light and fire.
Each one is a small light,
and all of us are a mighty light.
Away with darkness, away with blackness!
Away before the light.

—SARAH LEVY

"LIGHT, HEAT, ELECTRICITY, magnetism, chemism, energy, and matter are—in origin, nature, and destiny—one and the same thing.... There are endless changes in physical energy.... In one universe it appears as light, in another light plus heat ... in untold millions of years it may reappear as some form of restless, surging electrical energy or magnetic power; and still later on it may again appear in a subsequent universe as some form of variable matter going through a series of metamorphoses...."[1]

Partly due to their birth in the plant's metabolic reaction to light, essential oils are able to function in our beings on many light levels. On the physical level, light that strikes the engineering marvels we know as leaves becomes the energy source for food manufacturing in photosynthesis. Oils that are distilled from leaves hold some of the subtle imprints of that leafy process such as Spearmint *(Mentha spicata)*, Tulsi or holy basil *(Ocimum basilicum sanctum)*, and Bay laurel *(Laurus nobilis)*. In reality, all oils hold the traces of the process. On the highest level, we are beings of light and energy. We all contain spirit luminosity. When we use the oils for spiritual upliftment, we see that this magical liquid, more than water or oil, is capable of enlivening our energy body as molecules of light.

Pictures of people's auras have been taken before and after using essential oils with Kirlian photography. They show a change of color and light due to the revitalizing effect of the oils. Valerie Worwood said, "Using essential oils in the auric field brings a new [light] energy to the field. The colors of the aura become brighter and clearer.... If the vibration of a person is low for any reason, such as a depressed mental state or ill health, the essential oils can stir or agitate the auric field, stimulating it to reorganize itself into a state of harmony."[2]

Just as light is energy that can manifest as heat, electricity, and magnetic power, on a smaller emotional scale in our humble lives light is constantly changing form:

It can reappear after the dark storms of the disturbing, wailing of our pain bodies. As the light enters our consciousness, love floods our hearts and lifts us up to a place of compassion and forgiveness. It's like being dunked in a tub of beautiful Bulgarian Rose oil diffused in water.

Another gift of light can come when we feel toxic and polluted. A shaft of light energy can lead you to craving a healthier diet and seeking to move for better lymph drainage. The light shaft is like a shower of shimmering Grapefruit and cleansing Fennel to detoxify your body and your emotions.

The light emerges in a different form at the end of a long, dark tunnel of struggle, discipline, and work. The light floods your mind with a sense of satisfaction and fulfillment. It's like bathing in the nurturance of Roman chamomile and the joyful release of Bay laurel.

Sometimes a transmutation of light molecules becomes an uplifting guide. You are feeling lost and confused when suddenly a decision you make brings a spotlight of luminosity to beam down reassurance. It acts like a spritzer of Neroli and Sandalwood to recharge your spiritual awareness and renew your sense of true direction.

As friends of the light, we support Gaia, the mother of our loving planet Earth. Like a supportive parent, she is able to take much abuse from her thoughtless children. However, it's time we clean her streams, lakes, and rivers. It's time we eliminate petroleum gas pollution from her air. It's time we stop dumping plastic bags in her oceans and unbiodegradable garbage on her land. It's time we stop destroying so many bird, fish, and animal species from all the lands and seas. It's time we preserve her remaining plant genuses and stop burning forests that increase global warming. It's time we use natural sunlight and wind to create energy. Help us bring in the light and wake up in time!

Using plant medicines help us manifest more light molecules energetically in our bodies' cellular structure, since essential oils are a secondary metabolite of the plant's ability to utilize the sun's light energy. They are pro-life! Gaia likes our use of renewable essential oils harvested from her plants. Their proliferation leads to more gardens, trees, oxygen, health, and beauty.

We can develop our relationship with our angels. They will guide us to new opportunities when we make the right decisions. As written in *The Urantia Book*, "... these angels act to make the best possible use of the course you have chosen." The angels have gifted us with the use of this beautiful planet for the duration of our short lives. They delight in bringing people together to serve the planet's needs.

Molecules of light are related to the air element, energy. Molecules of essential oils are also close to the air element. Distillation brings them forth from the plant, using heat that turns them into a gas and then cools them down, converting the molecular substances back into a liquid and connecting them to the water element. There is continual energetic transformation in distillation as in the universe and in our bodies.

"We all tend to see our bodies as 'frozen sculpture'—solid, fixed, material objects—when in truth they are more like rivers, constantly changing, flowing patterns of intelligence,"[4][?] Deepak Chopra wrote. We experience the pulsation, the vibrancy of the body as the cells are constantly being born, presented, and passing away. We can feel universes within us coming into existence and passing away, just as we can discover them in the heavens. This is similar to essential oils that are captured through the alchemy of distillation. They remain volatile and escape into the air if not contained in a bottle. They resemble precious jewels for our empowerment in the moment. These cycles of our bodies and essential oils are like the universal light energy that goes through continual change.

As we experience all the transformations of our lives, essential oils are miraculous tonics of light to keep us close to homeostasis and balance. They will be even more effective as we continue to evolve into spiritually awake people, seeking a closer connection to the divine light within us.

Notes

Part One: Eleven Women Who Used Essential Oil Therapy for Healing

Chapter One: Hatshepsut, the First Female Pharaoh of Egypt

1. Catherine H. Roehrig, Renée Dreyfus, and Cathleen A. Keller, eds. *Hatshepsut: From Queen to Pharaoh* (New York: Metropolitan Museum of Art, 2005), 3.
2. Janet R. Buttles, *The Queens of Egypt* (London: Archibald Constable, 1908), 90.
3. Evelyn Wells, *Hatshepsut* (Garden City, NY: Doubleday, 1969), 52.
4. Michal Dayagi-Mendels, *Perfumes and Cosmetics in the Ancient World* (Jerusalem: Israel Museum, 1989), 113.
5. Lise Manniche, *An Ancient Egyptian Herbal* (Austin: University of Texas Press, 1989), 49.
6. Ibid., 52–53.
7. Wells, *Hatshepsut*, 88.
8. Roehrig, *Hatshepsut*, 84.
9. William Kaufman, *Perfume* (New York: Dutton, 1974), 33.
10. Wells, *Hatshepsut*, 106.
11. Ibid., 123.
12. Ibid., 150.
13. Nicolas Grimal, *A History of Ancient Egypt*, trans. Ian Shaw (Oxford, UK: Blackwell, 1992), 209.
14. Eduard Naville, *The XVIII Dynasty Temple of Deir el-Bahri* (London: Egypt Exploration Fund, Memoir 28, 1907), 14.
15. Joyce A.Tyldesley, *Daughters of Isis: Women of Egypt* (New York: Viking, 1994), 146.
16. Naville, *The XVIII Dynasty Temple of Deir el-Bahri*, 49.

Chapter Two: Esther, the Persian Queen Who Saved the Jews

1. Esther 1:6, *The Layman's Parallel Bible,* Modern Language version (Grand Rapids, MI: Zondervan, 1973), 1220.
2. Bonnie S. Anderson and Judith P. Zinsser, *A History of Their Own: A Comprehensive Survey from Prehistoric Times to the Present Day,* vol. 1 (New York: Harper & Row, 1988), 27.

3. Ibid.

4. Roy Genders, *Perfume through the Ages* (New York: Putnam, 1972), 42.

5. Exodus 30:22–25, *New International Version of the Holy Bible* (Grand Rapids, MI: Zondervan, 1978), 93.

6. Song of Solomon 4:12–15, *The Layman's Parallel Bible,* 1640.

7. Paul Frischauer, *So Great a Queen: The Story of Esther, Queen of Persia* (New York: Scribner, 1950), 96.

8. Esther 2:15-17, *The Layman's Parallel Bible,* 1224.

9. Molly Cone, *Purim* (New York: Crowell, 1967), 10.

10. Esther 3:8, *The Layman's Parallel Bible,* 1226.

11. Esther 5:34, *The Layman's Parallel Bible,* 1228.

12. Esther 7:3, *The Layman's Parallel Bible,* 1232.

13. Esther 7:6, *The Layman's Parallel Bible,* 1232.

14. Esther 8:6, *The Layman's Parallel Bible,* 1234.

Chapter Three: Cleopatra, the Queen of Kings

1. Lucy Hughes-Hallett, *Cleopatra: Histories, Dreams, and Distortions* (New York: Harper & Row, 1990), 211.

2. Richard Le Gallienne, *The Romance of Perfume* (New York: Hudnut, 1928), 15.

3. William Shakespeare, *The Complete Works of Shakespeare* (London: Collins Clear Type Press, 1923), 915.

4. Michal Dayagi-Mendels, *Perfumes and Cosmetics in the Ancient World* (Jerusalem: Israel Museum, 1989), 44.

5. Lise Manniche, *An Ancient Egyptian Herbal* (Austin: University of Texas Press, 1989), 44.

6. Ibid., 46.

7. Dayagi-Mendels, *Perfumes and Cosmetics in the Ancient World,* 36.

8. Hughes-Hallett, *Cleopatra,* 94.

9. Ibid., 23.

10. Gaston Delayen, *Cleopatra* (New York: Dutton, 1934), 86.

11. Shakespeare, *The Complete Works of Shakespeare,* 106.

12. Roy Genders, *Perfume through the Ages* (New York: Putnam, 1972), 20.

13. Delayen, *Cleopatra,* 103.

14. Eleanor Sinclair Rohde, *The Scented Garden* (London: The Medici Society, 1931), 3.

15. Genders, *Perfume through the Ages,* 30.

Chapter Four: Women in the Life of Jesus

1. Tsevi Zohar, "The status of women in Jewish law," *Nashim* 5764:7 (Spring 2004), 242.

2. Urantia Foundation, *The Urantia Book* (Chicago: Urantia Foundation, 1955), 1612.

3. Ibid., 1698.

4. Ibid.

5. Ibid.

6. Ibid.

7. John 12:3, *The Layman's Parallel Bible,* Modern Language version (Grand Rapids, MI: Zondervan, 1955), 2592.

8. Roy Genders, *Perfumes Through the Ages* (New York: Putnam, 1972), 50.

9. Patricia Davis, *Subtle Aromatherapy* (Essex: C. W. Daniel, 1991), 222.

10. Urantia Foundation, *The Urantia Book,* 1879.

11. Mark 14:3, *The Layman's Parallel Bible,* 2448.

12. Urantia Foundation, *The Urantia Book,* 1652.

13. Mark 6:12–13, *The Layman's Parallel Bible,* 2420.

14. Urantia Foundation, *The Urantia Book,* 1678–79.

15. Ibid., 1679.

16. Ibid.

17. Jeanne Rose, *375 Essential Oils and Hydrosols* (Berkeley: Frog, 1999), 87.

18. Urantia Foundation, *The Urantia Book,* 1680.

19. Ibid., 2033.

20. Ibid., 1874.

Chapter Five: Zenobia, the Syrian Queen of the Palmyrene Empire

1. William Wright, *An Account of Palmyra and Zenobia: With Travels and Adventures in Bashan and the Desert* (London: Thomas Nelson 1895), 105.

2. Edward Gibbon quoted in *Palmyra and Its Empire: Zenobia's Revolt Against Rome* by Richard Stoneman (Ann Arbor, MI: University of Michigan Press, 1992), 6.

3. Richard Stoneman, *Palmyra and Its Empire: Zenobia's Revolt Against Rome* (Ann Arbor, MI: University of Michigan Press, 1992), 34.

4. Pliny the Elder, Chapter Five, "Roman Technology," in *Historia Naturalis,* vol. 2, John F. Healey, trans. (New York: Penguin Putnam, 1991), 83.

5. Jacqueline F. Long, "Vaballanthus and Zenobia," *De Imperatoribus Romanis,* (Chicago: Loyola University, 1997), 4.

6. William Ware, Zenobia, *Queen of Palmyra: A Tale of the Roman Empire in the Days of the Emperor Aurelian* (Boston: Dana Estes, 1912), 121.

7. Ibid., 60.

8. Wanda Sellar, *The Directory of Essential Oils* (Essex, UK: C. W. Daniel, 1992), 83.

9. Roy Genders, *Perfume through the Ages* (New York: Putnam, 1972), 60.

10. Ibid., 59.

11. Ibid., 60.

12. Athenaeus, *The Deipnosophistae* (Cambridge, MA: Harvard University Press, 1927), 78.

13. Trebellius Pollio, *Historia Augusta* (Augustan History), David Magie, trans. (New York: Loeb Classical Library, 1932), 136.

14. Eunapius quoted in Stoneman, *Palmyra and Its Empire*, 145.

15. *Ware, Zenobia, Queen of Palmyra*, 97.

16. Zosimus, *Historia Nova*, the Decline of Rome (San Antonio: Trinity University Press, 1967), 86.

17. Wright, *An Account of Palmyra and Zenobia*, 140.

18. Ibid., 168.

Chapter Six: Theodora, Empress of the Byzantine Empire

1. Roy Genders, *Perfume through the Ages* (New York: Putnam, 1972), 91.

2. Arnold James Cooley, *The Toilet in Ancient and Modern Times* (New York: Burt Franklin, 1970), 43.

3. Michal Dayagi-Mendels, *Perfumes and Cosmetics in the Ancient World* (Jerusalem: Israel Museum, 1989), 96.

4. John Vandercook, *Empress of the Dusk: A Life of Theodora of Byzantium* (New York: Reynal & Hitchcock, 1940), 52.

5. Ibid., 64.

6. Genders, *Perfume through the Ages*, 67.

7. Procopius of Caesarea, *Anekdota (Secret History)*, Richard Atwater, trans. (Ann Arbor: University of Michigan Press, 1961), 79.

8. Robert Browning, *Justinian and Theodora* (New York: Praeger, 1971), 85.

9. Ibid., 68.

10. Vandercook, *Empress of the Dusk*, 171.

11. Browning, *Justinian and Theodora*, 86.

12. Kathryn Degraff, *Aromatherapy and the Psychology of Fragrance* (San Francisco: New Century, 1996), 6.

13. Vandercook, *Empress of the Dusk*, 210.

14. J. A. S. Evans, *The Age of Justinian: The Circumstances of Imperial Power* (London: Greenwood, 1996), 38.

15. Ibid., 104.

Chapter Seven: Trota, the Wise Woman of Medicine

1. John H. Lienhard, *Engines of Our Ingenuity* (Oxford: Oxford University Press, 2003), 87.

2. Monica Helen Green, ed., *The Trotula: A Medieval Compendium of Women's Medicine* (Philadelphia: University of Pennsylvania Press, 2001), 135.

3. Ibid., 143.

4. Ibid., 161.

5. Ibid., 143.

6. Roy Porter, *Medicine: A History of Healing* (New York: Marlowe, 1997), 178.

7. Trotula of Salerno, *The Diseases of Women,* Elizabeth Mason-Hohl, trans. (Hollywood: Ward Ritchie, 1940), 29.

8. Green, 71–73.

9. Alma Gottlieb, "Menstrual cosmology among the Beng of Ivory Coast," in *Blood Magic: The Anthropology of Menstruation,* Thomas Buckley and Alma Gottlieb, eds. (Berkeley: University of California Press, 1988), 58.

10. Green, 85.

11. Green, 101.

12. Green, 167.

13. Green, 171.

14. Green, 60.

Chapter Eight: Hildegard of Bingen, Prophetess of the Rhine

1. Flona Bowie and Oliver Davies, eds., *Hildegard of Bingen* (London: SPCK, 1990), xiv.

2. Ibid., 9

3. Sabina Flanagan, *Hildegard von Bingen* (London: Universty of Adelaide), www.hildegard.org/documents/flanagan.html.

4. Sabina Flanagan, *Hildegard of Bingen* (1098–1179): A Visionary Life (London: Routledge, 1989), 4.

5. Ibid., 5.

6. Bonnie S. Anderson and Judith P. Zinsser, *A History of Their Own: A Comprehensive Survey from Prehistoric Times to the Present Day,* vol. 1 (New York: Harper & Row, 1988), 188.

7. Bowie and Davies, *Hildegard of Bingen*, 20.

8. Flanagan, www.hildegard.org.

9. Ibid.

10. Bowie and Davies, *Hildegard of Bingen*, 18.

11. Wighard Strehlow and Gottfried Hertzka, *Hildegard of Bingen's Medicine* (Santa Fe, NM: Bear, 1988), 72.

12. Jeanne Achterberg, *Woman as Healer* (Boston: Shambhala, 1990), 56.

13. Strehlow and Hertzka, *Hildegard of Bingen's Medicine*, 45.

14. Ibid., xxvi.

15. Ibid., 17.

16. Ibid., 72.

17. Ibid., 16.

18. Ibid., 28.

19. Columba Hart, trans., and Jane Bishop, trans. *Hildegard of Bingen: Scrivias* (Mahwah: Paulist, 1990), 71.

20. Strehlow and Hertzka, *Hildegard of Bingen's Medicine*, xxiii.

21. Hart and Bishop, *Hildegard of Bingen*, 18.

22. Bowie and Davies, *Hildegard of Bingen*, 21.

Chapter Nine: Catherine de Médicis, Queen of France

1. George Frederick Young, *The Medici* (New York, Modern Library, 1930), 393.

2. Mark Strage, *Women of Power: The Life and Times of Catherine de' Medici* (New York: Harcourt Brace Janovich, 1976), 43.

3. Milton Waldman, *Biography of a Family: Catherine de Medici and Her Children* (Boston: Houghton Mifflin, 1936), 13.

4. Ralph Roeder, *Catherine de Medici and the Lost Revolution* (New York: Garden City, 1939), 148.

5. William Kaufman, *Perfume* (New York: Dutton, 1974), 77.

6. Roeder, *Catherine de' Medici and the Lost Revolution*, 70.

7. Roy Genders, *Perfume through the Ages* (New York: Putnam, 1972), 128.

8. Richard Le Gallienne, *The Romance of Perfume* (New York: Hudnut, 1926), 30.

9. Strage, *Women of Power*, 129.

10. Jean Heriter, *Catherine de Medici* (New York: St. Martin's, 1959), 76.

11. Roeder, *Catherine de Medici and the Lost Revolution*, 240.

12. William Leeper Crain, *Balzac's Le Secret des Ruggieri: A Critical Edition* (Columbia: University of Missouri Press, 1970), xxiii.

13. Genders, *Perfume through the Ages,* 126–27.
14. Ibid., 128.
15. Heriter, *Catherine de Medici,* 377.
16. Strage, *Women of Power,* 297.
17. Le Gallienne, *The Romance of Perfume,* 41.
18. Jeanne Achterberg, *Woman as Healer* (Boston: Shambhala, 1991), 89–90.

Chapter Ten: Elizabeth I, the Virgin Queen of England

1. Mary Luke, *Gloriana: The Years of Elizabeth I* (New York: Coward, McCann & Geoghegan, 1973), xii.
2. Psalm 118:23, *The Layman's Parallel Bible,* Modern Language version (Grand Rapids: Zondervan, 1973), 1498
3. Luke, *Gloriana,* xii.
4. Lacey Baldwin Smith, *The Horizon Book of The Elizabethan World* (New York: American Heritage, 1967), 74.
5. Smith, *The Horizon Book of The Elizabethan World,* 96.
6. Ibid., 79.
7. Ibid., 86.
8. Arnold James Cooley, *The Toilet in Ancient and Modern Times* (New York: Burt Franklin: 1970), 65.
9. Roy Genders, *Perfume through the Ages* (New York: Putnam, 1972), 152.
10. Ibid., 154.
11. Ibid, 155.
12. Carolly Erickson, *The First Elizabeth* (New York: Summit Books, 1983), 222.
13. Ibid., 223.
14. Genders, *Perfume through the Ages,* 149.
15. Ibid., 142.
16. Ibid., 144.
17. Erickson, *The First Elizabeth,* 224.
18. Christopher Hibbert, *The Virgin Queen: Elizabeth I, Genius of the Golden Age* (New York: Addison-Wesley, 1991), 137.
19. Ibid., 189.
20. Eleanor Sinclair Rohde, *The Scented Garden* (London: David & Charles, 1989), 7.
21. Genders, *Perfume through the Ages,* 153.
22. Ruth Winter, *The Smell Book: Scents, Sex, and Society* (New York: Lippincott, 1976), 48.

23. Rohde, *The Scented Garden*, 8.
24. Cooley, *The Toilet in Ancient and Modern Times*, 68.
25. Genders, *Perfume through the Ages*, 155.
26. Luke, *Gloriana*, 184.

Chapter Eleven: Marguerite Maury, the Holistic Healer

1. Marguerite Maury, *The Secret of Life and Youth* (Essex: C. W. Daniel, 1989), 19.
2. Robert Tisserand, *Aromatherapy: To Heal and Tend the Body* (Santa Fe, NM: Lotus, 1988), 44.
3. Christine Wildwood, *Aromatherapy: Massage with Essential Oils* (Rockport, MA: Elements, 1991), 17.
4. Maury, *The Secret of Life and Youth*, 9.
5. Daniele Ryman, *The Aromatherapy Handbook* (Essex: C. W. Daniel, 1984), ix–x.
6. Maury, *The Secret of Life and Youth*, 1.
7. Ibid., 202.

Part Two: Honoring the Work of Contemporary Aromatherapists

Chapter Twelve: The Sense of Smell and the Limbic Brain

1. Gerhard Buchbauer et al.," Fragrance compounds with sedative effects upon inhalation," *Journal of Pharmaceutical Sciences* 82 (1963), 660–65.
2. P. Badia et al., "Responsiveness to olfactory stimuli presented in sleep," *Physiological Behavior* 48 (1990), 87–90.
3. S. Torri et al., "Contingent negative variation and the psychological effects of odor," in *Perfumery: The Psychology and Biology of Fragrance* by Steve Van Toller and George H. Dodd (London: Chapman & Hall, 1988), 107–20.
4. P. Rovesti, *In Search of Perfumes Lost* (Venice: Blow-up, 1980), 9.

Chapter Thirteen: Modern Methods of Using Essential Oils

1. Jager et al., "Skin absorption of linalool and linalyl acetate," *Neuropsychopharmacology* 29 (1992), 1925–32.
2. Robert Tisserand and Tony Balacs, *Essential Oil Safety* (Edinburgh: Churchill Livingstone, 1995), 63.
3. Liz Earle, *New Vital Oils: The Ultimate Guide to Radiant Beauty and Health* (London: Random, 2003), 45.

4. Tisserand and Balacs, *Essential Oil Safety*, 32.

5. Ibid., 24–25.

6. Kurt Schnaubelt, *Medical Aromatherapy: Healing with Essential Oils* (Berkeley: Frog, 1999), 223–24.

7. De La Motte et al., "German chamomile for children with diarrhea," *Arzneimittel Forschung* 47 (Munich: Harrison Clinical Research, November 1997), 1247–49.

Chapter Fourteen: The Importance of Chemical Makeup

1. Kurt Schnaubelt, *Medical Aromatherapy: Healing with Essential Oils* (Berkeley: Frog, 1999), 80.

2. Igimi et al., "Limonene can dissolve gallstones," *Digestive Diseases and Science* 36 (1991), 200–08.

3. Elson, Maltzman, Boston, Tanner, and Gould, "d-limonene, anti-carcinogenic activity," *Carcinogenesis* 9:2 (1988), 331–32.

4. Safyh et al., "Chamazulene in German chamomile," *Planta Medicine* 60 (1994), 410–13.

5 A. Ultee et al., "Mechanisms of action of carvacrol," *Applied and Environmental Microbiology* 65:10 (1999), 4606–10.

6. A. Ramanoel, "Thyme, great anti-bacterial vs. *Staphlococcus* and *E. Coli*," *Arch Institute of Pasteur* 76 (1987), 59.

7. S. Dean, "Oregano is anti-viral," *Flavor and Fragrance* 5 (1990), 51–53.

8. J. Stiles, "Anti-fungal property of oregano vs. candida," *Journal of Applied Nutrition* 47 (1995), 96–102.

9. Tantaoui, "Anti-parasitical oregano vs. *Aspergillus parasiticus*," *Environmental Pathology, Toxicology and Oncology* 13 (1994), 67–72.

10. Pierre Franchomme and Daniel Pénoël, *L'Aromatherapie Exactement* (Limoges, France: Roger Jollois, 1990), 383.

11. Carson and Riley, "Terpin-4-ol and linalool were effective," *Journal of Applied Bacteriology* 78:3 (1995), 264–69.

12. Sivropoulou et al., "Oregano is effective anti-bacterial vs. larynx carcinoma," *Journal of Agriculture Food Chemistry* 44:5 (1996), 1202–05.

13. A. Ultee et al., "Carvacrol causes increased permeability to H and K ions," *Journal of Dairy Science* 90 (1999), 2580–96.

14. Cabo et al. "Caryophyllene is anti-spasmolytic," *Planta Medicine Phytotherapy* 20:3 (1986), 213–18.

15. Franchomme and Pénoël, *L'Aromatherapie Exactement*, 180.

16. Buchbauer et al., "Essential oils with sedative effects upon inhalation," *Journal of Pharmaceutical Sciences* 82:6 (1993), 660–64.

17. V. Nikolaevski, "Esters are hypotensive with sedative action on the heart," *Patol Fiziol Eksp Ter* 5 (1990), 52–53.

18. F. Occhiuto et al., "Bergamot reduces coronary dilator action," *International Journal of Pharmacology* 23:2 (1996), 225–30.

19. G. Roulier, *Les Huiles pour Votre Sante* (Paris: Dangles, 1990), 74.

20. F. Occhiuto et al., "Bergamot is sedative medicine for cns," *International Journal of Pharmacology* 33:3 (1995), 198–203.

21. Sylla Shepherd-Hangar, *Aromatherapy Practitioner Reference Manual*, vol. 1 (Tampa: Atlantic Institute of Aromatherapy, 1995), 167.

22. S. Zaynoun et al., "Bergamot is phototoxic," *British Journal of Dermatology* 96 (1977), 475–82.

23. Randy Zirtls et al., "Limonene has an anti-tumoral effect," *Cancer Research* 53:17 (1993), 3849–52.

24. M. Gould, "Prevention of mammary cancer by monoterpenes," *Journal of Cellular Biochemistry* 22 (1995), 139-44.

25. Elizabetsk et al., "Anti-infectious and sedative effect of linalool on cns," *Fitoterapia* 66:5 (1995), 407–14.

26. F. Occhiuto et al., "Bergamot helps with coronary spasm and arrhythmias," *International Journal of Pharmacology* 23:2 (1996), 128–33.

27. Joy Bowles, *The Chemistry of Aromatherapeutic Oils* (Crows Nest, Australia: Allen & Unwin, 2003), 86.

28. Robert Tisserand and Tony Balacs, *Essential Oil Safety* (London: Churchill Livingstone, 1995), 192.

29. Pierre Franchomme and Daniel Pénoël, *L'Aromatherapie Exactement*, 294.

30. Tambe et al., "Beta-caryophyllene reduces stomach cell damage," *Planta Medica* 62:5 (1996), 469–70.

31. Go Onawunmiet et al., "Anti-bacterial activity of neral and geranial," *Journal of Ethnopharmacology* 12:3 (1984), 279–86.

32. N. K. Dubey et al., "Citral vs. P388 leukemia cells," *Current Science* 73:1 (1997), 22–24.

33. Tisserand and Balacs, *Essential Oil Safety*, 40.

34. Carson and Riley, "Alcohols," *Journal of Antimicrobial Chemotherapy* 50 (1995), 246–47.

35. H. Gobel et al., "Menthol reduces pain headaches," *Cephalalgia* 14 (1994), 228–34.

36. S. Pattnaik et al., "Ten oils vs. 22 bacteria," *Microbios* 86 (1996), 237–46.

37. Taddai et al., "Menthol inhibited muscle contraction," *Fitoterapia* 59:6 (1988), 463–68.

38. R. S. Leicester and R. H. Hunt, "Peppermint to relieve colonic spasm," *Lancelot* 2:8305 (1982), 989.

39. H. Gobel et al., "Essential oils and headache mechanisms," *Phytomedicine* 2:2 (1995), 93-102.

40. Asakura et al., "Alpha eudesmol, sesquiterpenol from cedarwood (*Juniperus virginiana*) inhibits omega-agatoxin IVA sensitive Ca2," *Brain Research* 823:1–2 (2004), 169–76.

41. Luft et al., "Farnesol reduced blood pressure," *Arteriosclerosis, Thrombosis and Vascular Biology* 19:3 (1999), 959–66.

42. Valerie Ann Worwood, *Aromatherapy for the Soul: Healing the Spirit with Fragrance and Essential Oils* (Novato, CA: New World Library, 1999), 287.

43. Franchomme and Pénoël, *L'Aromatherapie Exactement*, 183.

44. T. Betts, "Study on epilepsy: Oils to make seizure free," *Aromatherapy Quarterly* (Spring 1994), 19–22.

45. A. Rioja et al., "Farnesol and leukemia cells," *FEBS Letters* 467:2–3 (2000), 291-95.

46. C. Violion et al., "Ylang as anti-fungal," *Fitoterapia* 67:3 (1996), 279–81.

47. C. Ontengco et al., "Ylang vs. staphylococcus aureus," *Aeta Manilana* 43 (1995), 19–23.

Chapter Fifteen: Case Studies

1. John Nunn, *Ancient Egyptian Medicine* (Norman, OK: University of Oklahoma Press, 1996), 144.

Chapter Sixteen: Essential Oils for the Treatment of Infection

1. Kurt Schnaubelt, *Medical Aromatherapy: Healing with Essential Oils* (Berkeley: Frog, 1999), 4.

2. Jean Valnet, *The Practice of Aromatherapy: A Classic Compendium of Plant Medicines and Their Healing Properties* (New York: Destiny Books, 1980), 44.

3. Paul Belaiche, *Traite de Phytotherapie et Aromatherapie* (Paris: Maloine S.A., 1979).

4. Pierre Franchomme and Daniel Pénoël, *L'Aromatherapie Exactement* (Limoges, France: Roger Jollois, 1991).

5. Rideal et al., "Germicidal powers and capillary activities of certain essential oils," *Performance of Essential Oil Record* 19 (1928), 285–304.

6. S. L. Malowan, "Essential oil ability to influence cell metabolism," *Der Parfinneur* 4 (1930), 20.

7. Robert Tisserand and Tony Balacs, *Essential Oil Safety* (London: Churchill Livingstone, 1995), 58.

8. Harris and Harris, "Essential oil effect on cell membrane," *Aromatherapy Quarterly* 44 (1995), 25–27.

9. Savino et al., "Antimicrobial activity of essential oil of boldo," *Bolettino di Micro-biologia e Indagini Lab.* 14:1 (1994), 5–12.

10. Philippe Goeb, "Bronchi-pulmonary pathologies," *Les Cahiers de L'Aromatherapie Records* (1995), 65.

11. Kelner and Kober, "Moglichkeiten der verwendung atherischer ole zur raumdesinfektion," *Arzneimittel Forschung* 5:4 (1954), 224–29.

12. J. M. Schmidt et al., "Essential oils against Candida," *Oral Microbiology Immunology* 20:2 (1936), 101–05.

13. Herman and Kucera, "Anti-viral substances in mint family plants," *Proceedings of the Society for Experimental Biology and Medicine* 124 (1967), 865, 874.

14. Inouye et al., "Antisporulating and respiration inhibitory effect on filamentous mycoses," 41:9–10 (1998), 403–10.

15. Galal et al., "Evaluation of certain volatile oils for their antifungal properties," *Journal of Drug Research* 5:2 (1973), 235–45.

16. P. Belaiche, "Treatment of vaginal infections of Candida albicans with essential oils of *Melaleuca alternifolia*," *Phytotherapy* 15 (1985), 13–14.

17. N. Cuong, "Antibacterial properties of Vietnamese cajeput oil," *Journal of Essential Oil Research* 6 (1994), 63–67.

18. H. Wagner, *Plant Drug Analysis* (Berlin: Springer-Verlag, 1984).

19. Jane Buckle, *Clinical Aromatherapy: Essential Oils in Practice* (Philadelphia: Churchill Livingstone 2003), 188–189.

20. Shirley Price and Len Price, eds., *Aromatherapy for Health Professionals* (London: Churchill Livingstone, 1995), 61–62.

21. Zakarya et al., "Antimicrobial activity relationships of eucalyptus essential oils," *Plantes Medical Phytotherapy* 26:4 (1993), 319–31.

22. Caelli et al., "Tea tree oil for *Staphylococcus aureus*," *Journal of Hospital Infections* 46:3 (2001), 236–37.

23. B. Kedzia, "Antimicrobial activity of chamomile," *Herba Polonica* 37:1 (1991), 29–38.

24. M. Roberts, *Biology: A Functional Approach*, 4th ed. (Walton on Thames, UK: Nelson Thornes, 1986), 74.

25. James A. Duke, *A Handbook of Medicinal Herbs* (Boca Raton, FL: CRC Press, 1985), 450.

26. C. Mathias, "Contact urticaria from cinnamic aldehyde," *Archives of Dermatology* 116:1 (1980), 74–76.

27. G. May and G. Willuhn, "Antiviral activity of aqueous extracts from medicinal plants in tissue cultures," *Arzneimittel-Forschung Drug Research* 28:1 (1979), 1–7.

28. Franchomme and Pénoël, 239.

29. Ibid., 243.

30. Price and Price, *Aromatherapy for Health Professionals*, 167.

31, Christian Duraffourd, "Essential oils' three actions vs. respiratory infections," *Journale de la Plante Medicinole* 33 (Perigny, France: Enforme Tous Les Jours, 1987), 82.

32. Schilcher in *Aromatherapy for Health Professionals* by Price and Price, 68.

Chapter Seventeen: Immune Stimulating Effect of Essential Oils

1. Michael A. Schmidt, "Antibiotics: The Promise and the Peril," Pacific Institute of Aromatherapy Conference, 1995.

2. Chris Highland, ed., *Meditations of John Muir: Nature's Temple* (Berkeley: Wilderness, 2001), 11.

3. Ann Percival, *Aromatherapy: A Nurse's Guide for Women* (Surrey: Amberwood, 1995), 36.

4. Ibid., 37.

5. Anthony L. Komaroff, ed., *Harvard Medical School Family Health Guide* (New York: Simon & Schuster, 1999), 867.

6. H. Wagoner, *Economic and Medicinal Plant Research*, vol. 1 (London: Academic, 1985).

7. Daniel Pénoël. "The Immune System of Mankind," *Aroma 93 Conference Proceedings* (Brighton, UK: Aromatherapy Publications, 1993).

8. Elaine N. Marieb, *Essentials of Human Anatomy and Physiology*, 7th ed. (San Francisco: Benjamin Cummings, 2003), 374.

9. Schmidt, "Antibiotics," 84.

10. Wighard Strehlow and Gottfried Hertzka, *Hildegard of Bingen's Medicine* (Santa Fe, NM: Bear, 1988), 55.

11. T. Komori et al., "Effects of citrus fragrance on immune function and depressive states," *Neuroimmunomodulation* 2 (1995), 174–80.

Chapter Eighteen: Achieving Optimal Health with Essential Oil, Nutritional, and Herbal Therapy

1. Deepak Chopra, *Creating Health: How to Wake Up the Body's Intelligence* (Boston: Houghton Mifflin, 1987), 131.

Chapter Nineteen: Essential Oils and the Mind-Body Connection

1. Bill Moyers, *Healing and the Mind* (New York: Doubleday, 1993).

2. Deepak Chopra, forward to *Molecules of Emotion: The Science Behind Mind-Body Medicine* by Candace B. Pert (New York: Simon & Schuster, 1997), 9–10.

3. Candace B. Pert, *Molecules of Emotion: The Science Behind Mind-Body Medicine* (New York: Simon and Schuster, 1997), 147.

4. T. Umezo, "Anti-conflict clinical trial of rose," *Pharmacology, Biochemistry and Behavior* 64 (1999), 35–40.

5. I. Ceccarelli et al., "Citrus oil-induced increase of hippocampal acetylcholine," Neuroscience Letters 330 (2002), 25–28.

6. E. Elizabetsky et al., "Effects of linalool on glutamatergic system," *Neurochemical Research* 20:4 (1995), 461–65.

7. Peter Damian and Kate Damian, *Aromatherapy: Scent and Psyche.* (Rochester, VT: Healing Arts, 1995), 143.

8. Bruce H. Lipton, *The Biology of Belief: Unleashing the Power of Consciousness, Matter, & Miracles* (Santa Rosa, CA: Mountain of Love, 2005), 163.

9. Ibid., 181.

10. G. Seth et al., "Effect of essential oil of Cymbopogan citratus on the CNS," *Indian Journal of Experimental Biology* 14:3 (1976), 370–71.

11. H. Gobel et al., "Effect of peppermint and eucalyptus oil preparations on neurophysiological headache parameters," *Cephalalgia* 14 (1994), 228–34.

12. René-Maurice Gattefossé, *Gattefossé's Aromatherapy* (Essex: C. W. Daniel, 1993), 7–10.

13. R. Fujiwara, "Effects of a long-term inhalation of fragrances on stress-induced immunosuppression," 5 (1994), 318–22.

14. F. Occhiuto et al., "Effects of *Citrus bergamia* on the CNS," *International Journal of Pharmacognosy* 33:3 (1995), 198.

15. A. Al-Hadder and Z. Hasan, "Rosemary and diabetes," Journal of Ethnopharmacology 43 (1994), 217–21.

16. Jane Buckle, *Clinical Aromatherapy: Essential Oils in Practice* (Philadelphia: Churchill Livingstone, 2003), 300.

17. John R. Lee and Virginia Hopkins, *Dr. John Lee's Hormone Balance Made Simple: The Essential How-to Guide to Symptoms, Dosage, Timing, and More* (New York: Warner, 2006), 74.

18. Buckle, *Clinical Aromatherapy,* 295.

19. Ibid.

20. A. Hardcastle, "Influence of peppermint oil on absorptive processes in rat small intestine," *Gut* 39 (1996), 214–19.

21. M. Albert-Puleo, "The effect of fennel on uterine contraction," *Journal of Ethnopharmacology* 76 (2001), 299–304.

22. M. Albert-Puleo, "Fennel and anise as estrogenic agents," *Journal of Ethnopharmacology* 2:4 (1980), 337–44.

23. Paul Belaiche, *Traite de Phytotherapie et d'Aromatherapie* (Paris: Maloine S.A., 1979), 65.

24. John E. Sarno, *Healing Back Pain: The Mind-Body Connection* (New York: Warner, 1991), 184.

25. N. Hadfield, "Aromatherapy massage to reduce anxiety," *International Journal of Palliative Nursing* 23 (2001), 50.

26. E. Feher et al., "Thyme oil's effects on nerve fibers," Programme Abstracts, 24th *International Symposium on Essential Oils* 78 (1992), 47.

27. Steve Van Toller, ed., *Fragrance: The Psychology and Biology of Perfume* (New York: Springer-Verlag, 1993), 225.

28. T. Komori et al., "Effects of citrus fragrance on immune function and depressive states," *Neuroimmunomodulation* 2 (1995), 174–80.

29. Elizabeth Kübler-Ross, *On Death and Dying* (New York: Touchstone Books, Simon & Schuster, 1969), 240.

30. Joan Borysenko, *Minding the Body, Mending the Mind* (Reading, MA: Bantam, 1987), 4.

31. Urantia Foundation, *The Urantia Book* (Chicago: Urantia Foundation, 1955), 1216.

32. Larry Dossey, *Healing Words: The Power of Prayer and the Practice of Medicine* (San Francisco: HarperCollins, 1993), 164.

Part Three: Future Prospects for Aromatherapists

Chapter Twenty: Energetic Medicine

1. Albert Einstein, *The Collected Papers of Albert Einstein*, Vol. 2, *The Swiss Years: Writings, 1990–1909* (Princeton, NJ: Princeton University Press, 1990).

2. Barbara Ann Brennan, *Hands of Light: Guide to Healing through the Human Energy Field* (New York: Bantam, 1987).

3. John C. Pierrakos, *Core Energetics: Developing the Capacity to Love and Heal* (Mendocino, CA: Life Rhythm, 1990).

4. Dennis Willmont, *Aromatherapy in Chinese Medicine* (Marshfield, MA: Willmountain, 2003).

5. Philip M. Chancellor, *Handbook of Bach Flower Remedies* (Essex: C. W. Daniel, 1971).

6. Dana Ullman, *Homeopathic Educational Services* (Berkeley: Homeopathic Educational Services, 2007).

7. Patricia Davis, *Subtle Aromatherapy* (Essex: C. W. Daniel, 1991), 32.

8. Richard Gerber, *Vibrational Medicine: New Choices for Healing Ourselves* (Santa Fe, NM: Bear, 1988).

9. Wighard Strehlow and Gottfried Hertzka, *Hildegard of Bingen's Medicine* (Santa Fe, NM: Bear, 1988), 123.

10. Eva-Marie Lind, "Aromatherapy and reflexology," *American Alliance of Aromatherapy* 4 (Winter 1997), 44.

11. Laura Norman, *Feet First: A Guide to Foot Reflexology* (New York: Simon & Schuster 1988).

Chapter Twenty-One: Integrative Medicine

1. http://www.ourcivilisation.com/medicine/usamed/deaths.htm.

2. Bill Moyers, *Healing and the Mind* (New York: Doubleday, 1993), 31.

3. Andrew Weil, Life and Wellness Conference, October 20–22, 2006, Mammoth Lakes, California.

4. Scott Morcott quoted in Karrie Osborn, "Hospital Spas," *Associated Bodywork and Massage Professionals* (April–May 2005), www.massagetherapy.com/articles/index.php/article_id/910.

5. Y. Miyazaki et al., "Essential oils increase speed of performing a mental task," *Mokuzai-Gakkaishi* 38:10 (1992), 903–908.

6. C. H. Manley, "Psychophysiological effect of odor," *Critical Reviews in Food Science and Nutrition* 33:1 (1993), 57–82.

7. Rachael McGraw, "Aromatherapy Oils Could Stamp Out Spread of mrsa Superbug," *Medical News Today* (East Sussex: MediLexicon International, 2004), www.medicalnewstoday.com/articles/18188.php.

8. C. F. Carson, "Study on essential oils and mrsa infections," *Journal of Antimicrobial Chemotherapy* 37:6 (1995), 1177–181.

9. Jane Buckle, "How to integrate clinical aromatherapy in a hospital setting," Centre for Complementary Health Care and Integrated Medicine (St. Petersburg, FL: Aromatherapy Conference Tours, March 2006).

10. Jane Buckle, *Clinical Aromatherapy: Essential Oils in Practice* (Philadelphia: Churchill Livingstone, 2003), 378.

11. Aurora Ocampo, Department of Integrative Medicine, Beth Israel Medical Center, 2007, http://www.healthandhealingny.org/complement/aroma_pract.asp.

12. Simon Scott, Tree of Life Rejuvenation Center, www.treeoflife.nu/spiritual-retreats/spiritual-fasting/.

13. Andrew Weil, *Mind-Body Workbook* (Boulder, CO: Sounds True, 2005), 1.

Chapter Twenty-Two: Aromatic Gardens

1. Sabina Flanagan, *Hildegard of Bingen (1098–1179): A Visionary Life* (London: Routledge, 1989), 63.

2. Marcel Lavabre, *Aromatherapy Workbook* (Rochester, VT: Healing Arts, 1997), 11.

3. Wendy Johnson, *Gardening at the Dragon's Gate: At Work in the Wild and Cultivated World* (New York: Bantam, 2008), 101.

4. Eleanour Sinclair Rohde, *The Scented Garden* (Boston: Hale, Cushman & Flint, 1936), 6–7.

5. Johnson, *Gardening at the Dragon's Gate*, 314.

6. Evangeline Lausier, quoted in "A Healing Garden" by Mark Schreiner, *Inside Duke Medicine* (Durham, NC: Duke University Health System, 2008), http://www.dukehealth.org/HealthLibrary/HealthArticles/a_healing_garden.

Chapter Twenty-Three: Molecules of Light

1. Urantia Foundation, *The Urantia Book* (Chicago: Urantia Foundation, 1955), 472.

2. Valerie Ann Worwood, *The Fragrant Heavens: The Spiritual Dimensions of Fragrance and Aromatherapy* (Novato, CA: New World Library, 1999), 124–29.

3. Urantia Foundation, *The Urantia Book*, 1246.

4. Deepak Chopra, *Perfect Health: The Complete Mind/Body Guide* (New York: Three Rivers, 1991), 18.

Resources

High Quality Essential Oils

Elizabeth Van Buren
P.O. Box 7542
Santa Cruz, CA 95061
(831) 425-8218
(800) 710-7759
www.elizabethvanburen.com

Lifetree Aromatix
John Steele
(818) 986-0594

Original Swiss Aromatics
P.O. Box 6842
San Rafael, CA 94915
(415) 479-3998
www.originalswissaromatics.com

Analytical Services

Spectrix Labs
220 Country Estates Terrace
Santa Cruz, CA 95060
(831) 427-9336
www.spectrixlab.com

Education

College of Botanical Healing Arts
1821 17th Avenue
Santa Cruz, CA 95062
(831) 462-1807
(877) 321-7346
www.cobha.org

Clinical Aromatherapy for Health Professionals
R. J. Buckle
P.O. Box 868
Hunter, NY 12442
www.rjbuckle.com

Institute of Integrative Aromatherapy
Valerie Cooksley and Laraine Kyle
www.aroma-rn.com

Networking

Alliance of International Aromatherapists (AIA)
Suite 323, 9956 W. Remington Place, Unit A10
Littleton, CO 80128
(877) 531-6377

Integrative Health Centers

Tree of Life Rejuvenation Center
P.O. Box 778
Patagonia, AZ 85624
(866) 394-2520

Nature Photography

Avonel Jones
avoneljones@yahoo.com

Bibliography

Achterberg, Jeanne. *Women as Healer.* Boston: Shambhala, 1991.

Anderson, Bonnie S., and Judith P. Zinsser. *A History of Their Own: A Comprehensive Survey from Prehistoric Times to the Present Day,* vol. 1. New York: Harper & Row, 1988.

Athenaeus. *The Deipnosophistae.* Cambridge, MA: Harvard University Press, 1927.

Battaglia, Salvatore. *The Complete Guide to Aromatherapy.* Queensland, Australia: Perfect Potion, 1995.

Belaiche, Paul. *Traite de Phytotherapie et d'Aromatherapie.* Paris: Maloine S.A., 1979.

Borysenko, Joan. *Minding the Body, Mending the Mind.* Reading, MA: Bantam, 1987.

Bowie, Flona, and Oliver Davies, eds. *Hildegard of Bingen: An Anthology.* London: SPCK, 1990.

Bowles, Joy. *The Chemistry of Aromatherapeutic Oils.* Crows Nest, Australia: Allen & Unwin, 2003.

Brennan, Barbara Ann. *Hands of Light: Guide to Healing through the Human Energy Field.* New York: Bantam, 1987.

Browning, Robert. *Justinian and Theodora.* New York: Praeger, 1971.

Buckle, Jane. *Clinical Aromatherapy: Essential Oils in Practice.* 2nd ed. Philadelphia: Churchill Livingstone, 2003.

Buckley, Thomas, and Alma Gottlieb. *Blood Magic: The Anthropology of Menstruation.* Berkeley: University of California Press, 1988.

Buttles, Janet R. *The Queens of Egypt.* London: Archibald Constable, 1908.

Capon, Brian. *Botany for Gardeners.* 2nd ed. Portland: Timber Press, 2005.

Chancellor, Philip M.. *Handbook of the Bach Flower Remedies.* Essex: C. W. Daniel, 1971.

Chopra, Deepak. *Creating Health: How to Wake Up the Body's Intelligence.* Boston: Houghton Mifflin, 1987.

Chopra, Deepak. *Perfect Health: The Complete Mind/Body Guide.* New York: Three Rivers, 1991.

Cone, Molly. *Purim.* New York: Crowell, 1967.

Cooksley, Valerie Gennarie. Aromatherapy: Soothing Remedies to Restore, Rejuvenate and Heal. Paramus, NJ: Prentice Hall, 2002.

Cooley, Arnold James. *The Toilet in Ancient and Modern Times.* New York: Burt Franklin, 1970.

Cousens, Gabriel. *Conscious Eating*. Berkeley: North Atlantic Books, 2000.

Crain, William Leeper. *Balzac's Le Secret des Ruggieri: A Critical Edition*. Columbia: University of Missouri Press, 1970.

Damian, Peter, and Kate Damian. *Aromatherapy: Scent and Psyche*. Rochester, VT: Healing Arts, 1995.

Davis, Patricia. *Aromatherapy: An A–Z*. Essex: C. W. Daniel, 1988.

Davis, Patricia. *Subtle Aromatherapy*. Essex: C. W. Daniel, 1991.

Dayagi-Mendels, Michal. *Perfumes and Cosmetics in the Ancient World*. Jerusalem: Israel Museum, 1989.

Degraff, Kathryn. *Aromatherapy and the Psychology of Fragrance*. San Francisco: New Century, 1996.

Dossey, Larry. *Healing Words: The Power of Prayer and the Practice of Medicine*. New York: HarperCollins, 1993.

Duke, James A. *The Green Pharmacy: New Discoveries in Herbal Remedies for Common Diseases and Conditions from the World's Foremost Authority on Healing Herbs*. Emmaus, PA: Rodale, 1997.

Duke, James A. *A Handbook of Medicinal Herbs*. Boca Raton, FL: CRC Press, 1985.

Earle, Liz. *New Vital Oils: The Ultimate Guide to Radiant Beauty and Health*. London: Random House, 2003.

Eidson, Deborah. *Vibrational Healing: Revealing the Essence of Nature through Aromatherapy and Essential Oils*. Berkeley: Frog Books, 2000.

Einstein, Albert. *The Collected Papers of Albert Einstein, Volume 2, The Swiss Years: Writings, 1990–1909*. Princeton, NJ: Princeton University Press, 1990.

Erickson, Carolly. *The First Elizabeth*. New York: Summit Books, 1983.

Evans, J. A. S. *The Age of Justinian: The Circumstances of Imperial Power*. London: Greenwood, 1996.

Flanagan, Sabina. *Hildegard of Bingen: A Visionary Life*. London: Routledge, 1989.

Franchomme, Pierre, and Daniel Pénoël. *L'Aromatherapie Exactement*. Limoges, France: Roger Jollois, 1990.

Frischauer, Paul. *So Great a Queen: The Story of Esther, Queen of Persia*. New York: Scribner, 1950.

Fuller, H. J., and O. Tippo. *College Botany*. New York: Holt, 1949.

Gattefossé, René-Maurice. *Gattefossé's Aromatherapy*. Essex: C. W. Daniel, 1993.

Genders, Roy. *Perfume through the Ages*. New York: Putnam, 1972.

Gerber, Richard. *Vibrational Medicine: New Choices for Healing Ourselves*. Santa Fe, NM: Bear, 1988.

Gibbon, Edward. *The History of the Decline and Fall of the Roman Empire*. London: Strahan & Cadell, 1776–1789.

Gibran, Kahlil. *The Prophet.* New York: Knopf, 1962.

Green, Monica Helen, ed. *The Trotula: A Medieval Compendium of Women's Medicine.* Philadelphia: University of Pennsylvania Press, 2001.

Grimal, Nicholas. Translated by Ian Shaw. *A History of Ancient Egypt.* Oxford, UK: Blackwell, 1992.

Harris, Bob, and Rhiannon Harris. *The Essential Oil Resource Database.* www.essentialoilresource.com.

Hart, Columba, trans., and Jane Bishop, trans. *Hildegard of Bingen: Scivias.* Mahwah, NJ: Paulist, 1990.

Heriter, Jean. *Catherine de Medici.* New York: St. Martin's, 1959.

Hibbert, Christopher. *The Virgin Queen: Elizabeth I, Genius of the Golden Age.* New York: Addison-Wesley, 1991.

Highland, Chris. *Meditations of John Muir: Nature's Temple.* Berkeley: Wilderness, 2001.

Holmes, Peter. *The Energetics of Western Herbs,* vol. 1 & 2. Boulder, CO: Snow Lotus, 1989.

Hughes-Hallett, Lucy. *Cleopatra: Histories, Dreams, and Distortions.* New York: Harper & Row, 1990.

Johnson, Wendy. *Gardening at the Dragon's Gate: At Work in the Wild and Cultivated World.* New York: Bantam, 2008.

Kaufman, William I. *Perfume.* New York: Dutton, 1974.

Komaroff, Anthony L., ed. *Harvard Medical School Family Health Guide.* New York: Simon & Schuster, 1999.

Lavabre, Marcel. *Aromatherapy Workbook.* Rochester, VT: Healing Arts, 1997.

Lawless, Julia. *Illustrated Encyclopedia of Essential Oils: The Complete Guide to the Use of Oils in Aromatherapy and Herbalism.* Rockport, MA: Element, 1995.

Lawrence, Brian M. *Monographs on Essential Oil.* Carol Stream, IL: Allured, 1975–1994.

The Layman's Parallel Bible (Modern Language version). Grand Rapids, MI: Zondervan, 1973.

Lee, John R, and Virginia Hopkins. *Dr. John Lee's Hormone Balance Made Simple: The Essential How-to Guide to Symptoms, Dosage, Timing, and More.* New York: Warner, 2006.

Le Gallienne, Richard. *The Romance of Perfume.* New York: Hudnut, 1926.

Lipton, Bruce H. *The Biology of Belief: Unleashing the Power of Consciousness, Matter, & Miracles.* Santa Rosa, CA: Mountain of Love, 2005.

Long, Jacqueline F. "Vaballanthus and Zenobia." *De Imperatoribus Romanis.* Chicago: Loyola University of Chicago, 1997.

Luke, Mary. *Glorianna: The Years of Elizabeth I.* New York: Coward, McCann & Geoghegan, 1973.

Mabberley, D. J. *The Plant-Book: A Portable Dictionary of the Vascular Plants.* Cambridge, UK: Cambridge University Press, 1989.

Manniche, Lise. *An Ancient Egyptian Herbal.* Austin: University of Texas Press, 1989.

Marieb, Elaine N. *Essentials of Human Anatomy and Physiology.* 7th ed. San Francisco: Benjamin Cummings, 2003.

Maury, Marguerite. *The Secret of Life and Youth.* Essex: C. W. Daniel, 1989.

Moyers, Bill. *Healing and the Mind.* New York: Doubleday, 1993.

Norman, Laura. *Feet First: A Guide to Reflexology.* New York: Simon & Schuster, 1987.

Nunn, J. F. *Ancient Egyptian Medicine.* Norman, OK: University of Oklahoma Press, 2001.

Percival, Ann. *Aromatherapy: A Nurse's Guide for Women.* Surrey: Amberwood, 1995.

Pert, Candace B. *Molecules of Emotion: The Science Behind Mind-Body Medicine.* New York: Simon & Schuster, 1997.

Pierrakos, John C. *Core Energetics: Developing the Capacity to Love and Heal.* Mendocino, CA: Life Rhythm, 1990.

Porter, Roy. *Medicine: A History of Healing.* New York: Marlowe, 1997.

Price, Shirley, and Len Price, eds. *Aromatherapy for Health Professionals.* London: Churchill Livingstone, 1995.

Roberts, M. *Biology: A Functional Approach.* 4th ed. Walton on Thames, UK: Nelson Thornes, 1986.

Robbins, Tom. *Jitterbug Perfume.* New York: Bantam, 1984.

Roeder, Ralph. *Catherine de' Medici and the Lost Revolution.* New York: Garden City, 1939.

Roehrig, Catherine H., Renée Dreyfus, and Cathleen A. Keller, eds. *Hatshepsut: From Queen to Pharaoh.* New York: Metropolitan Museum of Art, 2005.

Rohde, Eleanour Sinclair. *The Scented Garden.* London: David & Charles, 1989.

Rose, Jeanne. *375 Essential Oils and Hydrosols.* Berkeley: Frog, 1999.

Ryman, Daniele. *The Aromatherapy Handbook.* Essex: C. W. Daniel, 1984.

Sarno, John E. *Healing Back Pain: The Mind-Body Connection.* New York: Warner, 1991.

Sarno, John E. *The Mindbody Prescription: Healing the Body, Healing the Pain.* New York: Warner, 1998.

Schmidt, Michael A. *Beyond Antibiotics: 50 (or so) Ways to Boost Immunity and Avoid Antibiotics.* 2nd ed. Berkeley: North Atlantic Books, 1994.

Schnaubelt, Kurt. *Medical Aromatherapy: Healing with Essential Oils.* Berkeley: Frog, 1999.

Bibliography

Sellar, Wanda. *The Directory of Essential Oils*. Essex: C. W. Daniel, 1992.

Shakespeare, William. *The Complete Works of William Shakespeare*. London: Collins Clear-Type, 1923.

Sheppard-Hanger, Sylla. *The Aromatherapy Practitioner Reference Manual* (2 volumes). Tampa: Atlantic Institute of Aromatherapy, 1995.

Smith, Lacey Baldwin. *The Horizon Book of the Elizabethan World*. New York: American Heritage, 1967.

Stoneman, Richard. *Palmyra and Its Empire: Zenobia's Revolt Against Rome*. Ann Arbor, MI: University of Michigan Press, 1992.

Strage, Mark. *Women of Power: The Life and Times of Catherine de' Medici*. New York: Harcourt Brace Janovich, 1976.

Strehlow, Wighard and Gottfried Hertzka. *Hildegard of Bingen's Medicine*. Santa Fe, NM: Bear, 1988.

Tisserand, Robert. *Aromatherapy: To Heal and Tend the Body*. Santa Fe, NM: Lotus, 1988.

Tisserand, Robert. *The Art of Aromatherapy: The Healing and Beautifying Properties of the Essential Oils of Flowers and Herbs*. New York: Inner Traditions International, 1977.

Tisserand, Robert, and Tony Balacs. *Essential Oil Safety*. London: Churchill Livingstone, 1995.

Trotula of Salerno. *The Diseases of Women*. Translated by Elizabeth Mason-Hohl. Hollywood: Ward Ritchie, 1940.

Tyldesley, Joyce A. *Daughters of Isis: Women of Egypt*. New York: Viking, 1994.

Ullman, Dana. *Homeopathic Educational Services*. Berkeley: Homeopathic Educational Services, 2007.

Urantia Foundation, *The Urantia Book*. Chicago: Urantia Foundation, 1955.

Valnet, Jean. *The Practice of Aromatherapy: A Classic Compendium of Plant Medicines and Their Healing Properties*. New York: Destiny Books, 1980.

Vandercook, John. *Empress of the Dusk: A Life of Theodora of Byzantium*. New York: Reynal & Hitchcock, 1940.

Waldman, Milton. *Biography of a Family: Catherine de Medici and Her Children*. Boston: Houghton Mifflin, 1936.

Ware, William. *Zenobia, Queen of Palmyra: A Tale of the Roman Empire in the Days of the Emperor Aurelian*. Boston: Dana Estes, 1912.

Weil, Andrew. *Mind-Body Workbook*. Boulder, CO: Sounds True, 2005.

Wells, Evelyn. *Hatshepsut*. Garden City, NY: Doubleday, 1969.

Wildwood, Christine. *Aromatherapy: Massage with Essential Oils*. (Rockport, MA: Elements, 1991).

Willmont, Dennis. *Aromatherapy in Chinese Medicine*. Marshfield, MA: Willmountain, 2003.

Winter, Ruth. *The Smell Book: Scents, Sex, and Society.* New York: Lippincott, 1976.

Worwood, Valerie Ann. *Aromatherapy for the Soul: Healing the Spirit with Fragrance and Essential Oils.* Novato, CA: New World Library, 1999.

Worwood, Valerie Ann. *The Fragrant Heavens: The Spiritual Dimensions of Fragrance and Aromatherapy.* Novato, CA: New World Library, 1999.

Wright, William. *An Account of Palmyra and Zenobia: With Travels and Adventures in Bashan and the Desert.* London: Thomas Nelson, 1895.

Young, Geroge Frederick. *The Medici.* New York: Modern Library, 1930.

Image Credits and Permissions

Marjoram XV
Source: Avonel Jones, photographer

Hatshepsut as King 5
This file is licensed under the Creative Commons Attribution Share Alike 3.0 License.
Date: 15th century BC New Kingdom
Description: Limestone sculpture
Location: Metropolitan Museum of Art, New York, New York
Wikimedia Commons:
   http://commons.wikimedia.org/wiki/File:Hatshepsut_1.jpg

Hatshepsut's Temple at Deir El Bahri 12
This file is licensed under the Creative Commons Attribution Share Alike 2.5 license.
Date: October 2004
Location: Temple of Hatshepsut: Luxor West Bank, Egypt
Author Photo: Przemyslaw "Blueshade" Idzkiewicz
Wikimedia Commons:
   http://commons.wikimedia.org/wiki/File:Luxor_Temple_of_Hatshepsut_ Egypt

Queen Esther 16
This figure is in public domain because its copyright has expired.
Date: 1878
Description: Painting by Edwin Long
Location: National Gallery of Victoria, Melbourne
Wikimedia Commons: http://en.wikipedia.org/wki/File:Esther_haram.jpg

Cleopatra VII 25
This image is in public domain because its copyright has expired.
Date: 12 may 2007
Description: Photo of Cleopatra Statue at Rosicruian Egyptian Museum
Author: E. Michael Smith Chiefio

Wikimedia Commons:
http://commons.wikimedia.org/wiki/file:DSC093719.JPG

Jesus with Martha and Mary   35
This image is in public domain because its copyright has expired.
Date: before 1654-1655
Description: Christ in the House of Martha and Mary
Artist: Jan Vermeer van Delft
Location: National Gallery of Scotland
Wikimedia Commons:
http://commons.wikimedia.org/wiki/File:Jan_Vermeer_van_Delft_004.jpg

Queen Zenobia's last look upon Palmyra   46
This image is in public domain because its copyright has expired
Date: unknown, painter died in 1935
Description: Queen Zenobia's last look upon Palmyra
Painter: Herbert Schmalz
Source: www.illusionsgallery.com/Zenobia.html
Wikimedia Commons:
http://commons.wikimedia.org/wiki/File:Herbert_Schmaltz_Zenobia.jpg

Empress Theodora   59
This image is in the public domain because its copyright has expired
Date: year 547
Location: San Vitale in Ravenna
Artist: Meister Von San Vitale in Ravenna
Wikimedia Commons:
http://commons.wikimedia.org/wiki/File:Meister_Von_San_Vitale_
in_Ravenna_008.jpg

Trota of Salerno   65
This image is in the public domain because its copyright has expired.
Date: The late 12th or early 13th century
Description: Depiction of Trota of Salerno from a manuscript
Source: *Contraception and Abortion from the Ancient World
to the Renaissance* by John M. Riddle
Wikimedia Commons:
http://commons.wikimedia.org/wiki/File:Trotula_of_Salerno.jpg

Hildegard von Bingen 77

This image is in the public domain because its copyright has expired.

Date:

Description: Hildegard Von Bingen receiving Inspiration

Source: Minatures at the Rupertsberger Codex des Liber Scivias

Author: Original uploader was Robert Lechner at dė.wikipedia

Wikimedia Commons:

http://commons.wikimedia.org/wiki/File:Hildegard.jpg

Catherine de Médicis 88

This image is in the public domain because its copyright has expired.

Date: 1560

Description: Portrait of Catherine de Medici, chalk drawing

Artist: Francois Clouvet

Source: Moreau-Nélaton, Le Portrait en France à la cour des Valois, ..., 18.

Wikimedia Commons:

http://commons.wikimedia.org/wiki/File:Catherine1555.JPG

Elizabeth I 105

This image is in public domain because its copyright has expired.

Date: 1575

Description: The Darnley Portarait of Elizabeth I of England, oil panel

Artist: Unknown, perhaps Federico Zuccaro

Location: National Portrait Gallery, London

Source: *Tranya Cooper, A Guide to Tudor and Jacobean Portraits*

Wikimedia Commons:

http://commons.wikimedia.org/wiki/File:Elizabeth_I_Darnley_Portrait.jpg

Bay laurel 139

Source: Avonel Jones, photographer

Limonene 150

Source: Larry Jones, Spectrix Lab Data file

German chamomile 150

Source: Avonel Jones, photographer

Image Credits and Permissions

Index

Index

Burdock root *(Arctium lappa)*, 224
Burgess, Ruth, 43
B vitamins, 248

C

camphor-bearing oils, and homeopathy, 258
cancer. *See also* breast cancer; leukemia
  case study, 180–181
  holistic treatment of, 272
  integrative treatment approach, 272
  and the sesquiterpenols, 172
  and synthetic estrogens, 242
  Trota's remedy for, 67–68
Candida albicans (infection from)
  antifungal douche, 137, 164
  essential oil treatment, 203
Canon of Medicine (Avicenna), 70
carbon, the element, 148
carrier oils, 132–134
case studies
  emotional level, 189–194
  physical level, 179–189, 193–194
  spiritual level, 194–196
Castor oil *(Ricinus communis)*, 187–188
Cedarwood *(Cedrus atlantica)*, 9, 150, 172, 206, 226, 261
celibacy, 66, 103
cell membranes, essential oils' effect on, 200
central nervous system
  balancing, 189, 236–237, 248
  Bergamot, 157, 159, 240
  function and structure of, 234–237
  Lavender, 82, 181, 193, 233, 247
  relaxing, 167, 267
  Ylang-ylang, 175
chakras, 260–263
chamazulene, 151
Charles I (son of Catherine de Médicis), 91–92
chemical brain, the, 231–232
chemical structure and function of essential oils, 145–148
chi, 256
childbirth
  birth trauma, 232–233
  Catherine de Médicis' difficulties with, 87–88
  and pregnancy, oils for, 226
  Trota's remedies and recommendations, 71, 73

children
  early life patterning of, 236
  essential oils for, 225–226
Chopra, Deepak, 223, 231, 291
Cinnamon *(Cinnamomum verum)*, 20, 110, 152, 201, 202, 204, 226
circulatory system, 210
citrus oils. *See also specific citrus oils*
  for depression, 248
  for homeostatic balance, 220
Clary sage *(Salvia sclarea)*, xxi, 129, 152, 218, 243, 244, 263
Cleopatra, 23–31
clients, how to conduct a case study with, 178–179
Clove *(Syzygium aromaticum)*, 45, 152, 199, 201, 202, 242, 274
colds
  and constipation, essential oil blend, 218–219
  Ginger, 114
  Lavender, 82
  Peppermint, 169
  steam inhalation, 126
College of Botanical Healing Arts
  case studies from, 177
  curriculum, 276–277
  equipment for analyzing essential oils, 147
  organic chemistry, as requirement, 146
  steam-distillation process, 135–136
colon, the, 171, 218–219
communication network of the body mind, 231–232
compost piles, 285
compresses, 129, 275
cones of fragrance, ancient Egyptian, 6–7
conflict, Rose oil to release, 233
consciousness, altered states of, 26
Constantinople, 54–55
constipation, 81, 130, 161, 186, 216, 218–219
cooking with essential oils, 142
coptic jars, 9–10
cortisol, 240
cosmetics
  ancient Egyptian, 5, 6, 26–27
  Trotas recipes and suggestions for, 71–72
coughs, 9, 110, 114, 184–185, 200–201
Cousens, Gabriel and Shanti, 279
cranial sacral healing modality, 233
CRF (corticotrophin-releasing factor), 239–240

Index

Index

Index

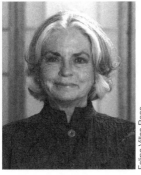

Felipe Villas Boas

About the Author

ELIZABETH ANNE JONES is a pioneer, leading educator, healer, formulator, and advocate of using therapeutic essential oils for integrative medicine. She has an extensive educational background from Skidmore College, University of California, Berkeley, and the California School of Herbal Studies. She has studied with top aromatherapists around the world including Marcel Lavabre, Kurt Schnaubelt, Pierre Franchomme, Robert Tisserand, and John Steele.

Jones has run a private aromatherapy practice for more than twenty-five years, and, with her husband, chemist Lawrence Jones, owns Elizabeth Van Buren, Inc., a company that manufactures high quality essential oil products for practitioners, spas, hospitals, massage schools, hospices, and nurses.

In 1997 she founded the College of Botanical Healing Arts in Santa Cruz, California, and has served as director and primary instructor since then. The college is a state-approved nonprofit with a 400-hour program to graduate essential oils practitioners. It is one of only a few schools in the United States that offers a comprehensive program of live classes.

Working on the education committee of the Alliance of International Aromatherapists (AIA), Jones helped to regulate the standards of aromatherapy education in the U.S. She has been a frequent speaker at northern California hospices, colleges, health conferences, and aromatherapy conferences. In addition, she wrote the definitive entry on aromatherapy for alt.MD.com, and was a contributor to the anthology *The World of Aromatherapy,* edited by Jeanne Rose and Susan Earle.

"When I met Elizabeth Jones, I knew she had the 'wisdom of the ages' and a deep connection with the spirit of essential oils which spins the magic that she has brought into so many lives."

— SHANTI GOLD COUSENS, MA, co-director of the Tree of Life Rejuvenation Center and former CoBHA student